MW00605645

THE

TRIFECTA

PASSPORT

THE TRIFECTA PASSPORT:

Tools for Mast Cell Activation Syndrome, Postural Orthostatic Tachycardia Syndrome and Ehlers-Danlos Syndrome

Amber Walker, PT, DPT, CFMP, CNPT

DISCLAIMER: The information contained in this book is intended to help readers make informed decisions about their health. This content is not a substitute for medical diagnosis and/or treatment by a professional healthcare provider. Please refer to your doctor for customized medical advice.

FIRST EDITION, January 2021
Copyright © 2021 by Amber Walker

All rights reserved. No portion of this book may be reproduced, stored in a retrieval system, or transmitted in any form or by any means—electronic, scanning, mechanical, recording, photocopy, or other—except for brief quotations in reviews or articles, without the prior written permission of the author.

Quotes from other authors/expert interviews have been reprinted/shared with permission and are also subject to copyright from the original source(s). The names and details of individuals in patient cases have been changed.

Published in the United States by Kindle Direct Publishing

ISBN: 978-1-7337117-2-2 (paperback)

ISBN: 978-1-7337117-3-9 (digital)

Editor: Jennifer Leopoldt Roop

Cover Art: Ryan Biore

Passport Workbook Graphic Design: Don Matthew

www.originwellnesscolorado.com/passport

To my patients, who teach me and inspire me every day.

Table of Contents

- Preface i

Part One: The Trifecta

- Chapter 1: Mast Cell Activation Syndrome (MCAS) 1
- Chapter 2: Postural Orthostatic Tachycardia Syndrome (POTS) 43
- Chapter 3: Ehlers-Danlos Syndrome (EDS) 67

Part Two: The Healing Plan

- Chapter 4: The Passport 101
- Chapter 5: Internal Health Stressors 127
- Chapter 6: External Health Stressors 171
- Chapter 7: Retraining the Nervous System 223
- Chapter 8: Nutrition 261
- Chapter 9: Structural and Musculoskeletal Issues 321
- Chapter 10: Movement 351
- Chapter 11: Detoxification 379
- Chapter 12: Summary & Case Examples 425

- Acknowledgments 441
- About the Author 443
- Bibliography 445
- Index 513

Preface

S everal months ago, just prior to the start of the coronavirus (COVID-19) pandemic, I found myself deep in a brainstorm session in a place where I seem to come up with all of my self-proclaimed bright ideas: the shower. Of course, the other place that I find myself brimming with new ideas is usually on a mountain trail somewhere, but on this particular day, I dashed to my office and, hair dripping, began to outline what I envisioned to be the content and theme for my next book.

My first book was entitled "Mast Cells United: A Holistic Approach to Mast Cell Activation Syndrome" and was published in early 2019. Some of the feedback I received was that, at 542 pages, the book was informative but sometimes too L-O-N-G to be read cover to cover by patients who were ill. My internal critic was also bothered by the fact that it had such a heavy focus on background information about mast cell activation syndrome (MCAS) and not enough useful tools for patients to use to work on holistic healing *on their own*. I felt that it was a solid overview and introduction to a lot of different topics, but it wasn't a super practical manual. (Of course, I also recognize that as humans, we can be our own worst critics.) However, I couldn't shake the feeling that my work in this arena was not finished yet.

In addition, on a personal note, in the years since I had finished writing the first book, I continued to find healing and reversal of symptoms in my own life from a number of resources not previously mentioned. My view on the approach to diet and other lifestyle factors has also evolved, both from personal experience and from additional professional training and certifications in functional medicine and nutrition.

Since the first book was published, I opened a practice called Origin Wellness, where I focus on wellness sessions with patients who are chronically ill. My goal in working with patients who have been sick for decades on average is to help provide them with the tools to "choose their own adventure" to healing. It can be an overwhelming road, with so much out there to pick from and so little guidance and framework on where to begin. For most patients, their predicament is further complicated by financial and relationship strain, severe day-to-day fluctuations in functional mobility, pain and fatigue, being homebound due to symptoms or extreme sensitivities to their environments, disability hearings or difficulty with employers or work duties, outrageously expensive medical bills... The list goes on.

I felt that as I worked with patients, the tools and resources I was able to share seemed somewhat random and disorganized, a mix of all sorts of different categories. My Type A personality yearned for something more concrete, more organized and more metaphorical to help patients connect the dots. For a while I used different acronyms to encompass the most important healing tools, but nothing seemed to stick.

So, let me introduce you to the concept of the healing passport. Why a passport? Well, anyone who knows me knows that I have a *slight* inclination to spontaneously book trips to another country. And as you'll soon see in Chapter 4, there's a lot that we can learn from passports. The beauty of the passport is that there is no "right" or perfect way to fill up the pages with immigration stamps and visas. Nor is there a perfect time frame; some people only fill up a page or two in 10 years, while others have a full book of different experiences very quickly.

Why the trifecta? MCAS, POTS (a form of dysautonomia called postural orthostatic tachycardia syndrome) and the hypermobile type of Ehlers-Danlos syndrome (hEDS) tend to go hand in hand in patients with chronic illness. The estimates of prevalence are all over the map, but there's a very good chance that any reader picking up this book will know someone who is suffering from one, two or all three of these issues, regardless of whether they have been diagnosed yet. There's so much overlap in symptoms between these three conditions, so the goal of this book is to shift the focus from "treating MCAS", "treating POTS" or "treating EDS" as singular entities to an approach that focuses on restoring proper systemic immune function, reducing inflammation, resetting the nervous system, etc. The ultimate goal is to help patients uncover the root issues behind these conditions so that the symptoms subside or resolve on their own.

Some practitioners have expanded the trifecta to the concept of "the pentad" which encompasses MCAS, POTS, EDS, functional gastrointestinal issues and autoimmune disease. There are so many additional topics and conditions relevant to the chronic illness patient population, and I toyed with including more of them in this book, or perhaps expanding the book outline to include more in-depth information about other diseases. However, there seems to be a scarcity of nonmainstream resources for approaching the three conditions that make up the trifecta, and I wanted to provide a more focused and concise tool for these patients. Patients with other conditions may very well benefit from the content of this book too.

It's becoming increasingly clear that we have a tidal wave of issues in patients with chronic illness, and it's rarely just one/two/three conditions at play. Obviously, it's important to rule out certain issues with the help of a medical provider, but in the case of MCAS, patients can endure years of time pushing for the diagnosis to be confirmed via fairly unreliable blood and urine testing. In the meantime, for those seeking the diagnosis of these or other conditions, I encourage patients to consider prioritizing healing resources that may be beneficial—regardless of the official diagnostic label.

After I discuss a little background of each of the three conditions that make up the trifecta and seven different categories of strategies to find healing, I'll also include patient case scenarios so that readers can see what the holistic process can look like in clinical practice. Keep in mind that there's no blueprint for healing from chronic illness, and each patient has a unique set of factors and an individualized response to each trial and error resource that they chose to investigate. For most patients, the tools available in Part Two of the book will be valuable regardless of their exact diagnoses, labels or comorbidities. In my clinical experience, patients with MCAS, POTS or EDS (or some combination of all the above) struggle to find healing until they incorporate the holistic treatment outlined in Part Two. It's also my clinical experience that addressing one or two categories (such as diet and exercise) in isolation can be helpful, but more profound healing tends to occur when patients address all the different areas. Some of these tools are free and simple to implement, and some are quite expensive; thus, I will reiterate that the content shared in this book is truly a "choose your own adventure" set-up, and patients should decide what is the best road map for them with the help of their medical care team.

I throw around a lot of phrases in this book, including holistic, conventional, allopathic, naturopathic, alternative, complementary, integrative and functional medicine. What do these terms mean? They are certainly different from each other.

Holistic medicine is a concept based on the whole person and the focus of the mind, spirit and body as opposed to just focusing on the symptoms of a particular condition. The goal is to see the big picture and bring the mind, spirit and body into coherence, which leads to optimal health. Holistic medicine is an umbrella term that refers to the practitioner's style and *is not a separate entity in itself*. For example, conventional doctors, naturopaths, integrative providers and functional medicine doctors can all be holistic in their approach to patient care.

Conventional medicine is described as the science-based, modern system where medical doctors and other providers (like therapists, pharmacists and nurses) treat symptoms and diseases using drugs, radiation or surgery. For example, if you are found to have diabetes, you are typically placed on medications for it. Conventional medicine is used interchangeably with the terms allopathic medicine and traditional medicine.

Naturopathic medicine is an approach that uses natural remedies to help the body heal itself. This type of medicine aims to treat the whole person (mind, body and spirit) in order to heal the root causes of illness instead of masking the symptoms. Naturopathic doctors may utilize natural treatment approaches—some tried and true for centuries, and others that are more modern—like nutrition, herbs, fasting, intravenous therapies and sauna therapies. This approach focuses on the body's innate ability to heal itself when given the right tools.

Alternative medicine includes approaches for healing that are used in place of conventional therapies. Reiki, Ayurvedic medicine, homeopathy, aromatherapy, acupressure, acupuncture and other natural medicine approaches like herbalism, ozone therapy and reflexology are usually considered forms of alternative medicine. Some sources claim that while these approaches strive for healing, alternative medicine options typically lack adequate scientific testing (or in some cases are "proven ineffective"). This claim certainly depends on the modality in question; for example, many people turn a blind eye to the abundance of literature support behind acupuncture because of inherent bias or cultural factors. Other modalities such as aromatherapy or reiki are by nature more difficult to study or "prove" in a way that meets the standards for randomized controlled trials. And, many modalities that are considered alternative medicine can also be used as part of a treatment plan with an integrative, natural or functional medicine provider.

Complementary medicine is an approach where healing modalities are used to complement the traditional allopathic approaches. These types of medical therapies, such as osteopathy or acupuncture, may fall beyond the scope of conventional scientific medicine but are often used alongside it to treat disease. When approached properly, complementary medicine can be considered integrative.

Integrative medicine aims to address the full gamut of physical, environmental, mental, emotional, social and spiritual influences that influence our health. Integrative medicine is similar to functional medicine in that it strives to address the causes of illness through personalized care. Integrative medicine sees the patient and practitioner as partners in the healing process, which aims to tap into the body's innate healing potential and to modify certain lifestyle factors for long-lasting wellness. Integrative medicine strives to use interventions that are natural and less invasive when possible, giving attention to the prevention of illness and empowering patients with tools for lifelong healthy behavior. For example, an integrative plan may incorporate modern healthcare for diagnosis and treatment plus nutrition and exercise counseling and other tools like yoga, massage and acupuncture. Integrative medicine holds the core belief that poor lifestyle choices are underlying factors of many modern diseases.

Functional medicine is more concerned with the *how* and *why*—the dynamic processes that result in dysfunction—as opposed to the labels or names of diseases that we attribute symptoms to (the *what*). Thus, functional medicine aims to uncover the root cause of diseases and symptoms. According to the Institute for Functional Medicine, functional medicine is patient-centered, is personalized based on biochemical individuality, seeks a dynamic balance of gene and environmental interactions and is function- (vs. pathology-) focused.[1] Functional medicine views health as a positive vitality and not simply the absence of disease.[1]

Functional medicine providers often look at tests evaluating for things like the causes of gastrointestinal dysfunction (dysbiosis, bacterial infections, small intestinal bacterial overgrowth, candida, parasites, etc.). They may order tests looking at hormone dysfunction, adrenal issues, mold or biotoxins, genetic factors, nutrient deficiencies, environmental toxins and causes of liver stress, inflammation, infections and viruses, immune dysfunction, and structural and neurological dysfunction. They may also incorporate information about factors like electromagnetic pollution, mitochondrial dysfunction and emotional trauma into a healing plan that aims to eradicate or reverse the root issues. Thus, functional medicine embraces much of the philosophy of integrative medicine but takes it a step further by utilizing a systems-based approach to understand the root causes of illness as part of a partnership with the patient.

Functional medicine, naturopathic medicine and integrative medicine all treat the individual rather than the disease. Some providers may blend different types of medicine within their practices. For example, a naturopathic doctor may also practice functional medicine, and a functional medicine provider may integrate aspects of natural medicine into their patient care. When it comes to chronic illness, there is no silver bullet approach, but patients who stay open-minded to the different possibilities will have a great toolbox to experiment with in determining what their body responds best to.

Finding the right provider often entails trial and error, particularly for patients with the trifecta. Some integrative providers have an approach that focuses on taking many supplements that have multiple ingredients, and this approach may need to be modified significantly for patients who have sensitivities. Not every provider may recognize this or be equipped to work with complex patients who react to natural agents. If you've had a bad experience in the past with a naturopathic or functional medicine provider, keep in mind that no two practitioners are exactly alike. Just as we often need to try several mainstream medical providers before finding the right fit, the same concept applies to the natural and functional medicine world.

I designed this book with a patient audience in mind. The patients who have chronic conditions who I've been blessed to know over the years are some of the most informed and educated people I've ever met; I hope that the content of this book has the right depth to speak to both the newly diagnosed and those who have been on their healing journey for a long time. I also hope that this book will be useful for medical providers looking to better familiarize themselves with the trifecta and caregivers aiming to support loved ones.

A few things to remember as you read along: This is not individualized/customized medical advice and it is by no means intended to substitute for medical care. This is not all-inclusive, and I'm sure in the months and years following its publication I will uncover more tools from personal experience, professional experience and research. This book will not focus heavily on sharing the research behind these conditions. There's a lot of research out there, and if you're interested in those types of details, please refer to my first book, "Mast Cells United" (2019), which cites hundreds of studies, many of them related to the trifecta. I also want readers to know that I will not beat around the bush with certain topics. I have certain views and opinions that differ greatly from mainstream medical advice, and I hope you will stay open-minded to the idea of a blend of integrative and functional medicine, natural medicine and certain undeniably important tenets from the mainstream approaches for these conditions. Lastly, I will try to spare you too many cheesy travel metaphors along the way... though I can't make any promises!

PART ONE:
THE TRIFECTA

Chapter 1:
MAST CELL ACTIVATION SYNDROME (MCAS)

Mast cell activation syndrome (MCAS) is a complex topic that's very difficult to summarize concisely. The purpose of this chapter is to provide a condensed overview of the condition.

Very little prevalence data is currently available, but two research studies in Germany found the general population prevalence of MCAS to be 14%-17%.[1,2] In contrast, the prevalence among first-degree relatives may be closer to 33%, suggesting strong genetic and/or environmental ties.[2] Multiple sources have noted that epigenetic processes appear to be connected to the transgenerational transmission of MCAS.[3,4] More research is needed with laboratory diagnosis of MCAS, as opposed to symptom report in the general population, to confirm the true overall prevalence. The take home message is this: MCAS is very common!

MCAS more consistently affects people assigned female at birth, with a predominance estimated to be between 69%-94% across five different studies.[1,2,5-7] Gender-specific hormonal factors and differences in gene expression may be connected to the disparities.[8] The lifespan for those with MCAS appears to be normal, but the quality of life can range from mildly impaired to very poor.[4] There exists a large spectrum of experiences within this diagnosis and an array of individual responses to treatment over time.

Mast Cell Terminology

Mast cell activation disease (MCAD) is an umbrella term that refers to a group of disorders characterized by:[9]

- The accumulation of pathological mast cells in potentially any or all organs and tissues and/or
- The aberrant (abnormal) release of variable subsets of mast cell mediators

In other words, MCAD involves either too many mast cells around the body, and/or the abnormal release of too many chemicals by mast cells. *Abnormal sensitivity levels and release of chemicals by mast cells* with a normal quantity of mast cells is characteristic of MCAS, whereas an *abnormal quantity of mast cells* is consistent with a condition called mastocytosis, which is much less common and has several subtypes. There are also rare forms of cancer that are considered types of MCAD.

The term MCAD is sometimes (incorrectly) used interchangeably with mast cell activation syndrome (MCAS). MCAD describes the physiological state of disruption in different mast cell properties; *MCAS is one of the several types of MCAD.*

Figure 1. Mast Cell Activation Disease[9]

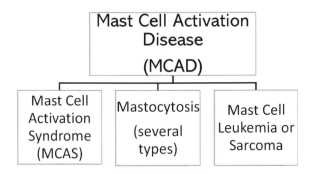

"Mast cell activation" is sometimes abbreviated "MCA" in the literature, and describes symptoms of mediator release, but is *not* the same as a *diagnosis* of MCAS or MCAD. Symptoms of mast cell activation can occur with a large number of conditions and issues.

"Clonal mast cell disease" is often distinguished in the literature and includes either mastocytosis or monoclonal mast cell activation syndrome (abbreviated MMCAS or MMAS, depending on the author). MCAS and MMCAS and systemic mastocytosis all have evidence of genetic mutations that likely contribute to the disease process, but the *KIT* mutation at codon D816V is much more common in patients with clonal disease, including systemic mastocytosis and MMCAS.[3] Essentially, patients with monoclonal MCAS meet the criteria for MCAS and also partially meet the criteria for systemic mastocytosis.

Mast Cell Overview

Mast cells are a type of white blood cell that serve as an important part of the body's immune system. Mast cells are present in nearly all types of tissue. Researchers often suggest that mast cells are akin to immune system watchdogs. They are also described as the "jack-of-all-trades immune cells" that can interact with and modulate the function of many different cells throughout the entire body.[10] Mast cells have receptors for allergens, pathogens, neurotransmitters, neuropeptides and hormones. Compared with other innate immune cells, mast cells can release a substantially higher number and diversity of substances.[11]

Mast cells are especially prominent in boundary tissue that is located near the external world, such as the skin, lung mucosa, digestive tract, eyes, nose and mouth. They are found in all tissues, including the brain, bone marrow, fat tissue, liver, spleen and lymph nodes.[12] They are present in most tissues that surround blood vessels and nerves.

Mast cells contain granules that they release when signaled, and these granules contain compounds that stimulate other processes to occur.

Compounds or *mediators* are biologically active chemical molecules that are released by mast cells. *Degranulation* refers to the process of mast cells releasing compounds into the circulatory system. The release of these mediators is a normal occurrence when the body perceives a threat, but it's the *excess number* of mast cells releasing granules at once (mastocytosis) or the *degree of sensitivity to which the cells are getting triggered* to release granules (mast cell activation syndrome) that ultimately creates problems.

When a reaction occurs, mast cells immediately release histamine, heparin, proteases and tumor necrosis factor-alpha in response to a stimulus. Over the next several minutes, the release of prostaglandins and leukotrienes is generally observed. Over the next several hours, cytokines and interleukins add to the inflammatory cascade.[13] In addition to releasing chemical mediators, mast cells also affect the endocrine and energy systems by their DNA secretion.[13] These important mechanisms can also inflict collateral damage on the tissues they were designed to protect when mast cells are improperly activated.[14]

Some sources estimate that there are over 200 identified mast cell mediators that are released in response to different triggers.[15] This is one of the reasons that it's difficult to "catch" or diagnose mast cell activation disease based on blood or urine samples; there are many mediators released and every patient is a little bit different in regards to which chemical mediator may be high at a given time, depending on the day and a multitude of internal and external factors. Each mediator has its own specific response down the chain, which can explain the wide range of symptoms experienced by patients.

Table 1. Common Mast Cell Mediators: Actions and Symptom Correlation[16,17]

MEDIATOR	ACTION	SYMPTOMS TRIGGERED WHEN IN EXCESS
Heparin	Angiogenesis, nerve growth factor stimulation	Swelling, anaphylaxis, inflammation, inhibited clotting, easy bruising, menorrhagia; long-term effects may decrease bone mineral density
Histamine	Vasodilation, angiogenesis, mitogenesis, pain, bronchoconstriction	Headache, low blood pressure, redness, swelling, itching, intestinal cramping, diarrhea, increased gastric acid, urticaria (rash), activation of leukocytes, throat symptoms
Leukotriene	Vasoconstriction, pain	Narrowing of blood vessels, constriction of airways, increases in vascular permeability and contractibility
Prostaglandin D2	Bronchoconstriction, vasoregulation, pain	Constriction of airways, flushing, itching, low blood pressure, runny nose/mucus secretion, arrhythmias, low bone mineral density
Serotonin	Vasoconstriction, pain	Raises blood pressure, increases breathing rate and heart rate, impacts mood, increases appetite, suppresses insulin release from pancreas

Tryptase	Tissue damage, inflammation, pain; level indicates mast cell numbers, not severity of disease	May impact cholesterol levels, degrades tissue, causes inflammation

Mast cells play a crucial role in many important bodily processes that occur continuously, including the generation of new blood vessels, the body's ability to repair wounds, the function of the blood-brain barrier, and the immune system's reactions and defenses against intruders. Anaphylaxis or an allergic reaction that can trigger life-threating complications sometimes occurs among patients with MCAS, although not every patient experiences these types of reactions. There are numerous stimuli that can induce mast cell activation on the cellular level.

Examples of triggers reported to induce mast cell activation include:[13,18-20]

- airplane or car travel
- alcohol
- caffeine
- certain foods, particularly foods that have been aged, cured, fermented or smoked
- chemical toxins found in cleaning supplies, swimming pools, etc.
- direct sunlight
- extreme temperatures (in the air or in water submersion, like a hot tub)
- fevers, bacterial infections, the influenza virus, fungal infections, parasites and other viruses

- food additives/preservatives such as carrageenan, citric acid and "natural flavor"
- ingredients in personal health and beauty products (such as chemicals/toxins in nail polish, shampoo, deodorant, lipstick, sunblock, etc.)
- insect stings/bites
- invasive medical/surgical procedures
- mechanical vibration (such as vibration experienced while sitting on a bus, subway or roller coaster)
- medications and supplements
- mold and water-damaged buildings
- occupational environmental factors
- pesticides and other food source contamination
- pharmaceutical drugs
- physical or emotional stress
- physical stimuli (pressure and temperature changes)
- radiation and exposure to electromagnetic fields
- radiocontrast media
- secondhand smoke
- surgical implantations and hardware

This list is certainly not all-inclusive. Triggers tend to vary between patients and will sometimes vary within the same patient over time. "Typical" culprits like pets, dust and seasonal allergens may or may not be regular triggers. Many patients experience spontaneous reactions to food; often, food that they've considered "safe" in the past will suddenly trigger a reaction. Foods that are high in things like histamine, oxalates, sulfur or salicylates can be problematic for some patients. Emotional stress has been cited as the most common trigger in patients with mastocytosis[21] and also appears to play a substantial role in the MCAS population.

Some of the medications connected to mast cell activation include: NSAIDs (nonsteroidal anti-inflammatory drugs), morphine, muscle relaxants, vancomycin, estradiol and adenosine.[13] Hormonal medications including combined estrogen-progestin birth control pills and contraceptive injections may be triggers for some patients. For those patients using medication for high blood pressure, ACE-inhibitors interact with mast cells through influence on the angiotensin/renin system, and beta-blockers may increase the risk of anaphylaxis.[22]

When a thorough patient history is evaluated, mast cell-associated symptoms are often traced back to the early years in patients who have MCAS and flares are sometimes precipitated by stressful life events and trauma. It can be useful to write out a timeline of major life events and to examine whether they seem to coincide with a change in physical issues. This is not to say that stress causes MCAS, but it may be one of the early factors that contributed to the perfect storm of immune dysregulation. In many cases, the symptoms (and even subsequent experiences within the medical system) trigger a great deal of stress, leading to a vicious cycle of stress and inflammation.

Symptoms of MCAS

Note: For some individuals, these details can be triggering. The following sections describe MCAS symptoms, anaphylaxis management and comorbid conditions. This information can be overwhelming, so feel free to skip ahead to the diagnosis or treatment sections.

The response to mast cell degranulation can vary widely among patients. Acutely, most patients experience an individual and unique spectrum from a mild reaction to a full-blown anaphylactic response that requires epinephrine and other drugs alongside an emergency room visit. The more common acute episodes that fall somewhere in the middle will typically include flushing or redness of the face, itching with or without hives on the skin, blood pressure changes, difficulty breathing, abdominal cramping, nausea, vomiting or diarrhea, nasal and eye symptoms, throat tightness or soreness and headaches. There are extreme and rare cases where patients need to be hospitalized and treated with continuous intravenous mast cell stabilizers and monitored constantly due to persistent anaphylaxis. Clinically, while the rare case experiences anaphylaxis, most patients experience milder anaphylactoid reactions.

On top of these episodic symptoms, patients with MCAS typically experience dozens of problems that fall into their symptom list on a chronic, continual basis—a baseline of instability. Symptoms tend to wax and wane, to migrate, and are generally very hard to nail down and diagnose. Many patients can relate to thousands upon thousands of dollars of medical bills, time spent with doctors investigating one of their symptoms under a narrow lens, and the inevitable labeling as a "hypochondriac" or person who has somatization of symptoms when multiple or recurrent medical conditions are present with no discernible cause. Many patients feel disrespected and belittled from their experiences with the medical system when doctors, family members or friends have insinuated that their confusingly recurrent ailments—which repeatedly test negative for distinct diagnoses—are all in their head. Patients frequently experience a wide range of emotions such as anger, anxiety, depression, frustration, and even self-loathing when they are disrespected in this manner.

Table 2. Symptoms Commonly Experienced in Patients Who Have MCAS[13]

System	Symptoms
Cardiovascular	tachycardia (high heart rate), blood pressure irregularity (both high and low blood pressure), flushing (especially of the face), syncope (fainting) or pre-syncope (near-fainting), heart racing and blood pressure responses to positional changes, heart disease, intermittent chest pain
Cutaneous	Urticaria/hives (rash), flushing, efflorescence (spots on skin) with/without pruritus (itching), telangiectasia (red lines on skin from small blood vessels), angioedema (swelling of the lower layer of the skin), abnormal bleeding, frequent bruising, delayed skin healing from injury, abnormal sweating, abnormal body odor, hair loss
Gastrointestinal	bloating, diarrhea and/or constipation, nausea, vomiting, abdominal pain, intestinal cramping, abdominal distention, heartburn, malabsorption of nutrients, delayed gastric (stomach) emptying, H. pylori-negative gastritis (stomach lining inflammation), oropharyngeal burning pain (in middle part of the throat), aphthae (canker sore), ileocecal valve (valve separating small and large intestine) dysfunction, food sensitivities, irritable bowel syndrome, median arcuate ligament syndrome or "MALS" (structural compression of the celiac artery and possible neural structures resulting in abdominal ischemia and pain), microbiome bacterial issues including SIBO (small intestinal bacterial overgrowth)

Miscellaneous	fatigue, asthenia (feeling weak), fever, environmental sensitivities (odors, chemicals, vibration, animals, etc.), interstitial cystitis (bladder pain and increased urinary frequency), unexplained weight loss or gain, poor tolerance to exercise, idiopathic anaphylaxis, sensitivity to sunlight and/or extreme cold and heat, odd reactions to insect stings, difficult menses, thyroid and adrenal issues, poor tolerance to medications or anesthesia, poor tolerance to alcohol, poor tolerance to fermented foods and/or processed foods, poor tolerance to foods high in histamine, oxalates or salicylates
Musculoskeletal	muscle pain and aches, osteoporosis/osteopenia (decreased bone mineral density), bone pain, migratory arthritis, fibromyalgia
Neurological	difficulty with memory and concentration, anxiety, depression, insomnia (difficulty sleeping), lightheadedness, vertigo (sensation of the room spinning), headache and/or migraine, neuropathic pain (abnormal nerve-related pain sensations), numbness and tingling, lower attention span, tinnitus (ringing in the ears)
Ophthalmologic	conjunctivitis (pink eye), difficulty focusing with vision, increased floaters in eye, intermittent blurred vision, general eye irritation and redness, decreased oxygen to optic nerve resulting in decreased ability to differentiate between contrasting shades
Respiratory	asthma-like symptoms, sinus inflammation, unexplained shortness of breath, recurrent unexplained cough, rhinitis (nose mucous inflammation), frequent upper respiratory infections and/or pneumonia, shallow breathing patterns, impaired use of diaphragm muscle for breathing

Experts note that physical examination and certain blood/lab work and imaging abnormalities may also be present in some cases of MCAS. These can include hepatic splenomegaly (enlargement of liver and spleen), hyperbilirubinemia (elevated bilirubin in the blood), elevation of liver transaminases (enzymes), hypercholesterolemia (high cholesterol in the blood), splenomegaly (enlarged spleen) and lymphadenopathy (lymph nodes enlarged, abnormal consistency or abnormal number).[13]

The plethora of varying clinical presentations and characteristics leads one to conclude that there's really no "hallmark" set of signs and symptoms for mast cell activation disease. MCAS is highly variable; no two patients present with the exact same history, triggers, and type of reactions. Some experts believe that the wide array of manifestations is dependent upon which chemical mediator or mediators seem to be driving the symptoms in a patient. Some point to genetics and epigenetic factors. Problems with detoxification and mast cell reactivity to different viral and bacterial loads may also be the key to why this condition presents in so many ways. Patient-specific comorbidities (presence of other diseases), the variety of organ sites that can become infiltrated with mast cells, the wide range of triggering stimuli, local- and organ-specific factors, and the magnitude of the release reaction are all factors that impact the unique patient picture.[23]

Experts note that there are many conditions that are often comorbid with mast cell disease:[23]

- Chronic inflammatory response syndrome (CIRS) from biotoxin exposure
- Fibromyalgia syndrome (FMS)
- Ehlers-Danlos syndrome (EDS)
- Gulf War illness (GWI)
- Interstitial cystitis/bladder pain syndrome (IC/BPS)
- Irritable bowel syndrome (IBS)
- Kounis syndrome
- Multiple chemical sensitivity (MCS) syndrome
- Myalgic encephalomyelitis/chronic fatigue syndrome (ME/CFS)
- Post-Lyme syndrome
- Postural orthostatic tachycardia syndrome (POTS)
- Post-traumatic stress disorder (PTSD)
- Small intestinal bacterial overgrowth (SIBO)

Anaphylaxis

While anaphylaxis is not experienced by every patient who has MCAD, it's important to be aware of its signs and how to respond. Anaphylaxis is a serious and acute allergic reaction where chemical mediators cause several physiological responses. This usually occurs in response to a predictable trigger, such as getting a bee string, taking a medication or ingesting a food that's a known allergen, but can also occur "idiopathically" or for unknown reasons. Anaphylaxis can occur very rapidly—in a matter of seconds from exposure to a trigger—so it's crucial that each patient and their families, caregivers or housemates are aware of what to do in the event of an emergency. Anaphylaxis typically affects multiple body areas and can be life-threatening if proper treatment is not administered. Epinephrine injections are usually necessary to stop the reaction.

It's important to emphasize that you should not rely on waiting for emergency medical services during anaphylactic episodes. Life-saving decisions can come down to a number of seconds, and you cannot assume there will be time to drive to the hospital or wait for an ambulance to arrive.

The signs and symptoms of anaphylaxis can include:[24]

- Cardiovascular: low blood pressure*, fast or slow pulse rate
- Central nervous system: anxiety/sense of doom, confusion, headache, loss of consciousness, lightheadedness, change in mood in children (quiet or irritable)
- Eyes: swelling or redness of the conjunctiva, itching or tearing of the eyes
- Gastrointestinal: crampy abdominal pain, diarrhea, vomiting
- Genitourinary: loss of bladder control, pelvic pain, uterine cramps
- Nose: runny nose, nasal congestion, sneezing
- Respiratory: wheezing, shortness of breath, coughing, clearing throat, hoarseness, pain with swallowing, difficulty swallowing
- Skin: hives, itching, flushing, swelling of mouth or tongue, angioedema

Note: occasionally blood pressure is elevated instead of lowered

The presence of syncope (fainting) or the absence of hives during anaphylaxis may be indicative of more serious reactions and a more serious potential underlying condition.[25] One study noted that patients with clonal mast cell disorders were most likely to experience anaphylaxis following an insect sting (Hymenoptera venom), whereas patients with non-clonal MCAS more often had drugs as a trigger preceding anaphylaxis.[25]

Anaphylaxis is likely to occur in any of the following three scenarios:[26]

1. Acute onset of an illness (minutes to hours) with involvement of:
   - skin, mucosal tissue or both
   - <u>and at least one of the following:</u> respiratory compromise (shortness of breath, wheezing, stridor, coughing, hypoxemia) or decreased blood pressure or end organ dysfunction (such as collapse, incontinence, or fainting)
2. <u>Two or more</u> of the following occur suddenly after exposure to a likely allergen or other trigger for that patient (minutes to several hours):
   - symptoms in skin/mucosa (generalized hives, itching/flushing, swollen lips/tongue/uvula), respiratory compromise, sudden gastrointestinal symptoms (crampy abdominal pain, vomiting), decreased blood pressure/end organ dysfunction (such as collapse, incontinence or fainting)
3. After exposure to known allergen for that patient (minutes to several hours): <u>low blood pressure (BP)</u>
   - Infants and children: low systolic BP (age specific) or greater than 30% decrease in systolic BP.
   - Adults: systolic BP of less than 90 mmHg or greater than 30% decrease from patient's baseline

The American Academy of Allergy, Asthma & Immunology's guidelines for management of anaphylaxis includes intramuscular epinephrine injected into the anterolateral thigh as an "immediate intervention."[27] This is the first-line treatment, based on strong evidence.[27] There are no substitutes for epinephrine (with the except of a few special scenarios where epinephrine is contraindicated). Antihistamines including diphenhydramine, breathing treatments, steroids and other medications may be used in conjunction with epinephrine, but are *not* considered first-line treatment and do not work fast enough.[27,28] Several further subsequent interventions are recommended that would take place in a hospital setting.

A biphasic reaction is a two-phase anaphylactic event that occurs after the anaphylaxis is treated and the symptoms resolve. Even when the trigger has been removed and the patient is not re-exposed to the allergen, some patients experience a delayed second reaction that may be more or less severe or similar to the first.[26] This risk increases in patients who originally need more than one dose of epinephrine and/or who had severe anaphylaxis the first time around, and it's important to be aware of this possibility.[26] Again, most patients with MCAS do not experience regular anaphylactic emergencies, but it's good to be aware of what they can look like.

Diagnosis of MCAS

Mast cell activation syndrome is a relatively new diagnosis that has only been recognized more widely in the past 12 or so years. There are multiple groups of researchers/clinicians who have published recommended diagnostic criteria for MCAS, but there is no current universally determined gold standard. This challenge is a major pitfall in the advancement of MCAS awareness and acceptance in the medical community. Currently, the basics of diagnosis consist of the presence of typical symptoms, abnormal laboratory markers of mast cell activity and a symptomatic response to mast cell-targeting treatment.

The diagnosis of MCAS is somewhat controversial. Some experts worry that it's turning into the new fibromyalgia-type label and there's concern of overdiagnosis, misdiagnosis or improper clinical diagnosis without objective confirmation. Other experts voice concern that, due to poor diagnostic testing options, many patients with MCAS are being missed and subsequently lose access to treatments that could help them. There's also a possibility that MCAS is another label for systemic inflammation triggered by a bunch of underlying root issues. Many of the issues that can result in mast cell-associated global inflammation will be discussed individually throughout Part Two of this book.

As a whole, most experts agree that the diagnostic process should include the following components: thorough patient history, questionnaire evaluation, differential diagnosis consideration, physical examination, tissue or bone marrow biopsy when certain criteria are met, baseline laboratory tests, specific chemical mediator testing of the blood and urine, consideration of additional imaging or testing if appropriate, classification of the specific type of MCAD, medication trials and patient education.

Diagnostic Criteria

One group of published recommendations have traditionally involved a combination of certain symptoms, results from extracutaneous tissue and/or bone marrow biopsies, elevated levels of certain mast cell mediators in the blood and urine, and (eventually) symptomatic response to mast cell-targeting treatments.[9] Their diagnostic criteria have been modified various times over the years to a new set of most recent guidelines explained in a 2020 publication by Weinstock, Pace, Rezaie, Afrin and Molderings.[29]

Another group has traditionally focused on the presence of typical clinical symptoms, a response to mast cell mediator–targeting drugs, the absence of another disorder that could account for symptoms, and either an increase in tryptase levels or—more recently—another established mast cell mediator for diagnosis.[30] Updated recommendations were published in a 2019 article by Weiler, Austin, Akin, Barkoff, Bernstein, Bonadonna, Butterfield, Carter, Fox, Maitland, Pongdee, Mustafa, Ravi, Tobin, Vliagoftis and Schwartz as part of a working group AAAAI (American Academy of Allergy, Asthma & Immunology) committee report.[31]

Table 3. Proposed Diagnostic Criteria for MCAS

	Weinstock et al. (2020)[29]	Weiler et al. (2019)[31]
Major Criteria	After excluding of mimickers or alternative explanations of symptoms (differential diagnosis), the patient meets the major criterion of characteristics of mast cell activation in two or more systems. See Table 4 for a list of systems and symptoms that qualify for this criterion.	If patients meet the following criteria: Recurrent symptoms consistent with mast cell activation with involvement of two organs,* AND Elevation of one or more validated mast cell mediators [serum tryptase (utilizing the "20% +2" formula), urinary n-methyl histamine, urinary 11 beta-prostaglandin F2 alpha and urinary leukotriene E4],

		AND Response to targeted therapeutic interventions
Minor Criteria	Elevation in the blood and/or urine of mediators relatively specific to the mast cell: (1) plasma prostaglandin D2 and histamine, (2) serum tryptase and chromogranin A, and (3) 24-h and/or random urine N-methylhistamine, leukotriene E4 and 2,3- dinor-11-ß- prostaglandin-F2-α. - Clinical improvement using mast cell-directed medical therapy. Greater than or equal to 20 mast cells per high- power field in extracutaneous tissue (luminal gastrointestinal tract or bladder) biopsies.	Then the patient should be evaluated for: A genetic mutation in KIT** or TPSAB1 alpha- tryptase** (via blood test or buccal swab; bone marrow biopsy may be last resort in certain scenarios). Gene- by-Gene is a company that tests for the tryptase mutation with a cheek swab.[32]
Conclusions	Diagnosis of MCAS is made by the major criterion plus any one of the minor criteria.	If the patient tests positive for these tests, they should be classified to have Primary MCAS with a somatic or germ line genetic mutation. If the genetic testing is negative, the patient would be classified to

		have MCAS without a known mutation.

* Weiler et al. (2019)[31] defined symptoms consistent with mast cell activation to include different cardiovascular, dermatologic, respiratory and gastrointestinal signs.

**TPSAB1 alpha-tryptase is a test for hereditary alpha tryptasemia. KIT mutations are part of the diagnostic criteria for systemic mastocytosis.

Previously published laboratory considerations including spindle-shaped mast cells and CD25 expression are no longer advised for MCAS testing because they are more specific for mastocytosis.[29]

Weinstock et al. (2020)[29] described the major criterion for diagnosis including symptoms from at least two or more of the following systems:

Table 4. Systems and Symptoms Considered in the Diagnosis of MCAS[29]

SYSTEM	SYMPTOMS
Constitutional	Fatigue, fevers, weight loss or gain
Dermatological	Flushing, pruritus, urticaria, rashes
Esophageal	Heartburn, dysphagia, globus pharyngeus (sensation of something stuck in throat), chest pain
Eyes, Ears, Nose, Throat	Conjunctivitis, tinnitus, hearing loss, rhinitis, sinusitis, sore throat
Hepatic	Elevated transaminases, hepatomegaly
Lymphatic	Lymphadenopathy
Musculoskeletal	Myalgia, arthralgia, edema
Neurological	Headaches, migraines, brain fog, anxiety, flushing, nausea
Salivary Glands	Swelling
Small & Large Intestine	Abdominal pain/discomfort, diarrhea, constipation
Stomach	Dyspepsia
Urogenital	Frequency, urgency, dysuria

The publication by Weinstock et al. (2020) supports the use of the validated Mast Cell Mediator Release Syndrome (MCMRS) questionnaire that factors in the patient's medical history, symptoms, laboratory assessment, biopsy results and radiographic changes.[29]

These two groups of experts differ in certain points, such as whether it's appropriate to use chromogranin A or tissue biopsies for testing, whether a response to targeted therapeutic interventions is necessary prior to diagnosis and whether hereditary alpha tryptasemia (HAT) and/or anaphylaxis should be a part of the conversation. For now, it seems that the community has tentatively accepted multiple diagnostic approaches until more time provides adequate assessment of the validity of the different proposed options.

Testing Summary

Table 5. Chemical Mediators Tested in Patients with Suspected MCAS[29]

MAST CELL MEDIATOR	TESTING CONSIDERATIONS
Histamine: 24-hour Urine *N*-methylhistamine (NMHIN) and/or Plasma Histamine	Keep sample chilled continuously; Diet can influence histamine level by ~30%; DAO supplementation, vitamin C and antihistamine medications can affect this test result (avoid 5 days prior if appropriate)
Prostaglandins: 24-hour Urine Prostaglandin D2 (PGD2), and/or 24-hour Urine Prostaglandin 9a,11b-F2 (PGF2a), and/or Plasma Prostaglandins	Keep sample chilled continuously; PGF2a is (more stable) metabolite of PGD2 (PGF2a believed to be superior for MCAS detection); Aspirin and other NSAIDs can affect this test result (avoid 5 days prior if appropriate); Urine more accurate than blood test
Tryptase (serum)	High levels encountered with MCAD in approximately 15% of patients;[5,9] Baseline testing at least 24 hours after acute episode; Baseline level (0.2) + Baseline Level + 2 ng/ml = Cutoff for MCAS criterion via tryptase level during a symptomatic episode by Weiler et al. (2019)[31]

MAST CELL MEDIATOR	TESTING CONSIDERATIONS
24-hour Urine Leukotriene E4 (LTE4)	Keep sample chilled continuously; Zileuton/Zyflo medication may affect this test result (avoid 5 days prior if appropriate); Urine Leukotriene B4, C4 and D4 may also be ordered[4]
Serum Chromogranin A Note: this testing is supported by some but not all experts	High levels may also indicate heart conditions, kidney problems, liver failure, chronic atrophic gastritis or neuroendocrine tumors; Proton pump inhibitors (PPIs) can affect this test result (avoid 5 days prior if appropriate)

For the above mediators, levels higher than the reference range are considered positive while low levels are not clinically significant in terms of diagnosis. Experts recommend that the mediator testing occur at baseline (when the patient is not experiencing an acute mast cell reaction) and be repeated within 1–6 hours of an acute attack if the original testing is negative and the suspicion of MCAS remains high.[29] At current, negative mediator test results do not necessarily exclude the diagnosis.

One of the major drawbacks to mediator testing is that some labs do not recognize the importance of keeping the plasma and urine samples continuously chilled, potentially resulting in false negatives. For example, urine collection containers should be kept on ice or in a refrigerator, transported to the laboratory on ice and frozen before they are shipped out.

Some authors assert that chromogranin A is a problematic marker because it resides in neuroendocrine cells. Heparin was previously mentioned by some researchers as a potentially useful mediator for MCAS testing, but limitations in commercial laboratory procedures in the United States currently prevent it from making the most updated diagnostic cut.[29,33] Further research is warranted to investigate whether platelet activating factor, heparin, chymase or carboxypeptidase A3 are suitable mediators to include in future MCAS testing.[31]

Experts agree that a thorough differential diagnosis process should occur with each patient, as outlined in Table 6.

Table 6. Differential Diagnosis Considerations for MCAS[9,13]

Endocrinological Disorders	adrenal disorders
	diabetes mellitus
	Morbus Fabry
	pancreatic endocrine tumors (gastrinoma, insulinoma, glucagonoma, somatostatinoma, VIPoma)
	parathyroid tumor
	thyroid gland disorders
Gastrointestinal Disorders	celiac disease or non-celiac gluten sensitivity
	congenital (or acquired) sucrase isomaltase deficiency
	eosinophilic esophagitis
	eosinophilic gastroenteritis
	GERD (gastroesophageal reflux disease)
	H. pylori-positive gastritis
	infectious enteritis
	inflammatory bowel disease (Crohn's disease, ulcerative colitis)
	intestinal obstructions
	irritable bowel syndrome
	microscopic colitis
	parasitic infections
	primary lactose intolerance
	vasoactive intestinal peptide-secreting tumor

Immunological / Neoplastic Diseases	any overload or depletion of a host of immunoglobulins carcinoid tumor/syndrome hereditary angioedema hypereosinophilic syndrome intestinal lymphoma pheochromocytoma primary gastrointestinal allergy vasculitis
Neurological and Psychiatric Conditions	anxiety autonomic dysfunction/dysautonomia chronic fatigue syndrome depression headaches multiple sclerosis
Skin Conditions	angioedema atopic dermatitis chronic urticaria scleroderma
Other Conditions	coronary hypersensitivity (Kounis syndrome) cholelithiasis fibromyalgia hepatitis hereditary hyperbilirubinemia porphyria POTS (postural orthostatic tachycardia syndrome)

It's important to note that in some cases, patients may present with true clinical diagnoses of MCAS and one or more of the above conditions. For example, many patients with MCAS also have clinical diagnoses of POTS, irritable bowel syndrome, anxiety and/or depression. Guidance from a skilled medical practitioner is important to ensure not only the validated presence of MCAS, but also that no other conditions are being missed in the MCAS diagnostic process.

Clinical Considerations

One frustration among the patient community is the tendency for medical providers to fixate on tryptase levels, ignoring other chemical mediators. Research indicates that tryptase—while still a good screening tool for mast cell neoplasia—poorly reflects mast cell activation.[5,34,35]

While elevated tryptase levels are certainly not telltale for MCAS, it's possible that a *small subgroup* of MCAS patients have a genetic predisposition to elevated tryptase. Research indicates that 4%-6% of the general population may have elevated tryptase levels.[36,37] A condition called hereditary alpha tryptasemia (HAT) has gained increasing attention in recent research and, as mentioned above, is now part of the MCAD diagnostic discussion.

Numerous studies have noted episodes of idiopathic anaphylaxis and anaphylaxis as the result of a sting by an insect in the Hymenoptera order (such as wasps, bees, hornets and yellowjackets) to be more prevalent in patients with MCAD (specifically, systemic mastocytosis) than in the general population.[13,38-40] One study found that out of all patients who had allergic reactions to Hymenoptera venom, nearly 14% were found to have underlying mastocytosis or mast cell activation syndrome.[40]

The majority of patients with MCAS do *not* present with high tryptase or an allergy to Hymenoptera venom, but there is a subgroup of patients who do present with these characteristics, which may warrant ruling out systemic mastocytosis. While tryptase is an easy, relatively cheap test with clinical value in patient screening, it should not be the only line drawn in the sand for diagnostic consideration. This is a common frustration point for many patients who end up having to argue with their doctor in order to have other mast cell mediator tests ordered.

Many patients are initially drawn in the direction of MCAS investigation after first learning about histamine intolerance from a medical practitioner or website. Histamine is one of the more recognized mast cell mediators that is a notorious culprit in the production of certain distinct allergy-like symptoms, but it is only *one of the many* chemicals released by mast cells.

Histamine intolerance (HIT) and MCAS are not the same thing. However, it's very possible that patients who have signs of HIT actually have an underlying case of MCAS, and it's also possible that certain patients with MCAS struggle with histamine issues more so than with other chemical mediators. Histamine intolerance is believed to be linked to certain genes that may contribute to an individual's difficulty processing histamine, specifically HNMT, DAO, MAO, PEMT and NAT2.[41]

If any of these genes or the particular enzymes, B vitamins or minerals that support them aren't working properly, the individual may experience a buildup or overload of histamine that can trigger a number of symptoms. Gastrointestinal issues, hormonal dysregulation and a deficiency in the DAO enzyme are also tied to HIT.[42] Common triggers are ingested foods and beverages and sometimes exercise. Individuals may experience many symptoms of MCAS, including headaches, fatigue, swelling, hives, difficulty breathing, nasal congestion, flushing, abdominal symptoms, anxiety, fast heart rate, difficulty sleeping and high blood pressure.[42] Histamine intolerance is not a formal medical diagnosis; rather, it's an informal description.

Patients with MCAS may note some initial symptomatic improvement with a low histamine diet, but this change alone is not typically sufficient to counteract the root issue of inappropriate mast cell degranulation to non-food triggers on a chronic basis, as occurs with MCAS. For patients with MCAS, the symptom chronicity, triggers, intensity and wide scope of problems look distinctly different from HIT because MCAS involves several different chemical mediators—not just histamine—that are perpetually reacting inappropriately to factors beyond the narrow lens of diet.

Conventional IgE allergy testing may be inaccurate or inconclusive in this patient population. IgE testing aims to determine allergies for foods and other environmental factors that the patient is currently exposed to. Foods that have been avoided may test (falsely) negative because the body may not have sufficient antibodies for them. Some believe that the testing may also be inaccurate in patients who have dermatographia ("skin writing" or skin redness in response to pressure or a scratch) even if control areas are utilized. Others assert that food allergy testing may be inaccurate in patients who have a leaky gut, where they tend to test positive to the foods that they consume the most.

Some patients with MCAD describe reacting to nearly everything on testing and others appear to have no skin prick abnormalities. Some patients also report that skin prick testing has resulted in symptom flares. Some patients with MCAD reflect that their "true" allergens that consistently trigger anaphylactoid reactions will test negative on skin prick testing and blood allergy testing, while others come back with dozens of IgE-positive "allergies" to previously benign foods. Some patients also report that their IgE-positive test results are completely different every time they are tested.

Recent research concluded that conventional allergy IgE testing overestimates the rate of true clinical allergy, resulting in overdiagnosis and adverse impacts on quality of life.[43] Allergy testing should be performed with care in this patient population and should be discussed with your medical team on a case-by-case basis. It appears that new testing may be coming out in the near future to test for not only allergies but for other markers and indicators of MCAS.[43]

When a patient finally receives a diagnosis of MCAS, it's tempting to blame *everything* on the new diagnosis. However, it's important to avoid the slippery slope of attributing every condition on your medical resume to MCAS. When MCAS is diagnosed on top of another condition, it doesn't mean that the other condition is not necessarily there. Likewise, it's also essential to avoid the temptation to associate every new symptom or problem that pops up with MCAS.

Conventional Treatment of MCAS

Over-the-counter and prescription medication usage, in addition to trigger avoidance, are classic approaches to conventional management of MCAS. First-line therapy approaches for MCAS typically include H1 and H2 antihistamines, disodium cromoglycate (also known as cromolyn), vitamin C and ketotifen.[44] There is high value in the medications that are considered first-line therapy for MCAS, and many patients find that they do not need to pursue other classes of medications because these medications create a substantial improvement in symptoms. The use of immunosuppressive drugs, omalizumab, inhibitors of tyrosine kinase and other kinases, investigational drugs, cytoreductive drugs and polychemotherapy are also reported in the literature for MCAS treatment if first-line approaches are exhausted.[44]

The trial and error process can take months to find the right combination, dosage and brand of medication (or supplement). Patience and attention to detail are crucial in this process. It's important to make ONE change at a time—this applies not just to *types or brands* of medications, but also to the *dosage* and *frequency* per day. According to the experts, for most medications a one-month trial will generally be adequate to determine if the current medication/dosage will be of significant benefit.[9,45] This time frame is dependent on the particular medication, however. (For example, ketotifen and cromolyn trials generally take longer—up to several months—to determine efficacy. When in doubt, check with the prescribing doctor.)

If less than optimal treatments are continued while other new meds are added, unmanageable polypharmacy can develop; this should be avoided.[46] A quality—rather than quantity—approach to treatment with medications and supplements is ideal.

Keep in mind that many patients react to fillers/dyes/additives and may need to trial many versions of the same active ingredient before ruling it in or out. For example, a patient may tolerate the generic H1 blocker cetirizine but react to the brand name Zyrtec medication. That same patient may do better with the brand name Allegra and react more to the generic versions of the same active ingredient. Patients may even react to the capsule itself. It may be beneficial to try compounding pharmacies that have hypoallergenic filler options. Certain supplements and medications (including aspirin and quercetin) may contain plant-based substances called salicylates, which can also be the source of sensitivity in some individuals.

Many supplements and medications also contain grains like gluten and corn, even though these ingredients may not be obvious from reading the label. Some companies have been found to falsely advertise ingredients and the true quantity of an active ingredient, so caution is warranted with online purchases. Reputable companies can be more expensive but may be better options for patients with sensitivities to ensure that the appropriate ingredients and dosage are being obtained. The source of the supplement may also be vaguely explained on the label; patients with allergies to shellfish and nuts should be especially careful, as some supplements may be derived from or cross-contaminated with such ingredients. For example, the cheapest sources of quercetin are derived from peanut shells and fava beans, and when they are in a "proprietary blend" with questionable purity, they could trigger reactions in patients with G6PD deficiency or peanut allergies.[47]

Many patients will experience side effects from medications and/or supplements, some of which have been reported to disappear over time, while others may persist. It's also important to be clear on what types of reactions can be tolerated and what types necessitate immediate cessation of a medication. It's very helpful to discuss all of the above with your medical team.

It's common for patients to report reactions to the additives found in certain medications and supplements. Excipients are inactive substances that serve as a vehicle for the medication or supplement and can include fillers, binders and dyes. When a patient experiences a paradoxical reaction to something (such as feeling hyperactive instead of sedated with Benadryl®), it's worth investigating whether the excipient could be the cause. In these cases, dye-free or compounded versions may be better tolerated.

Patients may also experience times where they suddenly react to a medication (or supplement) they have been taking for a while without issues. In this case, it can be helpful to assume detective-mode as it's possible that the pharmacy may have changed brands or excipients in the medication without notifying the patient. If no explanation can be found, ultimately any medication or supplement that is ineffective or harmful should be immediately stopped.[9] It's also helpful to be aware of certain classes of medications that tend to trigger mast cell mediator release.

Table 7. Medications that May Trigger Reactions for Patients with MCAD[44]

TYPE OF MEDICATION	DRUGS THAT HAVE PROVEN OR THEORETICAL RISK
antibiotics	cefuroxime, gyrase inhibitors, vancomycin
anticonvulsive agents	carbamazepine, topiramate
cardiovascular drugs	ACE inhibitors, ß-Adrenoceptor antagonists
intravenous narcotics	methohexital, phenobarbital, thiopental
local anesthetics	amide-type: articaine, lidocaine; ester-type: procaine, tetracaine
muscle relaxants	atracurium, mivacurium, rocuronium
opioid analgesics	codeine, meperidine, morphine
peripheral-acting analgesics	acidic NSAIDS such as ibuprofen
peptidergic drugs	cetrorelix, icatibant, leuprolide, octreotide, sermorelin
plasma substitutes	gelatin, hydroxyethyl starch
selective dopamine and norepinephrine reuptake inhibitors	bupropion
selective serotonin reuptake inhibitors	all
X-ray contrast material	gadolinium chelate, iodinated contrast medium

Many patients with MCAS report regular use of pharmaceuticals in the above table without issues. Selective serotonin reuptake inhibitors (SSRI's) are an example of common medications that in some cases can be lifesaving, and factors like individualized tolerance and benefit play a big role in determining the proper approach.

Natural Treatment of MCAS

Not all patients tolerate synthetic medications, and likewise, not all patients tolerate natural supplements. Both can have additives, drug interactions, unwanted side effects and multiple ingredients that make it tricky to determine what exactly is triggering reactions.

Some patients find that taking conventional over-the-counter and prescription medications improve quality of life in the long-term with minimal or no adverse reactions. Others do better with non-conventional treatment options like herbal supplements and botanicals. An increasingly common trend is a blend of both options for the management of MCAS. Just as no two patients have identical symptom clusters, no two patients have the same treatment preference or tolerance.

It's important that once a stable baseline has been established, the treatment plan also includes trigger reduction and investigation of the root issues. By investigating and addressing root issues, many patients find that they are then equipped to alter their medication and/or supplement usage.

Natural supplement options that target mast cell pathways are extremely abundant in the literature and an all-inclusive review would expand beyond the scope of this book. Chapter 8 has several tables describing foods and herbs that may help boost the immune system and reduce/prevent symptoms in patients with MCAS.

The natural supplements most frequently described in the MCAS literature include aloe vera, alpha lipoic acid, Baikal skullcap, black cumin, boswellia, butterbur, camu camu, cannabinoids, chamomile, curcumin, EGCG (green tea), evening primrose oil, feverfew, gingko biloba, holy basil, khellin, licorice root, luteolin, mangosteen, melatonin, moringa, nettle, perilla extract, pycnogenol, quercetin, resveratrol, rutin, silibinin, silymarin, and vitamins/minerals (including vitamin D, vitamin C, zinc, magnesium and others).[48-74] These options and others will be elaborated on in the nutrition section in Chapter 8. Hormone-regulating supplements, Chinese herbal formulas and IV fluids are other approaches useful for some patients with MCAS. Supplements that help to heal the lining of the gut or improve digestive or pancreatic enzymes may also be useful adjuncts.

Probiotics can be helpful for patients with MCAS, but specific strains sometimes increase symptoms in certain individuals. Many probiotics contain fillers and added ingredients or poor shelf life, so it's important to carefully research brands and types. For the general MCAS population, experts tend to recommend *Bifidobacterium (bifidum, breve, infantis, longum)* and *Lactobacillus (gasseri, plantarum, rhamnosus, salivarius).*[75-78] Coexisting conditions also impact probiotic tolerance; for example, patients with small intestinal bacterial overgrowth (SIBO) find that some of the probiotics recommended for MCAS can flare up gastrointestinal symptoms. *Sacharomyces boulardii is* often used with patients who have either gliotoxin or ochratoxin mold exposure or SIBO, but individual tolerance varies.[77] Some patients also do well with spore-based probiotics containing *bacillus coagulans* and *bacillus subtilis.*[77]

To empower the patient to find underlying issues triggering the systemic inflammation and mast cell overactivation of MCAS, it is of the utmost importance to pay adequate attention to additional factors such as detoxification, emotional stress and trauma, exercise, health stressors like mold or viral infections, hydration, nervous system regulation, nutrition, sleep, stress, and toxin exposure. These topics will all be discussed at length in other chapters of this book.

Are We Barking Up the Wrong Tree?

Over the years, I've asked myself the question, "Are we barking up the wrong tree by focusing on MCAS?" Are we too busy focusing on the diagnosis or label of MCAS? Does the diagnosis even really matter?

There are a few concepts supporting that the diagnosis really does matter. One is that the diagnostic process helps rule out the scary stuff that could require immediate treatment... things like pheochromocytoma and carcinoid tumors. That being said, these conditions are very rare. And the overwhelming majority of conditions on the "differential diagnosis" consideration lists that are published in the literature are conditions that are often chronic comorbidities in patients with MCAS—things like thyroid disorders, celiac disease, GERD, parasitic infections, eosinophilic esophagitis, anxiety and depression, headaches, chronic fatigue syndrome, chronic urticaria, fibromyalgia and POTS, to name a few. Most patients with true lab-confirmed MCAS have a smattering of these true, test-confirmed additional conditions by the time they are diagnosed with MCAS or in the months following diagnosis.

Another—possibly more relevant—argument for the importance of "getting the diagnosis" figured out is that patients need the validation of having a name for their often widespread and chronic suffering. They may feel that they need something concrete to show their family members and friends (and sometimes even themselves) that they aren't crazy. They may need an overarching diagnosis, one that zooms away from the focus of one system, to explain why so many of their physiological organs and systems are in disarray simultaneously. Finally having answers can be extremely empowering.

Because many patients find themselves unable to work due to disabling symptoms, the diagnosis is also hugely relevant in terms of patients applying for disability and other supportive benefits to keep them afloat. Further, a subgroup of patients does not respond to over-the-counter medications like antihistamines and is limited in terms of more invasive treatment options to get things calmed down without an official diagnosis. I completely understand these perspectives and empathize with fellow patients.

But—outside of these scenarios—is focusing on diagnosing MCAS doing us a disservice in the long run? Are we wasting too much time and energy on the diagnosis when we could be focusing instead on finding the root issues and healing? Do we have tunnel vision in our perception of the role of mast cells? (These are rhetorical questions that I now ponder after having seen incredible patient results with holistic care, but I am obviously biased.)

One could argue that MCAS is not really a separate disease, but rather a state of system-wide inflammation triggered by the perfect storm of epigenetic changes and environment, involving dramatic mast cell dysfunction... in addition to a plethora of other cells that are likely not functioning properly. Have we spent too much time and energy in the quest to demonize mast cells? While targeting them may undeniably help mask symptoms, is this really the right approach? Which leads me to my next question....

Is a mainstream medicine approach to MCAS right for everyone? Obviously, there's a huge spectrum of patient scenarios here, and there are patients who are continually in a state of anaphylaxis, seizures and other issues that require very careful supervision and monitoring. The mainstream approach is to make the diagnosis and then find medications that alleviate symptoms, but it does not typically unearth WHY the symptoms are there in the first place. Of course, there are exceptions to this statement, and many doctors do search for factors like celiac disease, functional gastrointestinal issues and chronic infections as opposed to solely focusing on medications.

But is a functional medicine approach the best route? When we look at functional medicine, we find an approach that evaluates different health stressors in order to tease out what the underlying issues are, so that patients can focus on the root problem and decrease their inflammatory cascade—and subsequently see a reduction in mast cell activation, normalization of blood glucose and hormones, healing of the gut, etc. Many functional medicine providers investigate the following areas: toxic burdens, infectious disease in the form of bacterial and viral infections, gastrointestinal health (including candida, SIBO, leaky gut, parasites, protozoal infections, and more), metabolic and hormonal abnormalities, endocrine issues, nervous system and neurotransmitter abnormalities, nutrients and genetic/methylation factors.

When it comes to functional medicine, is identifying these issues one by one truly the best and most cost-effective approach that will unlock the most healing potential? A lot of these tests are expensive; for example, one round of testing may cost the patient $500-$1,000 out of pocket, only to affirm that yes, the patient does indeed have SIBO and other gut issues. Functional medicine testing can certainly be helpful if it determines the appropriate treatment approach for eradication of the root issue. For example, some strains of candida or bacteria may be more susceptible to certain products and may also be resistant to others, and it's helpful to use this information to guide treatment decisions. However, following the diagnoses, the patient may then need more money (and discipline) to embark on treatment and subsequent testing and may spend several months (or even years) focusing on that particular issue before moving on to the next one. What further complicates these efforts in some cases is the tendency to encounter barriers to treatment when working with providers who don't understand the complexity of the trifecta or the concept of medication/supplement intolerances.

Don't get me wrong, I am a huge fan of functional medicine and highly value my postgraduate training in this area. But what I've noted in clinical practice is this: Most patients with MCAS don't just have one or two functional medicine diagnoses—they often have a dozen of them all at once. So, where do we even start? What is the best approach to restore homeostasis to the entire system and subsequently alleviate or eliminate mast cell activation in the process?

Allostatic mechanisms are designed to maintain homeostasis, and they involve the neurological system, the immune system, and the endocrine system (and their complex interactions). Some consider allostatic load to be the "wear and tear" on the body that results from chronic stress. Proponents of the allostatic load response theory suggest that making changes like eliminating toxins and having a perfect diet will force the patient to live in a glass box; conversely, they believe that no single stressor is more important than the other. For example, they may claim that too much gluten is not more inflammatory than a single negative thought; all the different factors influence our system equally.

Thus, in order to restore homeostasis in the body, practitioners ought to help patients in a number of ways simultaneously: reducing environmental stressors and avoiding toxins is not a bad place to start, but it's also essential to instigate lifestyle changes, dietary changes, etc., that will address key metabolic imbalances seen within the systemic allostatic load in patients who are chronically ill. This could also include dealing with insulin resistance, inflammation, acidosis, emotional trauma, patterns triggering dysautonomia, nervous system factors, micronutrient deficiencies, etc., that contribute to the global dysfunction.

Embracing the concept of allostatic load could also mean addressing concepts like loneliness/isolation and high social stress. Research indicates that the influence of social relationships is comparable to risk factors such as alcohol consumption and smoking for risk of death; further, high social stress exceeds the mortality risk factors of obesity and physical inactivity![79] Addressing all the angles is of the utmost importance.

To me, this equates to a "modified functional medicine" approach in patients who are chronically ill—an approach that gently rebalances the emphasis on the diagnosis or label and empowers the patient to restore homeostasis with a number of different tools way beyond the scope of mast cells. Intrigued? We will dive much deeper into this approach soon. But first, let's review the two other conditions that make up the trifecta: POTS and EDS.

MCAS: TAKE-HOME MESSAGES

- Mast cells are a type of white blood cell, are present all over the body and engage in complex interactions with their environment. They are an important type of immune cell that can both suppress and add to inflammation, depending on the circumstances.
- Mast cells have receptors for allergens, pathogens, neurotransmitters, neuropeptides and hormones.
- Mast cells contain chemical mediators in vesicles that are released when signaled, a process called degranulation.
- These chemical mediators influence a vast number of processes throughout the body, and when in excess, can lead to system-wide symptoms. Tryptase, histamine, leukotrienes and serotonin are examples of well-known mast cell mediators.
- Mast cell triggers are patient-dependent and generally tend to include environmental toxins, dietary factors, exposure to an "invader" (like insect venom or a virus), medications and physical/emotional stress.
- While over 200 types of mediators exist, laboratory testing for patient diagnosis is limited to a handful of mast cell mediators.
- Mast cell activation disease (MCAD) is an umbrella term for several diseases including forms of mastocytosis, mast cell leukemia, mast cell sarcoma, as well as mast cell activation syndrome (MCAS).
- Patients with MCAS typically have multisystem symptoms and a generalized, widespread inflammatory pattern. Symptoms are often noted in the skin, eyes, major organs, gastrointestinal, respiratory, genitourinary, neuropsychiatric and musculoskeletal

systems. Patients may or may not present with signs of acute allergic reactions/anaphylaxis.

- MCAS is a disease that involves a normal number of mast cells that are "misbehaving" or reacting inappropriately to a wide range of triggers.
- MCAS is typically diagnosed by the presence of elevated chemical mediators in blood and/or urine testing, and some providers also consider the presence of abnormalities on tissue biopsy as diagnostic. Factors including a thorough differential diagnosis, the presence of mast cell-associated symptoms, and a clinical response to mast cell-targeting medications are also utilized in the diagnostic process.
- Research supports the possibility that MCAS has underlying somatic (acquired) and/or germline (inherited) mutations that contribute to disease etiology. Epigenetic factors also likely play a role.
- Anaphylaxis is a true medical emergency and it's important to have a written emergency plan, readily available auto-injectors of epinephrine (as appropriate) and a medical identification bracelet. Patients and family members should be well-versed in the signs of anaphylaxis.
- There's no shortage of medication options to address MCAS. Most patients are initially prescribed a combination of H1- and H2-receptor antagonists and should follow a stepwise approach to trialing other pharmaceutical drugs with the assistance of their medical team.
- Medication and supplement trials should be meticulously isolated to one substance at a time. In general, one month is usually sufficient to determine the efficacy of a single substance on symptoms.

- There are many natural substances that can also help manage MCAS. A natural approach to MCAS and other chronic conditions will be further elaborated on in Part Two of this book.
- An approach that emphasizes additional factors such as detoxification, emotional stress and trauma, exercise, health stressors like mold or viral infections, hydration, nervous system regulation, nutrition, sleep, stress, and toxin exposure are crucial for empowering the patient to find lasting healing from MCAS.

Chapter 2:
POSTURAL ORTHOSTATIC TACHYCARDIA SYNDROME (POTS)

Postural orthostatic tachycardia syndrome, also known as "POTS," is a condition where the heart rate increases abnormally in response to changes in position (typically, standing up). The word *orthostatic* refers to something caused by upright posture, and *tachycardia* means a fast heart rate. It can also occur when going from lying down to sitting. This condition is frequently reported in patients who have MCAS and/or EDS and is more common in individuals assigned female at birth between the ages of 15 and 40.[1] There are different types of POTS. As a syndrome, POTS is considered a cluster of symptoms that are frequently seen together (much like MCAS and EDS) as opposed to a disease.

Overview of POTS

The autonomic nervous system controls the background bodily functions that do not require conscious thought or action.[2] POTS is classified as a type of dysautonomia, where the autonomic nervous system is not working properly. Dysautonomia is fairly common and many conditions fall under its umbrella. It's often associated with autoimmune conditions.

Types of Dysautonomia include:[2]

- Autoimmune autonomic ganglionopathy
- Autonomic dysreflexia
- Diabetic autonomic neuropathy
- Familial dysautonomia
- Inappropriate sinus tachycardia
- Multiple system atrophy
- Neurally-mediated hypotension
- Neurocardiogenic syncope
- Orthostatic intolerance
- Pandysautonomia
- POTS
- Pure autonomic failure

Patients who experience POTS often report an intense heart-pounding sensation in addition to a rapid heart rate. Palpitations and dizziness are also experienced. Some people get light-headed and some people experience near fainting or fainting in conjunction with episodes. The onset is typically sudden and can sometimes be connected to a trigger such as trauma, emotional stress, infection, pregnancy, surgery, vaccination, virus or exposure to toxins.[3] Symptoms may be exacerbated around the time prior to the menstrual cycle.[3]

Tremors have also been reported in conjunction with episodes.[4] While near fainting is common, only about 30% of patients will actually pass out, according to one article.[3] There is some discrepancy in the literature in terms of whether fainting is consistent with POTS vs. other coexisting comorbidities, and syncope itself is not considered diagnostic.

One study noted that patients with POTS had greater difficulty with memory and concentration and scored higher on an attention deficit hyperactivity disease (ADHD) rating scale.[5] Symptoms may be more pronounced in the morning compared to the evening.[6] Acrocyanosis (discoloration of the legs) and coldness of the skin to the touch is noted in some patients with POTS.[3]

Many patients are wheelchair bound and/or homebound due to poor standing tolerance. Basic everyday activities such as bathing, cooking, housework and walking can be compromised in more severe cases. Approximately 25% of POTS patients are disabled and unable to work,[7] and one study found that the quality of life when living with POTS was comparable to that of patients on dialysis for kidney failure.[8,9] Patients are often misdiagnosed with anxiety or panic disorders before POTS is ever mentioned or considered. POTS alone can have a dramatic influence on a patient's quality of life.

Historically, POTS was described as early as the 1860s and was sometimes referred to as "Civil War Syndrome" and "Soldier's Heart." POTS was coined and first gained traction in being attributed to autonomic dysfunction in the 1990s.[10,11] In 2009, researchers theorized that additional mechanisms including cardiovascular deconditioning, neuropathy and cardiac beta-adrenoreceptor hypersensitivity could be responsible.[12] More recently, theories also expanded to include mechanisms related to blood volume, autoimmune conditions and inflammatory disorders.[13-15]

A 2020 review noted that several illnesses are now becoming part of the POTS landscape, including MCAD, chronic fatigue syndrome, gastroparesis, EDS and autoimmune disorders like Sjögren's syndrome.[16] Reversible conditions including the side effects/impacts of certain medications are now included in the POTS conversation.

Conditions Often Associated with POTS[2,16-18]

- Anxiety/depression
- Arthritis: rheumatoid; juvenile-onset rheumatoid arthritis
- Autoimmune disease (often positive ANA, but does not meet specific diagnosis)
- Celiac disease
- Chiari malformation
- Chronic immune deficiency
- Complex regional pain syndromes
- Diabetes
- Ehlers-Danlos syndromes (EDS) and joint hypermobility syndromes
- Endometriosis
- Epstein-Barr virus
- Fibromyalgia
- Gastroparesis and associated gastrointestinal diagnoses
- Heavy metal toxicity
- History of chemotherapy
- History of concussion
- Interstitial cystitis
- Irritable bowel syndrome (IBS)
- Lupus erythematosus
- Mast cell activation syndrome (MCAS)
- Median arcuate ligament syndrome (MALS)
- Migraine headaches
- Multiple sclerosis
- Myalgic encephalitis/chronic fatigue syndrome (ME/CFS)
- Pelvic floor dysfunction

- Polycystic ovarian syndrome (PCOS)
- Raynaud's syndrome
- Sinus node disease
- Sjögren's syndrome
- Small fiber neuropathy
- Small intestinal bacterial overgrowth (SIBO)
- Thyroid disease: Graves' disease and Hashimoto's thyroiditis

Some experts theorize that median arcuate ligament syndrome (MALS) is connected to dysautonomia and POTS symptoms. This condition, which commonly affects thin individuals between the ages of 20 and 40,[19] involves compression of the celiac artery and possibly the celiac ganglia by the median arcuate ligament, resulting in narrowing (stenosis) of the blood vessel that can be noted on ultrasound and CT imaging on exhale. This compression is believed to cause ischemia downstream to the abdominal tissues, spleen and liver, an audible epigastric bruit sound, vomiting, weight loss, gastroparesis and other symptoms.[19] Positioning can affect the median arcuate ligament, and it tends to relax when you are positioned on one side or in the fetal position. MALS has also been connected to dysregulation of the autonomic nervous system due to the increased or continual neural impulses initiated by mechanical pressure on the celiac ganglia by part of the diaphragm.[19]

Some tumors and cancerous conditions may mimic POTS.[4] Paraneoplastic syndrome associated with lung, breast, ovarian or pancreatic cancer may present as POTS, and this condition produces autoantibodies that target acetylcholine receptors in the autonomic ganglia.[4]

POTS has also been noted as an adverse effect following the vaccine for human papilloma virus (HPV).[20] Some theorize that this could be from vaccine content toxins or activation of mast cells.[20] However, while some articles show compelling connections, other experts dispute that the connection exists.[21-25] Head trauma, gastric bypass surgery and other conditions have reported associations with POTS as well. However, it's important to note that more high-quality evidence is needed to deny or confirm all the theorized triggering factors associated with POTS.[10,12,18,26-32]

Various researchers express concern that the condition has expanded to encompass symptoms unrelated to abnormal orthostatic or autonomic measurements. Further, critics note that tachycardia is a symptom that can be present in many treatable (and serious) conditions that may be missed if symptoms are attributed to POTS. The symptoms of POTS outside of the heart rate response are often considered vague and nonspecific, further complicating diagnosis.

In recent years, more medical professionals have become aware of the presence of POTS. Postural symptoms most commonly reported in addition to orthostatic intolerance include palpitations, lightheadedness, weakness, tremor, blurred vision and exercise intolerance.[16] Non-postural symptoms often include gastrointestinal issues (bloating, nausea, abdominal pain, diarrhea) as well as brain fog, insomnia, fatigue and migraines.[16]

Table 8. Symptoms Considered Common among Patients with POTS[2,33]

SYSTEM	SYMPTOMS
Cardiovascular	Orthostatic intolerance, orthostatic tachycardia, palpitations, dizziness, lightheadedness, (pre-) syncope, exercise intolerance, poor perfusion, dyspnea, chest pain/discomfort, acrocyanosis, poor microcirculation to extremities such as Raynaud's syndrome, venous pooling, limb edema
Dermatological	Petechiae, rashes, erythema, telangiectasias, abnormal sudomotor regulation leading to excess sweating or the inability to sweat, pallor, flushing
Gastrointestinal	Nausea, dysmotility, gastroparesis, constipation, diarrhea, abdominal pain, weight loss
General	General deconditioning, chronic fatigue, exhaustion, heat intolerance, fever, debility, being bedridden, anxiety, depression
Musculoskeletal	Muscle fatigue, muscle pain, weakness
Neurological	Headache/migraine, mental clouding ("brain fog"), cognitive impairment, concentration problems, anxiety, tremulousness, light and sound sensitivity or intolerance, blurred/tunnel vision, neuropathic pain (regional), insomnia and sleeping disorders, involuntary movements

Respiratory	Hyperventilation, bronchial asthma, shortness of breath
Urological	Bladder dysfunction, nocturia, polyuria

POTS Classification

A quick review of scientific literature and websites reveals that there are some discrepancies in terms of the understanding of the different types and subcategories of POTS. In general, scientific literature agrees that there are two categories of POTS, Primary (Idiopathic) and Secondary POTS.

Primary (Idiopathic) POTS

Primary (Idiopathic) POTS is typically classified as having two distinct subtypes in the scientific literature—neuropathic and hyperadrenergic—though some resources describe a third category as hypovolemic POTS.

Neuropathic POTS (also referred to as "Partial Dysautonomia") is a type of POTS believed to be due to inadequate vasoconstriction of peripheral and splanchnic (internal organ) structures that occurs with orthostatic stress (upright positioning). This type of POTS is often associated with small fiber neuropathy, damage to the small fiber nerves that regulate the constriction of the blood vessels in the limbs and abdomen as well as regulation of the heartbeat. Due to damage, the peripheral blood vessels have difficulty maintaining normal blood pressure in certain against-gravity positions (such as standing up). Neuropathic POTS is believed to be caused by the veins in the legs not working properly, resulting in pooling of blood in the extremities, which then tells the brain that the blood pressure is low, which triggers a rise in heart rate to compensate. As blood pooling occurs (which is commonly noted in both POTS and EDS), the system tries to compensate for the drop in stroke volume so that the heart can continue to pump an adequate amount of blood to the body.

The "aldosterone paradox" describes the concept of the kidneys erroneously getting rid of fluids and electrolytes that the body needs because of neuropathic POTS-associated blood pooling in the lower part of the body, where the kidneys reside. In this scenario, it's believed that the kidneys detect too much blood volume and activate mechanisms to increase urinary output in order to compensate. However, what the kidneys don't realize is that the blood volume from their vantage point is not the same as the blood volume in the upper half of the body, and this mechanism leads to further dehydration in the upper body and a vicious cycle scenario.[2]

Patients with neuropathic POTS have been found to have less norepinephrine released (and less sympathetic nervous system activation) in their lower extremities when compared to their upper extremities.[34] This type of POTS is considered a mild peripheral autonomic neuropathy and 5:1 cases are female compared to male.[34] Neuropathic POTS development often occurs after surgery, trauma, sepsis, immunizations, pregnancy or a febrile viral illness.[4] Clinicians may observe an obvious darkening of the color of the legs while the patient is seated. There is also a developmental partial dysautonomic POTS that typically affects teenagers after they've experienced large growth spurts, though that type of POTS tends to naturally regress over time in 80% of cases.[4]

Hyperadrenergic POTS is associated with elevated levels of the stress hormone norepinephrine. This type of POTS is thought to be significantly less common in the general population (only comprising 10% of cases),[3] though sources indicate that it may be proportionally more common in patients presenting with mast cell activation issues.[35]

Hyperadrenergic POTS displays the other type of compensatory mechanism that can occur in response to abnormal blood perfusion via the release of adrenaline and noradrenaline from the sympathetic nervous system. Some patients wax and wane between hypovolemic and hyperadrenergic POTS, and experts maintain that for most patients, the designation does not necessarily change the treatment approach.[2] A condition called Morvan's syndrome results in antibody-based hyperadrenergic overdrive and can mimic some symptoms of hyperadrenergic POTS, though these patients typically do not have the degree of heart rate increase seen in POTS.[2]

Norepinephrine transporter deficiency (NET) is often discussed in relation to this patient population. NET describes the abnormality in a gene that leads to too much circulating norepinephrine. Certain antidepressants/anti-anxiety medications block this transporter, which can make heart rate responses and symptoms worse. Pheochromocytomas (norepinephrine-producing tumors) can mimic hyperadrenergic POTS and testing may be appropriate to rule this condition out.

Symptoms with standing typically involve tremors, cold and sweaty hands and feet, migraines, a sense of anxiety and an urge to urinate in patients with this subcategory of POTS.[4] Patients with hyperadrenergic POTS tend to present with elevated systolic blood pressure when upright, as opposed to the drop in blood pressure observed in patients with neuropathic symptoms.[35] This type tends to occur in a gradual and progressive manner. Doctors may order supine and upright testing of serum catecholamine levels if the hyperadrenergic type of POTS is suspected. Serum norepinephrine levels are typically >600 ng/ml (upright) with these patients.[4] Many believe that there is a strong influence of genetics in the development of hyperadrenergic POTS.

Hypovolemic POTS is a type of POTS that occurs due to abnormally low levels of systemic blood circulation (also known as hypovolemia). When patients change positions, a lower blood volume can result in a compensatory heart rate increase in order to help circulate the blood more adequately around the body, because there is less of it to go around. This is similar to the compensatory pattern described with neuropathic POTS, although the mechanisms between the two (low total blood volume causing heart rate compensation, compared to poor venous return in legs from neuropathy causing lower blood volume reaching the heart) are slightly different.

As the total blood volume falls, the heart must beat faster to compensate and maintain blood pressure. This is the main mechanism believed to be responsible for hypovolemic POTS, or "compensated neuro-cardiovascular dysfunction."[2] When this occurs *without* compensation, patients usually experience dizziness or fainting from the drop in blood pressure, known as orthostatic hypotension.[2]

Some sources assert that POTS patients often have several characteristics present, making the subcategories of Primary (Idiopathic) POTS irrelevant. For example, some patients may have low blood volume, small fiber neuropathy and elevated norepinephrine occurring simultaneously. Not all patients fit neatly into one categorical box.

Secondary POTS

Secondary POTS describes POTS that occurs in conjunction with another condition, including (but not limited to) lupus, Lyme disease and other vector-borne illness, Sjögren's syndrome, or diabetes or another condition that can cause neuropathy. For example, patients with Babesia, a condition associated with a tick bite, may have secondary POTS occurring due to the infiltration of parasitic infection.[36]

The most common cause of secondary POTS is believed to be type II diabetes, a condition that often has inherent peripheral neuropathy.[4] Patients with Parkinson's disease or multiple sclerosis and patients experiencing heavy metal toxicity or undergoing chemotherapy may also experience secondary POTS.[4]

Diagnosis of POTS

Similar to the disparities between published literature in regard to the diagnosis of MCAS, POTS authorities have also published slightly differing diagnostic criteria; there is no current set of universally accepted criteria.[16] Factors that muddy the waters include the presence of symptoms without any physiological findings, the poor reproducibility of physiological findings, and the response to various interventions. Reproducibility of tilt table vs. standing test options also remain unclear.

Critics question whether POTS is part of a bigger diagnosis and whether it should be considered a stand-alone label. The expansion of POTS to include concepts of hypovolemia, deconditioning and a hyperadrenergic state open the doors to an even wider (and less-sensitive) base of interpretation.

Limitations to current diagnosis include the lack of universal diagnostic criteria, the indication that many patients proceed with self-diagnosis in the absence of medical examination, the concern that a similar heart rate increase with standing is considered normal in some studies, and the fact that a one-time abnormal heart rate response can be diagnostic while lacking consistency to indicate an ongoing problem. Several factors may influence standing heart rate, including hydration, food selection and timing, glucose levels, salt intake, underlying health stressors including viral infections and length of time spent in recumbent position.[37-39]

The original diagnostic criteria were derived from head-up tilt table testing.[10] A Heart Rhythm Society (HRS) Expert Consensus Statement expanded the diagnostic criteria to the currently utilized 30/40 BPM heart rate increase and determined that tilt table testing was not required for diagnosis.[40,41] From then on, moving from recumbent to standing positions became an accepted method of testing for POTS[40,41] though it appears that these tests are not interchangeable.[42] What has remained constant across diagnostic recommendations, however, is that the raise in heart rate cannot be tied to a simultaneous drop in systolic blood pressure (>20 mmHg). However, some sources do voice concern that patients could truly have both conditions (POTS and orthostatic hypotension) occurring at once as separate entities.

At current, POTS is typically diagnosed in a medical clinic using a standing or tilt table test. A positive test is indicated by the presence of orthostatic intolerance symptoms associated with a sustained heart rate increase of 30 beats per minute (bpm) or absolute rate exceeding 120 bpm in adults within the first 10 minutes of shifting to an upright position.[4] In children, the diagnosis is made if the sustained heart rate increases by 40 beats per minute.[43]

When utilizing the standing test, the patient's heart rate should be taken after five minutes of resting supine (lying on their back), and then at two, five, and 10 minutes after quickly standing still. Blood pressure should be monitored after at least 30 seconds of standing to make sure it does not drop significantly. Patients with certain types of POTS tend to fidget when standing to help compensate for poor venous return or low blood volume, so it's important to instruct the patient to stand still. It may also be wise to have the patient stand with their back against a wall if they tend to faint or feel light-headed.[44]

For clinicians who have access to a tilt table, the patient rests supine for 20 minutes, and then the table is tilted upward to 70 degrees. The blood pressure and heart rate are monitored continuously and recorded at minutes two, five and 10. The patient is kept in the upright position for 40 minutes, or until they faint. A "normal" rise in heart rate is about 10 beats per minute from sit to stand. So, a rise of 30 beats per minute is considered clinically significant in adults.

The diagnosis of POTS can only be made if the patient has *not* been subjected to prolonged bed rest or medications that interfere with the autonomic nervous system (such as diuretics, vasodilators, anxiolytic agents and antidepressants). Dehydration, anemia and hyperthyroidism often cause tachycardia and must also be ruled out.[3]

The more conservative sources recommend repeat measurements of vital signs with standing or tilt table testing, with definitive and reproducible heart rate responses for at least 3–6 months, prior to diagnosis.

A 2020 review proposed the following diagnostic flowchart:[16]

- Symptoms of orthostatic intolerance AND
- Improvement of symptoms when supine AND
- Symptoms present for a minimum of 3 (preferably 6) months

PLUS

- Orthostatic Vital Signs
- Supine HR and BP followed by upright HR and BP (duration 5–10 minutes): Increase in HR >30 BPM (>age 19) or >40 BPM (<age 19) with no (or minimal) drop in BP (beginning >30 seconds after standing)

PLUS

- Secondary causes ruled out, specialist referral as needed to complete this process

The authors note some additional considerations: [16]

- Patients must NOT display any evidence of orthostatic hypotension (blood pressure drop with positional change).
- Fainting is not considered a diagnostic criterion.
- Symptoms of orthostatic intolerance include postural chest pain, exertional dyspnea (shortness of breath with movement), dizziness, dependent acrocyanosis (blue or purple discoloration from slow circulation), and lightheadedness with associated heart rate response abnormalities.
- Additional orthostatic symptoms such as chronic fatigue and brain fog are present for diagnosis.
- Additional autonomic symptoms such as bloating, constipation and sweating abnormalities are present for diagnosis.
- Orthostatic tachycardia must occur within 3–10 minutes of standing and/or tilt table testing.
- No other explainable cause for orthostatic tachycardia/tachycardia must exist.
- Symptoms alone do not make the diagnosis.

The review authors note that it's important to evaluate several orthostatic heart rate measurements over time and at various times of the day, with possible repeat testing on the same day. They compare POTS testing to the principles of hypertension diagnosis, where an isolated reading is not grounds for pharmacological intervention.[16] It's evident that more research is needed in this area, including the reproducibility of testing types and how to proceed in light of comorbid conditions and medications that could elevate or lower the heart rate.

Patients with the label of vasovagal syncope are sometimes described as having POTS, but some experts assert that that this type of fainting and POTS should not, by nature, go hand in hand.[16] Patients with vasovagal syncope experience initial tachycardia (high heart rate) followed by a drop in blood pressure and a slow heart rate, which is distinct from the elevated and sustained heart rate (in the absence of a drop in blood pressure) consistent with POTS.[16] When patients regularly feel as if they are going to faint, it's important to determine the exact physiological mechanisms occurring (by measuring vital signs) to aid in the diagnosis.

Deconditioning has been theorized to be connected to the development of POTS, with some going as far as to suggest that Primary POTS can be excluded if symptoms resolve rapidly after a short period of consistent exercise. Specifically, deconditioning appears to result in decreased stroke volume, decreased blood volume and cardiac atrophy, which can lead to sympathetic nervous system activation in the upright position.[18] However, many individuals in the general population are severely deconditioned and do not display symptoms of POTS, so this logic may be faulty and is generally not considered as part of the diagnostic process.

Some specialty clinics will also evaluate specific reflex testing, upright norepinephrine blood levels, sweat testing, blood volume measurement, exercise capacity, optic nerve function, vagus nerve function, brain MRIs, nerve conduction velocity, biofeedback and other metrics when considering the diagnosis of POTS, the potential subcategory of POTS, the baseline functional status and other contributing factors. Specifically, the Quantitative Sudomotor Autonomic Reflex Test, Thermoregulatory Sweat Test, gastric motility studies and skin biopsies looking at the small fiber nerves are sometimes utilized. Cardiologists may also include electrocardiograms and pulmonary function testing, three-day heart rhythm recording and exercise testing in their diagnostic work-up. Some providers also include a comprehensive laboratory evaluation of factors like hormones, mast cell activation markers, nutrients, autoimmunity, infectious disease and genetics.

Conventional Treatment of POTS

Conventional treatment of POTS focuses on the following areas:

- Guided exercise program
- Salt and water intake
- Compression garments
- Medications

A 2020 review found that there is little evidence supporting medications for reversing or shortening primary idiopathic POTS or improving outcomes when compared to placebo.[16] The authors noted that prospective studies supporting long-term benefits are lacking for all of the medications used with POTS.[16] Nonetheless, many patients are encouraged to try a prescription medication to manage POTS, such as a beta blocker, fludrocortisone, ivabradine, midodrine, or pyridostigmine.[2] Other medications such as alpha methyl-dopa, clonidine, droxidopa, methylphenidate, modafinil, octreotide, phenobarbital, serotonin reuptake inhibitors, vasopressin, and yohimbine may be considered.[16] These medications work to control the heart rate and cause peripheral vasoconstriction or volume expansion to reduce POTS symptoms. Out of all of the options, low dose propranolol has shown some improvement compared to placebo, although this was not as strong as the results of cardiovascular exercise alone.[45]

There are also certain drugs and medications that can worsen orthostatic intolerance and should be avoided, including: anticholinergics, alpha receptor blockers, beta blockers used indiscriminately/at higher doses, calcium channel blockers, central dopamine antagonists, diuretics, ethanol, ganglionic blocking agents, monoamine oxidase inhibitors, nicotine, nitrates, opiates, phenothiazines, tricyclic antidepressants (unless no other choice) and Viagra.[2] POTS triggers vary between patients, and common triggers to avoid include hot showers, large meals, alcohol, caffeine and activity in hot weather.

Conservative strategies (such as exercise programs and hydration) offer potential symptom relief without the possibility of medication side effects. Exercise has been cited as one of the most important treatments for dysautonomia.[2] Research supports the presence of tremendous benefits in patients who have POTS and perform rigorous cardiovascular exercise programs.[45,46] POTS-specific exercise programs typically begin in recumbent positions (such as supine, seated, or on a rowing machine). The Levine Protocol and the CHOP Modified Dallas Protocol are some of the more documented treatment approaches for exercise in patients with POTS; in-depth discussion of exercise approaches for POTS are presented in Chapter 10, "Movement."

Sodium intake, elevating the head of the bed 10–20 degrees at night for blood volume retention and compression garments may also offer some relief, though it's unclear what long-term effects these approaches may have on overall health. Patients who have hyperadrenergic POTS with high blood pressure are typically advised to avoid increasing their salt intake, while those presenting with low blood pressure may be instructed otherwise. Salt supplements are typically added directly into the water consumed to avoid concern over electrolyte disturbances. Typical dietary intake of salt is 3–5 grams per day; the general guidelines for recommended levels in patients with POTS are 6–9 grams total per day.[47,48]

For hydration, a minimum of 2–2.5 L per day is recommended, with higher levels when you are active and sweating.[49-51] Some resources cite extremely high intake of water for the management of POTS. It's important to note that caution should be taken here as too much water can cause electrolyte imbalances and potentially abnormal heart rhythms. While many POTS-specialty clinicians advocate for these approaches, many providers in the functional medicine or natural medicine world consider them a "Band-Aid approach" that does not address the underlying issue responsible for POTS.

Dietary modifications (including the avoidance of dairy, gluten, processed carbohydrates and alcohol) and eating smaller meals throughout the day are sometimes recommended. Some patients find that caffeine is helpful, while others find it can exacerbate symptoms. Some patients are advised to spend time in a zero-gravity position (such as a recumbent bike) or zero-gravity chair before, during and after eating in order to aid in digestion. Abdominal binders are also recommended for returning to the upright position while still digesting meals, though not all patients tolerate abdominal binders.

Other medical approaches for POTS are relatively undocumented. One case report noted that POTS resolved completely, and its remission was sustained, in a patient with MCAS who underwent a treatment plan combining low-dose naltrexone, intravenous immunoglobulin (IVIG) and antibiotic therapy for small intestinal bacterial overgrowth (SIBO).[52] The author concluded that the presence of SIBO may play an important role in POTS patients;[52] hopefully future research will investigate the role of the microbiome and gut health and specifically how it may relate to POTS. Another case report found favorable results with plasma exchange in a patient with POTS who did not have autoantibodies.[53] Vagal nerve stimulation from surgically implanted devices are being investigated as a treatment option for dysautonomia, but they may lead to a worsening of symptoms if not placed correctly.[2] Less invasive types of nerve stimulation like Transcranial Magnetic Stimulation and Retinal Tolerance Neuromodulation may offer alternative treatment options for this patient population.[2]

Dr. Diana Driscoll is the owner of the POTS Care clinic in Texas, and she offers comprehensive care that looks outside of the box to discover underlying reasons for POTS. Her book "The Driscoll Theory® Newly Revised: The Cause of POTS in Ehlers-Danlos Syndrome and How to

61

Reverse the Process" is an incredible resource for anyone looking to better the understand potential mechanisms behind POTS and how it may relate to EDS, MCAS, Arnold-Chiari ("Chiari") malformation, intracranial pressure issues and much more.[54]

Natural Treatment of POTS

There are so many types of dysautonomia and a variety of clinical presentations, and many people jump to the POTS conclusion (and subsequent medication-based treatment plan) without instigating further investigation of the cause. Sometimes it seems that POTS is simply another label indicating that there's a bigger picture issue going on in the body. Clinically, I've witnessed POTS symptoms disappear in my patients in days to weeks to months once triggers like mold, viral infections, and cervical spine issues were addressed (in the absence of other traditional interventions). It seems that patients with POTS are sensitive to many of the health stressors outlined in Chapters 5 and 6, and an approach that identifies and treats root issues is of the utmost importance with this patient population.

2017 research noted that nearly half of 624 patients with POTS were at high risk for suicide.[55] Health related quality of life, fatigue, pain and sleep quality were significantly impacted when compared to control subjects.[55] This highlights the dire need for improvements in comprehensive treatment options for this patient population.

Similar to the recommendations for a natural approach to MCAS, adequate attention to additional factors such as detoxification, exercise, emotional factors, hydration, nervous system regulation, nutrition, sleep, spine instability, stress, systemic inflammation and toxin exposure are also key for patients with POTS. Breathing exercises to enhance diaphragm muscle activation and improve function of the vagus nerve can also be helpful, alongside treatments that incorporate the polyvagal theory into nervous system retraining. (Chapter 7 will dive into these topics.) While exercise programs are considered conventional treatment of POTS, they are also an essential part of a comprehensive program and should be guided with the help of a professional who is well-versed in dysautonomia.

POTS: TAKE-HOME MESSAGES

- Postural orthostatic tachycardia syndrome, also known as POTS, is a condition where the heart rate increases abnormally in response to changes in position (typically, standing up). This condition predominantly affects individuals between the ages of 15 and 40.
- Postural symptoms most commonly reported—in addition to intolerance to standing—include heart palpitations, lightheadedness, weakness, tremor, blurred vision and exercise intolerance.
- Non-postural symptoms of POTS often include gastrointestinal issues (bloating, nausea, abdominal pain, diarrhea) as well as brain fog, insomnia, fatigue and migraines.
- The onset of POTS is typically sudden. Theorized triggers include trauma, infection, surgery, vaccination, pregnancy, emotional stress, exposure to toxins such as chemotherapy or heavy metals, female hormonal fluctuations and other triggers.
- POTS is a type of dysautonomia. The condition has two categories: Primary (Idiopathic) POTS and Secondary POTS.
- There are different classifications of Primary POTS including neuropathic and hyperadrenergic POTS. Some sources also consider hypovolemic POTS to be its own category of Primary POTS.
- Secondary POTS is tied to another known condition such as diabetes, lupus, tick-borne illness such as Babesia and Lyme

disease, Parkinson's disease, multiple sclerosis, Sjögren's syndrome and others.

- POTS is diagnosed with a tilt table or standing test, and the rise in heart rate must occur in the absence of a drop in the blood pressure.

- Conventional treatment of POTS typically focuses on medications, salt and water intake, compression garments and exercise programs. While the medication approach has poor literature support for the management of POTS, progressive exercise protocols have ample scientific backing for improving this condition.

- Medications, sodium consumption and compression garments may alleviate symptoms, but these strategies may also pose increased risk of long-term consequences on other aspects of health.

- Natural and integrative/functional medicine treatment approaches offer the greatest hope for remission of symptoms by addressing the causes. Comprehensive care that gives attention to factors like underlying health stressors, diet and nutrition, toxin exposure/detoxification, nervous system retraining, breathing, emotional health, sleep, hydration, stress management, exercise and systemic inflammation offer the greatest utility for patients with POTS.

Chapter 3:
EHLERS-DANLOS SYNDROME (EDS)

O ver the past decade, the terminology surrounding conditions with excessively mobile joints has been a bit murky. Joint Hypermobility Syndrome (JHS) is a term previously utilized in the literature, but it was difficult to distinguish JHS from the hypermobile type of Ehlers-Danlos syndrome in the research.

Hypermobility Terminology

Hypermobility Spectrum Disorder (HSD) is a newly utilized term to describe patients who have hypermobility and musculoskeletal manifestations that cannot be explained by another diagnosis, though formal diagnostic criteria have not been defined.[1,2] HSD is classified as a less-restrictive label for individuals who experience abnormalities in the degree of motion present at the joints, whereas the hypermobile type of Ehlers-Danlos syndrome is considered a more restrictive diagnosis.[1,2]

Before we dive too deep into hypermobility, let's zoom out a little to understand the full complexity of the Ehlers-Danlos syndromes.

Heritable disorders of connective tissue (HDCT) is an umbrella term for the following four conditions:

- Ehlers-Danlos syndromes (EDS)
- Marfan syndrome (MFS)
- Osteogenesis imperfecta (OI)
- Hypermobility Spectrum Disorders (HSD)

EDS describes hereditary disorders of the connective tissue that typically present with skin hyperextensibility, generalized joint hypermobility, and fragility of vascular and internal organ structures. In patients with EDS, defects in genes are responsible for abnormalities in the structure and biosynthesis of a protein called collagen. Similar to the fact that mast cells are present in nearly all body systems, collagen, too, can affect virtually every single body system. Also similar to MCAS, patients with EDS exist along a spectrum of severity, and individual stability and functioning can vary widely between patients, from mild impairments to life-threatening issues.

The prevalence of EDS varies depending on the type, with an average prevalence estimate of one in 2,500–5,000 people.[3,4] Once believed to be a rare condition, many clinicians currently feel that this number vastly underestimates the true prevalence of EDS.

EDS Classification

Since EDS was discovered, five different classification systems have been used by medical providers. The most recent set of guidelines was developed by the International Consortium on EDS in 2017 as an international classification of EDS that delineated 13 distinct clinical subtypes of the condition.[5]

Clinical EDS Subtypes

1. Classical EDS (cEDS)
2. Classical-Like EDS (clEDS)
3. Cardiac-valvular EDS (cvEDS)
4. Vascular EDS (vEDS)
5. Hypermobile EDS (hEDS)
6. Arthrochalasia EDS (aEDS)
7. Dermatosparaxis EDS (dEDS)
8. Kyphoscoliotic EDS (kEDS)
9. Brittle Cornea syndrome (BCS)
10. Spondylodysplastic EDS (spEDS)
11. Musculocontractural EDS (mcEDS)
12. Myopathic EDS (mEDS)
13. Periodontal EDS (pEDS)

At the same time, genetic classification was also proposed that separated the types of EDS into Groups A through F, based on the type of disordered mechanism involved (e.g., disorders of collagen folding and crosslinking, disorders of the complement pathway, disorders of glycosaminoglycan biosynthesis). However, hEDS was not included in this sub-typing since its mechanism is not yet understood.[5]

There appears to be a wide degree of symptom overlap between the subtypes and with other connective tissue disorders. Differential diagnosis is important for this population, and many patients need to be referred to a geneticist when EDS is suspected. The hypermobile type of EDS is the only type with a diagnostic grey area that relies on clinical diagnosis.[5]

The classical and hypermobile types of EDS account for more than 90% of cases.[3,4] The third most common type is vascular EDS, which has been estimated to affect 1 in 250,000 people.[6] Vascular EDS can have a big impact on lifespan because of the risk it poses for blood vessel problems such as an aneurysm (blood vessel that bursts). Classical EDS is more commonly characterized by difficulty with wound healing. All types of EDS tend to impact multiple systems.

Hypermobile EDS (hEDS)

Hypermobile EDS (hEDS) is believed to be an inherited connective tissue disorder that's caused by defects in collagen. This type of EDS is characterized by joint hypermobility, signs of faulty connective tissue throughout the body (such as hernias, prolapses and skin abnormalities), musculoskeletal pain/problems and a family history of similar characteristics. Several other types of symptoms are often noted in this patient population, such as digestive issues, pelvic floor and bladder problems, anxiety, dysautonomia and mast cell activation issues, though these symptoms are not part of the formal diagnostic criteria.

While hEDS is sometimes viewed as less severe than other types of EDS due to its decreased likelihood of internal organ issues, patients with hEDS often experience debilitating acute and chronic musculoskeletal pain and dysfunction. Spine pain, joint dislocations and subluxations are common, and many patients also find themselves considering surgical intervention.[4] The majority of this book will focus on hypermobile EDS (hEDS) as it is the type most frequently associated with dysautonomia and mast cell activation issues.

While several defects in connective tissue proteins have been noted, without a clear genetic explanation for hEDS, most experts believe that the pathophysiology of the condition is likely multifactorial. Some believe that chronic mast cell activation and excess chemical mediator release could be responsible for the abnormal connective tissue properties noted in hEDS. Mast cells help the body to create connective tissue and collagen in response to stress/strain and the presence of wounds. When mast cells become dysfunctional, it's possible that the results of excess degranulation or elevated concentrations of certain chemical mediators can have a negative impact on the body's normal connective tissue healing process, whether it be in lying down too much scar tissue, or by forming weak bonds with new collagen that result in weak connective tissue.

On the other side of the theory spectrum, it's also possible that a genetic mutation causes hEDS (though it hasn't been officially discovered yet) and as a result, connective tissues are innately abnormal. If connective tissues are not healing or lying down new collagen properly, this could also trigger subsequent mast cell activation as the mast cells perceive the abnormality as a threat that triggers a cascade of chronic degranulation. While research has indicated that the majority of patients with MCAS plus other comorbidities exhibit joint hypermobility, the definitions of hypermobility have varied in the literature and it's difficult to make direct connections to EDS, but hopefully research will continue to investigate this area.[7]

In terms of the connection with dysautonomia, some believe that the abnormal vascular structures in EDS could contribute to the vascular pooling noted with postural orthostatic tachycardia syndrome (POTS). Others theorize that abnormalities with the autonomic nervous system, vagus nerve, intracranial pressure and Chiari malformation may be more closely connected to hEDS than we realize.[8] Conditions such as Chiari malformation and craniocervical instability (CCI) are associated with EDS and appear to have a direct anatomic influence on the vagus nerve, which could trigger subsequent dysregulation of the autonomic nervous system.

Delayed diagnosis of EDS is common; 2018 research reported an average of 22 years from symptom onset to diagnosis.[9] The diagnosis of EDS can have a tremendous influence on social and emotional factors. A 2019 review on the lived experiences of people with JHS and EDS noted several consistent themes, including social stigmas, restricted lives, a lack of professional understanding regarding their condition, the need to gain

71

control, and an attempt to "keep up."[10] It's clear that the presence of EDS alone can have a profound impact on an individual's quality of life.

Orthopedic concerns with hEDS

Orthopedic symptoms are widespread and can range from mildly irritating to severely disabling in patients with hEDS. Common concerns noted by physical therapists in this patient population include muscle spasms, subluxations (partial dislocations) and dislocations, damage to muscles/tendons, bone injuries, nerve entrapment and myofascial restrictions.[11] Central sensitization is the process where the body perceives pain more quickly and severely than the general population, and this can occur when pain is unmanaged over time.[11]

Orthopedic pain is often related to abnormal movement patterns, joint instability, and overload of connective tissue (tendons and ligaments), muscles and joints.[12] With generalized joint hypermobility, all four limbs and the axial skeleton are typically involved, as opposed to a single hypermobile joint in one area.[5] Due to the nature of the hypermobility, some patients experience severe muscle guarding and myofascial pain because the muscles are acting as extra stability for the joints, which move around too much and lack tight ligamentous support. Tendons, bursae, ribs and surrounding nervous system structures may also be impacted. Increased ligamentous laxity is often accompanied by reduced proprioception, or a decreased kinesthetic ability to sense where the body or joint is located in space, and patients with hEDS appear to have decreased proprioception.[13,14] Decreased proprioception may result in clumsiness or compensatory patterns such as gripping objects forcefully or wearing tight clothing and footwear.

Spine pain is a frequent concern in patients with hEDS. Spondylosis of both the cervical and lumbar spine are common, and sometimes laminectomy, discectomy and spinal fusions are performed. However, experts give a word of caution for spinal fusions in this patient population, as the tendency for "next segment" issues (where the joints above and below the fusion site are overloaded following surgery, making other segment(s) rigid with fusion hardware) appear to have a higher incidence in patients with joint hypermobility.[15] Joint hypermobility may also be a relative contraindication for artificial disks.[15] Other conditions affecting the neck and brainstem including Chiari malformation and craniocervical instability (discussed later in this book) may warrant surgical intervention in this patient population, depending on the severity.

Temporomandibular (jaw) joint pain, inflammation and mobility issues are sometimes noted in patients with hEDS and often go hand-in-hand with cervical spine issues. If the upper neck vertebrae are not aligned well, the jaw and bite alignment can be off. The jaw can sublux, dislocate, and experience clicking and popping sensations. The small muscles around the jaw can change their tone, resulting in pain, abnormal joint mechanics and spasms. Likewise, when the jaw alignment is off for dental or hypermobility reasons, neck vertebral torsion and spinal misalignment can occur.[16] Grinding of the teeth and tongue thrusting can also influence headaches and head position. Clenching of the jaw activates a muscle responsible for pushing food down the throat, and this can reduce airway space by 50%, which can contribute to sleep apnea.[16]

Conditions commonly affecting the hip in patients with hEDS include trochanteric bursitis, iliotibial band issues, femoral acetabular impingement (FAI), labral tears, piriformis syndrome, sacroiliac (SI) joint instability and referral pain from the lumbar spine (particularly L4–L5).[15] The hip does not typically dislocate or sublux in patients with hEDS, but it does tend to translate anteriorly in the acetabulum which can lead to chronic labral irritation and fraying over time.[17] Conservative management via physical therapy is an excellent option for these conditions. Arthroscopic surgery for FAI and labral tears can provide significant short-term relief of pain, though long-term data is lacking for patients with hEDS.[15,18]

Common knee joint concerns in the hEDS population include subluxation or dislocation of the patella (kneecap), meniscal tears and ligamentous tears. Patellar issues typically respond well to physical therapy, occasionally requiring an external brace or knee support, particularly in the acute phase. More severe cases may go on to develop patellofemoral arthritis. Excess motion of the knee from hypermobility appears to increase the risk of surgical intervention for internal structure damage (meniscus and knee ligaments) in the hEDS population.[15] Physical therapy is an important consideration for restoring muscular stability around the knee joint both pre- and post-op, and in some cases can prevent the need for surgery.

Ankle and foot issues appear to be common in this patient population. Ankle instability, recurrent ankle sprains, bunions and metatarsal pain are frequently observed. Malalignment of the hindfoot is often associated with chronic inflammatory issues up the chain (in the knee, hip, back and even in the shoulder).[15] Soft tissue surgeries around the ankle have a high failure rate, and bunions should be left alone if they are not painful.[15] Most patients do well with a conservative approach to ankle/foot injuries including physical therapy, orthotics and bracing.[15]

Shoulder instability is one of the more common concerns in patients with hEDS. Recurrent subluxations and dislocations, rotator cuff tendinosis and tears, shoulder impingement, labral tears, bursitis and scapular dyskinesia are frequently observed. Often, the deltoid muscle overpowers smaller muscles such as the rotator cuff, leading to altered kinematics, and this imbalance can be addressed conservatively with a physical therapist. Surgery may be warranted for full thickness rotator cuff tears that remain painful.[15] Research indicates that while the Neer inferior capsular shift surgery can help stabilize the shoulder, there's a high failure rate in patients who have very loose shoulders and surgery should be approached cautiously.[15]

Elbow area issues in patients with hEDS often include medial and lateral epicondylitis and radial tunnel syndrome, all of which tend to respond well to physical therapy. Posterolateral rotatory instability of the elbow is also sometimes noted in patients with joint hypermobility/EDS.[15]

The wrist joint is often a problematic area for patients with hEDS. Recurrent sprains, fractures from falling on an outstretched hand, proximal median nerve entrapment with pronator teres syndrome, carpal tunnel syndrome, and instability of the pisiform bone, radiocarpal, midcarpal and distal radioulnar joints are often noted.[15]

With the high degree of hypermobility that tends to be noted in the thumb and fingers in patients with hEDS, it's no surprise that these areas are often characterized by pain and inflammation. Carpometacarpal joint instability, thumb metacarpophalangeal joint hyperextension instability, sesamoiditis, interphalangeal joint hyperextension instability, De Quervain's tenosynovitis and trigger finger are commonly reported.[15] Braces and ring style splints can be helpful; a well-versed hand therapist will be an important part of the care team for management of hand, finger and wrist issues.

Thoracic outlet syndrome (TOS) is another common concern within this patient population. The nerves and blood vessels that pass from the neck/chest into the arm can get compressed underneath the first rib, anterior scalene and pectoralis minor muscles. Glenohumeral joint instability with inferior shoulder subluxation, commonly noted in hEDS, can also put extra postural tension on this area. While the compression occurs in the trunk, TOS often causes symptoms in the hand and arm. Conservative management of this condition is typically effective with the help of a physical therapist.[15]

Patients with hEDS may be more likely to suffer from concussions and post-concussion syndrome. This may be due to the increased tendency to faint from coexisting dysautonomia, or to injure themselves clumsily from reduced proprioception, vertigo/dizziness, intracranial pressure issues or brainstem compression triggering coordination and motor control issues. Direct trauma to the head or instances such as whiplash from a car accident may also increase the risk of concussion due to poor connective tissue support in the skull.

Specific strategies to address orthopedic concerns with hEDS will be further discussed in Chapter 9, "Structural and Musculoskeletal Issues."

Systemic issues with hEDS

Patients with hEDS often also have system-wide symptoms that reside outside of the orthopedic spectrum. Systemic signs of a generalized connective tissue disorder, such as atrophic scarring, hyperextensibility of the skin and organ prolapse may be present. Patients with hEDS may experience heart valve problems, and many patients have orthostatic intolerance and dysautonomia.[12,19] Chronic pain, sleep disturbances, anxiety/depression, fatigue, dental issues, urinary incontinence, easy bruising and slow skin healing are commonly noted in the hEDS patient population.[12,19,20] Balance difficulties/falling, decreased coordination and fine motor control, difficulty with handwriting, poor awareness of the body in relation to other objects, deconditioning, and hypersensitivity to pain are also frequently observed.[12,19]

Neurological issues including seizures, movement disorders (dystonia, tremors), sensory disturbances, dizziness, neurogenic bladder, bowel problems and sensory disturbances such as alternation in vision and hearing are also noted in patients with hypermobility disorders.[21]

Many patients also experience gastrointestinal problems.[19] In terms of gut health, both functional issues (such as impaired gastrointestinal motility) and structural issues (including hiatal hernias, rectoceles, rectal prolapse, pelvic floor muscle prolapse and visceroptosis) are noted in patients with EDS. Patients with hEDS are reported to frequently meet the criteria for disorders such as irritable bowel syndrome and functional dyspepsia.[22]

Sagging of a structure (ptosis) is usually caused by disease, paralysis or a congenital connective tissue issue. Ptosis associated with hEDS can occur all over the body. For example, diaphragm-ptosis may be associated with impingement of the celiac plexus and median arcuate ligament syndrome (MALS); cerebroptosis could contribute to Chiari malformation; venoptosis could be connected to POTS; and heel fascia ptosis could be related to the presence of piezogenic papules.[23] Mandibuloptosis could lead to temporomandibular joint (TMJ) dysfunction and airway obstruction.[23] The compression of the renal vein and increased venous pressure noted in Nutcracker syndrome affects blood pressure and adrenal regulation which can also impact cortisol and adrenaline levels.[23] Ptosis is one of the theorized mechanisms as to why patients with hEDS tend to have multisystemic symptoms.

Hypermobile EDS appears to have subsets of symptoms that predominate during different phases of the life span. Earlier years (childhood and adolescence) are often characterized by coordination issues, delayed motor development, gastrointestinal dysfunction and fatigue.[24] Dislocations and sprains are also possible in youth. Late teenage years into the 30s are more characterized by recurrent muscle, joint and connective tissue pain.[24] Some patients also experience insomnia, urogenital issues and nerve-related pain.[24] Adult hEDS patients aged 40 and older often experience widespread chronic pain (often labeled as fibromyalgia) with fatigue and organ issues.[24]

Table 9. Symptoms Commonly Noted with hEDS[24]

SYSTEM	SYMPTOMS
Cognitive	Anxiety and panic disorders, memory or concentration problems, depression
Gastrointestinal	Irritable bowel syndrome, constipation or diarrhea, bloating, abdominal pain, gastroparesis, food sensitivities, gastroesophageal reflux, chronic gastritis, heartburn, prolapsed rectum, hernias (all types)
Heart/Circulatory	Varicose veins; mitral valve prolapse or aortic dilatation (not common), dysautonomia with orthostatic hypotension and/or postural orthostatic tachycardia syndrome (POTS) presenting with: tachycardia, presyncope/syncope, anxiety, chronic fatigue, disordered sleep, exercise intolerance, dependent edema, purple skin, temperature dysregulation, "brain fog," and trouble concentrating; Raynaud's syndrome
Immune	Mast cell activation syndrome (MCAS): hives, pruritus, flushing, chemical and environmental sensitivities, medication and food sensitivities, fatigue, trouble concentrating, migratory pain, excessive inflammatory response, trouble concentrating, anxiety

Neurological	Insomnia/sleep disturbances, motor delay (in children), proprioceptive and motor control deficits leading to clumsiness, frequent falls, trips, or bumping into things, fibromyalgia/central sensitization, hyperalgesia, headaches, migraines, dizziness, paresthesia and nerve compression disorders, restless leg syndrome
Orthopedic	Soft tissue: tendinosis, bursitis, fasciitis, tenosynovitis, tendon ruptures, trigger points, muscle spasms, muscle strains, tendon abnormalities resulting in instability Bone & joints: sprains, subluxations, dislocations, chronic joint pain, osteoarthritis, scoliosis, bone mineral density abnormalities, possibly increased fracture rate
Skin	Hyperextensible skin, slow healing or scarring, poor wound healing, easy bruising
Urogenital	Urinary incontinence, prolapsed bladder or uterus, urinary tract infections, dysmenorrhea, endometriosis, vulvodynia, pelvic pain, painful intercourse

Diagnosis of hEDS

The process for clinical diagnosis of hEDS must be completed with a healthcare provider and is as follows:[24]

- Complete a preliminary assessment with the Beighton score. (See more information, below.)
- Complete a physical exam and review the clinical history. Refer for genetic testing if vascular or classical EDS (or any other type aside from hEDS) is suspected.

- Rule out other conditions as appropriate.
  - Osteogenesis imperfecta is a condition with genetic defects in collagen resulting in brittle bones that fracture easily.
  - Marfan syndrome is a connective tissue disorder that affects the heart, eyes, blood vessels and bones with characteristically long extremities.
  - Loeys-Dietz syndrome also affects the connective tissue and is characterized by an enlarged aorta and increased aneurysm risk, skeletal problems, skin abnormalities and other systemic issues.
  - Heritable and acquired connective tissue disorders and autoimmune rheumatologic conditions may also need to be ruled out with the help of a rheumatologist.
- If hEDS is diagnosed, the patient should also consider the possibility of testing for POTS and MCAS.

Historically there have been some discrepancies in terms of what constitutes a clinical diagnosis of hEDS. The updated EDS Classification instructs providers to factor in patient age when conducting the Beighton scale, as joint range of motion naturally decreases with age.[19]

As of the 2017 updated consensus, there are three separate sets of qualifications for the diagnosis of hEDS, and all three criteria must be met for the diagnosis.

Criterion 1: Generalized Joint Hypermobility[19]

The Beighton evaluation assesses hypermobility of the thumbs (both sides), fifth metacarpophalangeal joints (both sides), elbows (both sides), trunk, and knees (both sides), with one point given for each of the joints that meet the specific criterion.

Figure 2. The Beighton Evaluation for hEDS Diagnosis

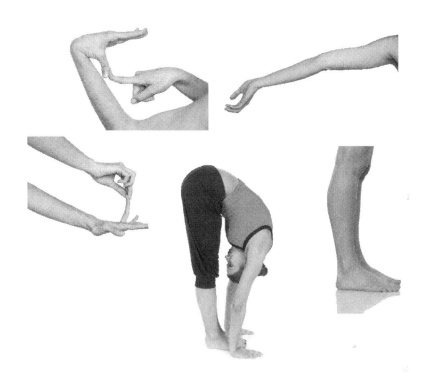

The Beighton evaluation is scored from a scale of zero to nine, and the following scores indicate a positive assessment for suspected hEDS:

Pre-pubertal patients: 6 or greater
Pubertal age to age 50: 5 or greater
Older than age 50: 4 or greater

Patients who score one point below the cutoffs for Criterion 1 should answer the following questions:

- Can you now (or could you ever) place your hands flats on the floor without bending your knees?
- Can you now (or could you ever) bend your thumb to touch your forearm?
- As a child, did you amuse your friends by contorting your body into strange shapes or could you do the splits?
- As a child or teenager, did your shoulder or kneecap dislocate on more than one occasion?
- Do you consider yourself double-jointed?

If two or more of these questions were answered with "yes," the patient is then considered positive for Criterion One.

Criterion 2: Characteristics of Heritable Systemic Connective Tissue Disorder[19]

For this criterion to be considered positive, patients must exhibit two or more features of a systemic connective tissue disorder:

- Feature A: 5 must be present
  - Unusually soft or velvety skin, mild skin hyperextensibility, unexplained striae (stretch marks), piezogenic papules (bumps noted while weight bearing) on both heels, recurrent or multiple abdominal hernias, atrophic scarring of multiple sites, prolapse of the pelvic floor/rectum/uterus, dental crowding with high or narrow palate, arachnodactyly (fingers/toes abnormally long and slender), arm span to height ratio >1.05, mitral valve prolapse, aortic root dilation with Z score>2

- Feature B:
  - Positive family history with at least one first-degree relative diagnosed with hEDS
- Feature C: 1 must be present
  - Musculoskeletal pain in 2+ limbs that recurs daily for at least 3 months, chronic widespread pain for >3 months, recurrent joint dislocations or frank joint instability without history of trauma

Criterion 3: Other Conditions Ruled Out[19]

For this criterion to be considered positive, all three bullets must be correct:
- Absence of unusual skin fragility (this would warrant investigation into other types of EDS).
- Exclusion of other heritable and acquired connective tissue disorders, including autoimmune rheumatologic conditions. (Patients who have an acquired connective tissue disorder like lupus or rheumatoid arthritis can be diagnosed with hEDS, but they must meet features A and B of Criterion Two.)
- Exclusion of alternative diagnoses that may also include joint hypermobility by means of hypotonia and/or connective tissue laxity. Examples include neuromuscular disorders (such as Bethlem myopathy), skeletal dysplasias (such as osteogenesis imperfecta) and other types of heritable connective tissue disorders (such as Marfan syndrome, Loeys-Dietz syndrome, and other types of EDS).

Genetic testing can help distinguish hEDS from other disorders and is used when the patient has a personal or family history of organ rupture like uterine rupture or aneurysms (where vascular EDS should be ruled out) and when the patient has symptoms involving skin or soft tissue findings (consistent with classical EDS).[20] A geneticist may also evaluate for other connective tissue disorders or conditions that can cause a dilated aorta.[20]

Complications Associated with EDS

Serious complications can occur with the hEDS patient population. Headaches are frequently reported with EDS, and the most common types are migraines, headaches generated by neck muscle tension and headaches triggered by jaw joint dysfunction. However, some headaches may have more serious causes. A headache that increases with strain such as a cough or a sneeze increases the index of suspicion for Chiari malformation.[25]

Chiari malformation is one of the most common complications and is theorized to occur with hEDS secondary to ligamentous laxity in the cervical spine (neck) and possible posterior gliding of the condyles.[25] An upright MRI is recommended to detect this condition, where the base of the cerebellum (brain) slips through the opening of the skull. This commonly presents clinically as pain, spasticity in the extremities, difficulty swallowing, paresthesia, chronic headaches and ataxia.[25] The exact incidence of Chiari malformation in EDS patients in unknown, although it has been noted that the female to male ratio is high (approximately 9:1).[26,27]

Spontaneous cerebrospinal fluid (CSF) leaking is often characterized by a worsening of headache while upright and a reduction in headache symptoms when lying down.[25] The cerebrospinal fluid surrounds the brain, but when there's a tear in the dura (the lining surrounding the spine), a slow leak can reduce the overall volume of CSF. This can cause an upright MRI to show signs of Chiari malformation. CSF leaks can occur spontaneously or after spinal taps and epidural anesthesia. They are sometimes accompanied by hearing abnormalities or a ringing or "underwater" feeling in the ears that may be more noticeable when the patient is upright. When the painful headache is triggered in the upright position, the sympathetic nervous system can trigger an increase in heart rate, so CSF leaks can sometimes mimic POTS symptoms. Seizure-like activity and zapping or shooting sensations in the head are also sometimes noted.[21] A brain MRI may detect a CSF leak in the first several weeks, but after that it becomes trickier to visualize, and contrast MRIs may assist.[21] Other tests such as MR myelogram, lumbar puncture to measure pressure, and CT myelogram are sometimes used with relatively poor diagnostic accuracy, and epidural blood patches may also be used to help confirm the diagnosis.[21]

Intracranial hypertension, a condition of elevated fluid levels and elevated pressure inside the brain, can occur in patients with EDS.[25,27] Headache, ringing or whooshing in the ears, feeling the heartbeat in the ears, visual disturbances, nausea/vomiting, and sensitivity to light may be noted with intracranial hypertension.[27] In this scenario, the headache is usually worse when the patient is lying down as opposed to being upright.[21] Intracranial hypertension occurs when something impedes the normal flow of the CSF, such as a Chiari malformation, certain medications, an infection or bleed in the brain, or blockage of the veins that drain blood out of the brain.[21] Intracranial hypertension can also cause swelling at the back of the eyes and pressure on the optic nerve and needs to be monitored carefully.[21] A lumbar puncture is often used to diagnose increased intracranial pressure. Medications, Chiari surgery, or the placement of stents or shunts are conventional treatment approaches for intracranial hypertension.

Tethered cord syndrome (TCS) is also associated with hEDS. A 2009 study found that 77% of patients who had symptoms of Chiari malformation also had TCS.[26] Tethered cord involves the conus of the spinal cord being yanked down, which pulls or pinches at the nerves at the base of the lumbar spine. This can be especially concerning for patients with Chiari who are already at risk for the upper part of the spinal cord and the brain being compressed.[25] Symptoms may include low back pain, leg weakness and/or sensory loss, and neurogenic bladder symptoms.[25]

Barre-Lieou syndrome (also known as craniocervical instability or CCI) can occur when a patient with anterior cervical spine (neck) instability experiences injury to the capsular ligaments. Without these ligaments functioning properly, the cervical spine can translate further forward than it should with movement, which results in the vertebrae pushing on the cervical sympathetic nervous system ganglion. In addition to dysautonomia, patients may also experience tongue numbness, blurred vision, ringing of the ears, dizziness and vertigo, headaches and neck pain.[25] Patients with EDS who experience a worsening of POTS symptoms in conjunction with neck and head positions may need to consider the diagnostic possibility of Barre-Lieou syndrome.[25] This concern will be discussed at length in Chapter 9.

Elongation of the styloid process or calcification of the stylohyoid ligament (typically noted on a CT scan), also known as Eagle syndrome, has been reported in patients with different types of EDS, most notably vascular EDS and hypermobile EDS. The styloid process is a small pointy bone near the ear that is an anchor point for several muscles that impact the function of the tongue and larynx (upper throat). Elongation of this bony prominence is often asymptomatic, but it can cause discomfort in the upper throat, voice changes and/or hoarseness, painful neck movements, earaches, headaches, painful tongue movements, and saliva secretion issues. The styloid bone is near several cranial nerves, including the glossopharyngeal nerve, vagus nerve, spinal accessory nerve, and hypoglossal nerve. In rare cases it has also been associated with carotid artery dissection resulting in strokes due to its proximity to vascular structures. Eagle syndrome is sometimes misdiagnosed as temporomandibular joint (TMJ) dysfunction and it may be seen clinically in patients who experience signs of craniocervical instability and Chiari malformation.

A compression of the nerves in the lower portion of the spinal canal, known as cauda equina syndrome, has also been noted in this patient population.[15] This condition is associated with a sudden onset of symptoms including incontinence (loss of bowel and/or bladder function), numbness in the groin area, sexual dysfunction, severe back pain, symptoms radiating into leg(s) and leg weakness. Constipation, urinary retention and difficulty initiating urination can also occur. While some patients recall some type of physical trauma precipitating symptoms, these symptoms often arise with no known mechanism of injury. Cauda equina is an emergency scenario that can require immediate surgery in order to prevent permanent paralysis or loss of bowel/bladder control.

Surgery is a tricky subject within the hEDS population due to slow tissue healing, and decisions should factor in the unique patient history, comorbidities and severity of the condition that is recommended for surgery. Conservative management including physical therapy and/or occupational therapy should be exhausted for non-emergent orthopedic conditions before considering surgery in most cases. One study found that patients who underwent physical therapy had a 66% success rate, compared to those who opted for surgery (33% success rate).[28]

If surgery is deemed necessary, it's recommended that the care team performs extra steps to minimize risk of skin- and tissue-related complications in patients with hEDS. Recommendations can include leaving the sutures in place for longer time frames, avoiding skin clips and using skin closure strips in addition to sutures.[29]

Bleeding symptoms are commonly noted in patients with both hypermobility and MCAS. Bleeding symptoms are often attributed to the abnormalities in the collagen of the vessel wall or connective tissues. The mechanism by which that occurs could be related to the interactions between platelets (cell fragments involved in clotting) and collagen. It appears that abnormalities in subendothelial collagen alter interactions with platelets and von Willebrand factor, which can result in a platelet plug formation.[30]

Patients with EDS (and in particular, vascular EDS) may be more predisposed to having complications during routine medical procedures and surgeries, such as bleeding and complications of anesthesia. Complications during pregnancy and labor/delivery have also been noted, so patients should work with an EDS-savvy care team when pregnant or considering surgery.[5]

Patients with EDS should be aware of the potential for addiction and side effects with opioid pain medications, as research has noted that this patient population is prescribed opioid medications at nearly double the rate when compared to the general population.[31] There's a large spectrum of limitations in activities of daily living within the hEDS patient community; on the severe end of the spectrum, some patients report 25-100 joint dislocations per day. For these patients, a comprehensive and holistic multidisciplinary pain management plan is essential. For patients who experience less severe and less frequent flare-ups of hEDS-related issues, the cons of opioid use may outweigh the benefits.

Trifecta Connections

What do we know about the trifecta of MCAS, POTS and hEDS? Are these connections legitimate and is there a scientific explanation? Many propose ideas about genetic mutations or the possibility of three different labels for one systemic diagnosis. Theoretically, dysfunctional blood vessels could be influenced by connective tissue abnormalities with EDS and could trigger abnormal blood pooling and blood pressure responses, which could influence autonomic nervous system function compensatory mechanisms and subsequent mast cell activation. Many mast cell mediators trigger vasodilation and a low blood pressure response and drops in blood pressure can trigger compensations in heart rate. Also, the symptom of flushing is commonly reported during episodes of dysautonomia, and this is also a sign of mast cell activation. However, opponents of this theory argue that long-standing genetic defects of collagen are not likely to trigger sudden overnight POTS symptoms. It's also difficult to discern whether mast cell activation represents the primary event or whether sympathetic activation ends up causing mast cell activation.[32]

A recent article noted that patients with hereditary alpha tryptasemia (HAT) appear to have higher rates of dysautonomia (including POTS) and Ehlers-Danlos syndrome, but the authors did not believe that these manifestations were caused specifically by MCAS.[33] The literature on this topic varies, with some authors concluding that the three conditions strongly co-segregate together,[34-38] and others denying connections or citing weak correlations.[39,40] One recent article described connections between Chiari malformation and the other trifecta conditions in children.[41] A 2019 review concluded that studies proposing a relationship between the three conditions were either biased or based on outdated criteria.[40] Thus, the scientific jury is still out on the potential prevalence of all three conditions occurring simultaneously as well as the mechanisms behind this connection.

However, several theories provide interesting potential insight into the connections between MCAS, EDS and POTS.

Figure 3. An Example of Proposed Mechanisms between EDS, MCAS and POTS

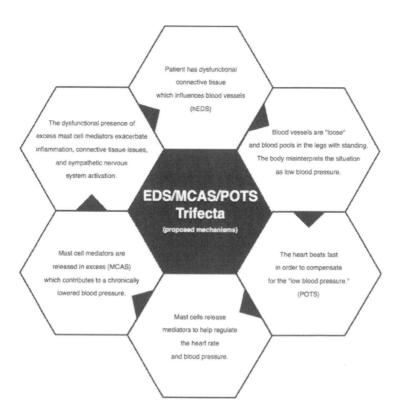

The above is a rather basic explanation that leaves out a very important factor impacting patients with the trifecta: the gastrointestinal system. In "Disjointed: Navigating the Diagnosis and Management of hypermobile Ehlers-Danlos Syndrome and Hypermobility Spectrum Disorders," Dr. Andrew Maxwell describes a Brain-Gut Axis Vortex connection that links MCAS and EDS with dysautonomia.[23] Specifically, Dr. Maxwell believes that vagus nerve dysfunction first triggers changes in gastrointestinal pH levels and motility, which is further compounded by the tendency for intestines to experience visceroptosis or sagging with hEDS.[23] From there, bacterial imbalances are more likely to occur in the gastrointestinal biome, which can lead to small intestinal bacterial overgrowth (SIBO).[23] Activation of mast cells in the gastrointestinal tract and the release of pro-inflammatory mediators may then trigger a cascade where a mast cell mediator called elastase-2 leads to leaky gut, in which bacterial and food particles leak into the subepithelial spaces and further activate mast cells.[23] Mast cell mediators can also influence the enteric nerves, which can lead to further disruption of gastrointestinal motility.[23] This process could also wreak havoc on the sensory nerve messages to the brain and the vagal motor messages, contributing to a vicious cycle of dysfunction.[23]

The presence of a high toxic burden is commonly noted in patients with the trifecta and is also known to negatively impact mast cells, nervous system regulation, inflammation in connective tissues and gut health. Stress and nutritional, viral, fungal, hormonal, parasitic and bacterial factors could also influence this vicious cycle of inflammation and dysregulation.

Conventional Treatment of hEDS

Mainstays of traditional medical management of hEDS typically focus on physical and occupational therapy, surgery, pharmacological pain management and external bracing devices to provide greater stability and to reduce dislocation risk. As previously mentioned, due to the nature of tissue healing impairments in patients with hEDS, experts generally recommend against surgery in cases where conservation management is an option.[15,24,42,43]

While many case reports exist, a 2018 review reported a lack of randomized controlled trials or scientific evidence for any specific rehabilitation approach with hEDS.[44] Part of the lack of evidence is related to the discrepancies in terminology and unclear criteria for "joint hypermobility" vs. "EDS" noted in the literature; very few studies utilized inclusion criteria consistent with the Ehlers-Danlos Society criteria for diagnosis of hEDS. One cohort study of 12 female patients supported the use of strength training, core stability exercises, body awareness/proprioception exercises and cognitive-behavioral therapy for patients with hEDS, noting improvements in muscle strength, endurance, self-perceived pain, activity participation and a reduction in kinesiophobia (fear of movement).[45]

A multifactorial approach to physical therapy in patients with hEDS is encouraged. Experts and existing evidence support physical therapy as an essential component of care.[24] Physical therapy strategies consist of exercise, patient/caregiver education, stress management, fatigue and pain management, splinting or bracing recommendations, self-management techniques and referral to other providers when appropriate.[24] Integration of manual therapy, modalities, neuromuscular reeducation, body mechanics and injury prevention/joint protection can also be useful.[24] Fear of movement tends to be high in this patient population, and patient education alongside external feedback, proprioception and motor control strategies can be extremely empowering.

Contrary to popular belief, joint mobilization is *not* an outright contraindication in this patient population. A 2018 case report noted the utility of focused joint mobilization and trigger point release as part of a comprehensive treatment plan for hEDS.[46] While global mobilization of hypermobile joints is not logical, *careful* manual therapy targeting very specific impairments in alignment and muscle balance may be appropriate for some patients demonstrating compensatory issues.

When it comes to proprioception, or the kinesthetic awareness of where a joint is positioned in space, training programs should include the hypermobile end range of the joint of concern.[47] This makes logical sense, as you would want to help a joint recognize and provide feedback on its position in space in order to prevent subluxations/dislocations as well as perform activities with proper biomechanics to reduce the risk of excessive joint impact and trauma. However, most experts recommend *against* performing joint loading/strengthening in the hypermobile end range, especially in open-packed positions.[24] Specific exercise strategies will be discussed in Chapter 10, "Movement."

Adaptive equipment including utensils and tools can modify activities to decrease stress on the hand and wrist joints.[24] Compression garments, braces, splints, orthotics and taping are often utilized to reduce joint stress and improve sensory input and proprioception.[24] Grabbers, shoehorns, special sponge devices for bathing, elastic shoelaces, sock donners and dressing sticks may also be helpful to protect the joints during dressing and other activities of daily living.[11]

Clinicians commonly use mechanical therapies such as splints and orthoses in the management of hEDS.[48] One study found that patients perceive splints and braces as effective components of treatment in the management of acute and chronic pain related to hEDS.[49] While there is a lack of evidence to support or refute the use of splints and braces in this patient population,[48] most experts agree that they can be helpful adjuncts to therapy. Clinical reasoning should assist in determining the duration of supportive mechanical therapies, as there is some concern that over-bracing or splinting for extended time periods can result in a worsening of the muscular stability and joint condition. This concern is not black and white, and patient-specific factors (such as the type and severity of dysfunction, the joint in question and the typical daily activities) should be considered in determining the plan for use of adaptive and supportive equipment.

Service dogs are sometimes utilized in patients with chronic conditions, including patients who have MCAS, EDS and POTS. Service dogs may support individuals with hEDS in several ways, including assisting with mobility, sensory issues, proprioception, episodes of brain fog/fatigue/dizziness, deep pressure therapy for anxiety, and alerting to events like seizures, fainting or migraines.[50]

Steroid injections, nerve blocks, lidocaine injections and prolotherapy are considered more controversial treatment options for patients with hEDS.[15] Injections of lidocaine may show positive results for short-term pain relief for patients with severe manifestations of hEDS, though high-quality research is needed.[51] Clinically, I've noted a recently increasing volume of patients who are considering prolotherapy. Prolotherapy, also called regenerative injection therapy, is a procedure where a natural irritant (typically dextrose) is injected into soft tissue in the hopes that it will trigger the body's natural immune response with new cellular proliferation and collagen deposition in tendons and ligaments. Prolotherapy for isolated sacroiliac joint issues is sometimes performed in patients with EDS, but it is considered a controversial treatment.[15]

To date, the bulk of the research surrounding prolotherapy and joint hypermobility has focused on the jaw joint. One study found that up to four sessions of prolotherapy improved pain, clicking, and mouth opening in patients with temporomandibular joint dysfunction (TMD).[52] A second study found that one to three prolotherapy injections showed reductions in symptoms in patients with hypermobility and TMD.[53] Other research noted positive TMD results sustained between one to four years post-prolotherapy.[54] However, two separate studies found no difference between the control group and different dextrose concentrations of prolotherapy for TMD.[55,56] A 2018 systematic review concluded that more research is needed, and it's unclear whether subluxations and dislocations are impacted by this treatment.[57] Other studies investigating its use for chronic musculoskeletal conditions beyond the jaw joint (such as tendinopathies, arthritis and spine/pelvic pain) indicate support in terms of subjective outcomes, though EDS-specific research is currently lacking.[58] Caution is warranted in interpreting these results, as few high-level studies were available regarding prolotherapy in patients with hypermobility concerns.

Natural Treatment of hEDS

Practitioners following a more natural or functional medicine approach tend to encourage patients to consider conservative management of symptoms first, as opposed to injections of substances that may negatively impact the tissues in the long-term and may be complicated by the presence of MCAS, dysautonomia and other factors. While the approach further outlined in this book may not reverse the innate properties of collagen that impact soft tissue function and joint hypermobility, addressing the root issues responsible for systemic inflammation can have a profound impact on musculoskeletal and organ function, reducing flare-ups.

Not all physical therapists, occupational therapists, chiropractors, osteopaths, or other healers are familiar with the management of hEDS, so it's important to research your local options. Combining this "underlying issues" approach and rehabilitation/prevention with a professional well-versed in EDS is essential. Well-planned exercise programs in conjunction with customized physical therapy, patient education and the tools outlined in subsequent chapters (such as addressing factors like nutrition, the nervous system and detoxification) can be profoundly helpful in preventing orthopedic and organ-level consequences of hEDS. Injections may provide a quick-fix form of pain relief, but they are not a long-term solution, and the jury is still out on prolotherapy. While pain and inflammation should certainly not be ignored, I encourage patients to avoid a Band-Aid approach to care when possible; a proactive approach to managing hEDS is key.

EDS: TAKE-HOME MESSAGES

- Ehlers-Danlos syndrome (EDS) describes hereditary disorders of the connective tissue that typically present with skin hyperextensibility, generalized joint hypermobility, and fragility of vascular and internal organ structures.

- The most recent classification of EDS identified 13 distinct subtypes. One of these subtypes, hypermobile EDS (hEDS), has no known genetic cause and is described as an inherited connective tissue disorder that's caused by defects in collagen.

- hEDS is characterized by joint hypermobility, signs of faulty connective tissue throughout the body (such as hernias, prolapses and skin abnormalities), musculoskeletal pain/problems and a family history of similar characteristics.

- Several other types of symptoms are often noted in this patient population, such as gastrointestinal issues, sleep disturbances, pelvic floor and bladder problems, anxiety, dysautonomia and mast cell activation issues, though these issues aren't part of the formal diagnostic criteria.

- Patients with hEDS tend to experience frequent injuries including subluxations, dislocations, tendon inflammation, joint sprains, arthritic pain, trigger point pain and muscular strains. Difficulty with balance and coordination are also commonly reported.

- The diagnosis of hEDS involves screening for generalized joint hypermobility using the Beighton scale, evaluating for characteristics of heritable systemic connective tissue disorders and ruling out other potential conditions that can mimic EDS. This process must be completed with a licensed healthcare provider.

- More serious concerns can occur with this patient population, including Chiari malformation, intracranial pressure issues and cerebrospinal fluid leaks, tethered cord syndrome, cauda equina syndrome, Barre-Lieou syndrome and bleeding abnormalities.
- Traditional medical management of hEDS typically focuses on physical and occupational therapy, surgery, pharmacological pain management and external bracing devices to provide greater stability and to reduce dislocation risk. Steroid injections, nerve blocks, lidocaine injections and prolotherapy are sometimes considered, though the literature has mixed results regarding these options and the potential long-term effects of these treatments are concerning.
- Due to the nature of tissue healing impairments in patients with hEDS, experts generally recommend against surgery in cases where conservative management is an option.
- While an integrative, natural or functional medicine approach may not reverse the innate properties of collagen impacting soft tissue function and subsequent joint hypermobility, addressing the root issues responsible for systemic inflammation can have a profound impact on musculoskeletal and organ function, reducing flare-ups.

PART TWO:
THE HEALING PLAN

Chapter 4:
THE PASSPORT PLAN

This chapter outlines beginning strategies for patients to get the most out of their healing journey. A PDF version of a downloadable passport workbook is available for free at www.originwellnesscolorado.com/passport.

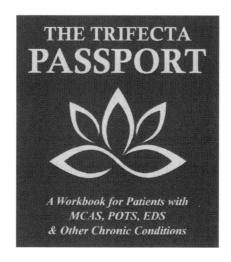

THE FUTURE

Who are you? Where are you going? What are your dreams? What will you do when you feel better?

Despite tending to have a meticulous and thorough picture of the past and what they have gone through, very few patients who are chronically ill give similar attention to the future. I've found through patient interviews that very few have an idea of what they truly want to do when they get better. It's as if they won't allow themselves to go there mentally. I encourage all my patients to dream big, have a vision and, most importantly, to write it down. Sending out your intentions and best-case scenario to the universe is an important first step to healing.

How can we heal if we don't have any idea of who we are, what we need or where we are going? A plan is key. Having a healing plan empowers you to shift away from any sentiments of learned helplessness that can occur as the result of being chronically unwell. Having a plan brings hope. Healing plans are not static but are constantly evolving over time as you have experiences that provide feedback and alter your symptomatic baseline.

I encourage patients to engage in an active exercise at the start of care in order to be intentional about documenting the plan for the future. Whether it's through journaling, sticky notes, creating a customized holistic healing paper passport, or handy reminders like cell phone screen savers, I encourage you to dig deep to express who you are, what you need, and the tools that you would like to try in order to find healing.

Focusing on the past often triggers anxiety and feelings of helplessness, and some patients even have PTSD from prior experiences with the medical system. Focusing on the future and things that you can control (like your self-care routine) can help to shift into a proactive mindset. It's helpful to refrain from over-identifying with the name of a particular diagnosis. In all reality, the three conditions that make up the trifecta are simply labels that describe a set of tendencies and symptoms.

I also encourage patients to limit time on social media, especially the Facebook patient groups. After all, we become what we are thinking about, and while those pages have many well-intentioned people running the show, the content and comments on there are sometimes inaccurate or excessively negative. Many patients feel invalidated and need to vent their emotions on those pages, and it's best to limit your own exposure to that type of energy, just as we may limit our exposure to too much stressful news on TV.

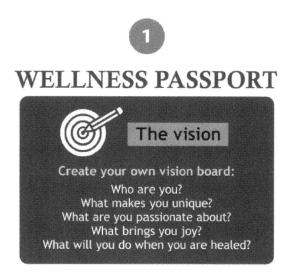

WELLNESS PASSPORT

1: THE PASSPORT COVER

Have you ever studied a passport closely? Do you own a passport? If so, grab it and take a closer look. My passport comes from the United States; hopefully there aren't too many anomalies within its contents for patients living in other countries.

The first thing I notice about the passport is that the cover is durable, built to withstand any bad weather, sweat and bending that it may encounter. Secondly, it has bold golden letters declaring the country. And lastly, the Great Seal of the United States is on the front cover, also in gold. The seal was approved by an Act of Congress in 1782 and is based on the concept that the original 13 colonies of the U.S. came together to become a single nation. You may recognize the seal from its placement on the dollar bill. The traditional motto of the United States, E pluribus unum, is Latin for "out of many, one."

As patients create their holistic healing plan on day one, I encourage them to create a metaphorical passport cover that they can strategically view every day, either as the printed first page in the PDF workbook or as a collage, vision board or e-collage image for their cell phone.

The cover of the passport is all about identity. The cover should embody a written or visual representation of the following: Who are you? What makes you unique? What are you passionate about? What brings you joy? What will you do (not if, but…) WHEN you experience better health?

Remember your "why." There will be many ups and downs within treatment, so it's important to never lose sight of this. The cover should also include your personal motto. This should be a short phrase that can be repeated. Some patients will use their favorite mantra or quote here.

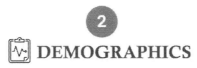

DEMOGRAPHICS

What does your stable baseline look like today?
What are the medications, supplements and other treatments that you have found helpful
to manage symptoms up to this point?
Take a picture of yourself to document your baseline.
This page is all about the starting point.

INSERT
PHOTO
HERE

NAME: _____

DATE OF BIRTH: _____

ALLERGIES: _____

Today's Date: _____

MEDICAL CONDITIONS:

CURRENT MEDICATIONS:

CURRENT SUPPLEMENTS:

2: THE DEMOGRAPHICS PAGE

The only laminated page in the passport, the demographics page contains your headshot and identifying information, such as your place of birth and date of birth. There are a few things I like to point out here about the United States passport.

The U.S. passport does not expire for 10 years. This is not what most patients want to hear, but the healing journey can take time and a lot of patience. It's important to have appropriate and realistic expectations. For most individuals, the holistic treatment approaches do not result in dramatic changes overnight, and patients report that it can take months to years to feel and see the progress.

All too often, patients make a change to something like diet but give up on the approach within a few weeks because they believe that it did not improve things for them. There's a difference between impatience and inefficacy. It's certainly more enticing to move along when the change requires extra grit and dedication, particularly when faced with negative mental chatter that's repeating messages like "This isn't working!" and "You'll never get better!" I have certainly been there on this one. It's important to commit to lifestyle changes full-heartedly and in some cases for the long haul. Are you ready for this commitment?

In terms of the headshot photo, taking a picture of yourself at the start of a new healing plan can be something that's beneficial to look back on later. Sometimes it's hard to "feel" healing, but photos can provide us with different snapshots in time that can reflect small and large changes in our well-being.

It's also helpful to visualize what your health will look like physically as you find healing. Perhaps certain physical traits like eczema, dark circles under the eyes and hives will be replaced with clear skin. Perhaps you envision yourself spending more time outdoors on mountain trails. Visualize what optimal health looks like for you physically and how that will impact your daily activities.

On the demographics page, paint a picture of your current "stable baseline." At this point in time, what are the medications, supplements and other treatments that you have found helpful to manage symptoms up to this point? This page is all about the starting point.

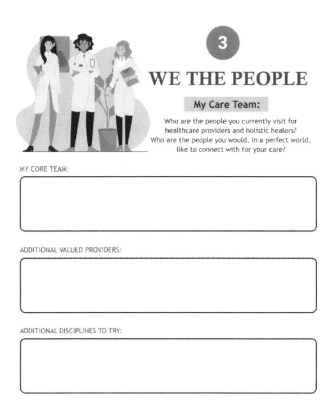

3

WE THE PEOPLE

My Care Team:

Who are the people you currently visit for healthcare providers and holistic healers? Who are the people you would, in a perfect world, like to connect with for your care?

MY CORE TEAM:

ADDITIONAL VALUED PROVIDERS:

ADDITIONAL DISCIPLINES TO TRY:

3: WE THE PEOPLE

Just above the demographics page, "We the People" represents a preamble from the United States constitution. For our holistic healing passport, this page serves as a place to outline the patient care team. Who are the people you currently visit in terms of healthcare providers and holistic healers? Who are the people you would, in a perfect world, like to connect with for your care?

For most patients, the existing care team includes a primary care provider and a handful of specialists, such as an allergist/immunologist, cardiac specialist, pulmonologist, nutritionist, etc. Some patients may also have physical/speech/occupational therapists, gynecologists and mental health specialists in this list.

This is where I encourage patients to create a holistic provider foundation based on a natural medicine or functional medicine approach. Specifically, patients with chronic illness can benefit tremendously from someone who can help to uncover the root issues that often trigger systemic dysfunction, instead of putting a Band-Aid on the symptoms. Don't write off an entire discipline if you've had a bad experience in the past; I encourage you to stay open-minded and to be selective about seeking a provider who has knowledge of the trifecta and other conditions.

I also encourage you to list types of alternative medicine that you have a curiosity about. Acupuncture, aromatherapy, Ayurveda, biofeedback, craniosacral therapy, guided meditation, herbalism, homeopathy, massage, osteopathic manipulation, Qi gong, reflexology, reiki, sound healing, traditional Chinese medicine, and visceral manipulation are examples of services that may benefit patients who are chronically unwell.

As an example, my own "We the People" page looks like this:

- Core team: my naturopath, my primary care provider, my allergist/immunologist
- Additional valued providers: my chiropractor who performs acupuncture and energetic medicine, my reiki master, my massage therapist
- Additional disciplines to try (I am curious about...): craniosacral therapy, visceral manipulation, reflexology, aromatherapy

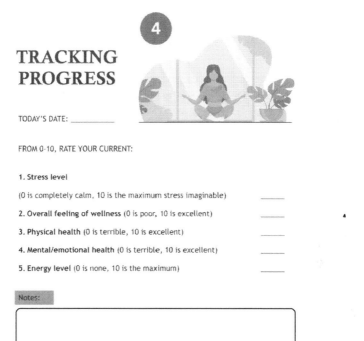

TRACKING PROGRESS

TODAY'S DATE: _____

FROM 0-10, RATE YOUR CURRENT:

1. Stress level

(0 is completely calm, 10 is the maximum stress imaginable)   _____

2. Overall feeling of wellness (0 is poor, 10 is excellent)   _____

3. Physical health (0 is terrible, 10 is excellent)   _____

4. Mental/emotional health (0 is terrible, 10 is excellent)   _____

5. Energy level (0 is none, 10 is the maximum)   _____

Notes:

4: TRACKING PROGRESS

At this point, I also encourage patients to record their baseline status for subjective questions as a reference that they can return to later.

The following questions are helpful to ask at the start (prior to beginning new treatment options), as well as periodically (with every monthly or quarterly check-in). There are several pages set aside in your passport download where you can record the date and answers to these questions to track them over time. It's best to answer them without looking at your prior answers each time you check in with the questions.

From 0–10, rate your

1. Stress level (0 is completely calm, 10 is the maximum stress imaginable)
2. Overall feeling of wellness (0 is poor, 10 is excellent)
3. Physical health (0 is terrible, 10 is excellent)
4. Mental/emotional health (0 is terrible, 10 is excellent)
5. Energy level (0 is none, 10 is the maximum)

Often, it's difficult to remember how bad things were as you adjust to new level of abundance and health. Keeping tabs on these areas can help show progress down the road.

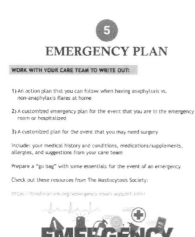

EMERGENCY PLAN

WORK WITH YOUR CARE TEAM TO WRITE OUT:

1) An action plan that you can follow when having anaphylaxis vs. non-anaphylaxis flares at home

2) A customized emergency plan for the event that you are in the emergency room or hospitalized

3) A customized plan for the event that you may need surgery

Include: your medical history and conditions, medications/supplements, allergies, and suggestions from your care team

Prepare a "go bag" with some essentials for the event of an emergency

Check out these resources from The Mastocytosis Society:

https://tmsforacure.org/emergency-room-support-info/

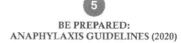

BE PREPARED:
ANAPHYLAXIS GUIDELINES (2020)

Anaphylaxis is likely to occur in any of the following three scenarios:

1. Acute onset of an illness (minutes to hours) with involvement of:
   × skin, mucosal tissue or both
   × and at least one of the following: respiratory compromise (shortness of breath, wheezing, stridor, coughing, hypoxemia) or decreased blood pressure or end organ dysfunction (such as collapse, incontinence, or fainting)

2. Two or more of the following occur suddenly after exposure to a likely allergen or other trigger for that patient (minutes to several hours):
   × symptoms in skin/mucosa (generalized hives, itch-flush, swollen lips-tongue-uvula), respiratory compromise, sudden gastrointestinal symptoms (crampy abdominal pain, vomiting), decreased blood pressure/end organ dysfunction (such as collapse, incontinence or fainting)

3. After exposure to known allergen for that patient (minutes to several hours): low blood pressure (BP)
   × Infants and children: low systolic BP (age specific) or greater than 30% decrease in systolic BP.
   • Age 1 month to 1 year: systolic BP less than 70 mmHg
   • Age 1-10 years: systolic BP less than (70 mmHg+ [2 x age])
   • Age 11-17 years: systolic BP less than 90 mmHg
   × Adults: systolic BP of less than 90 mmHg or greater than 30% decrease from patient's baseline

Know the signs and don't hesitate to use your emergency meds!

5: EMERGENCY PLAN

Often overlooked, the personal data and emergency contact page comes next. Patients with the trifecta (or some combination of it) are typically at higher risk of finding themselves in the emergency room due to anaphylaxis, joint dislocations, erratic heartbeats or fainting. While the goal is ultimately to bring greater systemic stability and fewer emergency scenarios, it can be helpful to write out an individualized emergency plan. This can reduce anxiety when obstacles do arise. Being prepared with written statements can assist the hospital team in the proper courses of action, given your medical history, allergies and suggestions from your care team.

To reduce anxiety, it can also be helpful to write out an action plan that you can follow when flared at home. For example, if you experience allergic reactions and feel unsure in how to proceed, reference the latest anaphylaxis guidelines (shared in Chapter 1) that are also in the "Emergency Plan" section of the Trifecta Passport so that you know when to use emergency medications like epinephrine or when to report to the emergency room. If you realize that what you are experiencing does not meet those guidelines, you may opt to manage symptoms with a different combination of medications or supplements approved by your care team.

Often when we are in a flare, all logic goes out the window as brain fog and anxiety kick in. An at-home flare plan should also touch on some other strategies as reminders. Write out specific examples of supplements or medications that you can increase (as per your care team) in terms of their frequency or dosage to help for a few days during a flare-up. Likewise, write out ideas for easily digested foods that are better tolerated during an exacerbation of symptoms. Create a list of self-care activities that you can prioritize on rough days. Set reminders for breathing exercises and meditation activities. Some patients also find it helpful to set up a chain of communication with loved ones to let them know when they are flared. If questions arise when you're feeling worse, write them down so that you can bring them with you to your next provider visit.

The Mastocytosis Society offers several free resources for patients, including a response plan, protocols and guides that are available for download at https://tmsforacure.org/emergency-room-support-info/. I encourage patients to fill these forms out, print them and email themselves a copy as well.

6

IMPORTANT INFORMATION

1. This process is all about trial and error. Do not expect overnight change, do not expect healing to be linear, and do not expect it to be easy.

2. Make sure that you start with a healthy mindset. When negative thoughts come, replace them with your positive motto.

3. Never lose sight of your goals, your vision, and your identity outside of illness.

4. Surround yourself with like-minded and positive individuals and reassess toxic relationships in your life.

5. Don't try to do everything at once. It's tempting to dive into every avenue simultaneously, but that can make it difficult to discern which treatment is actually helping. Patients who are sensitive often need to adjust protocols and plans to smaller steps, lower doses and a slower pace, and this is important.

6. Keep in mind that what works for so-and-so may not work for you. Try to avoid comparison.

7. Accept that there will be setbacks and bumps in the road, but also keep in mind that with the right tools, many symptoms are reversible. This too shall pass.

8. Remember that seeking help is empowerment, not weakness. Do no put off getting the mental health help you may need. Anxiety and depression are extremely common in chronic illness. They are not the cause, but they are a nearly universal outcome, and they need to be addressed to find full healing.

9. Stay in tune with your body and listen to those "gut" feelings. Honor your perspective and experiences. You know your body best!

10. Be compassionate toward yourself. Work on self-love. Believe that your healing is not a matter of if, but when.

What wisdom do you think is most relevant for your own situation? Create a list of important points and refer to them often.

6: IMPORTANT INFORMATION

The important information page in the passport is often overlooked, but it includes some tips and tricks for travelers.

Here is my version for the patient who experiences symptoms from the trifecta or other chronic conditions:

1. This process is all about trial and error. Do not expect overnight change, do not expect healing to be linear and do not expect it to be easy.

2. Make sure that you start with a healthy mindset. When unhealthy negative self-talk occurs, replace it with a positive truth about yourself.

3. Never lose sight of your goals, your vision and your identity outside of illness.

4. Surround yourself with like-minded and positive individuals and reassess relationships that deplete you.
5. Don't try to do everything at once. It's tempting to dive into every avenue simultaneously, but that can make it difficult to discern which treatment is actually helping. Patients who are sensitive often need to adjust protocols and plans to smaller steps, lower doses and a slower pace, and this is important.
6. Keep in mind that what works for so-and-so may not work for you. Try to avoid comparison.
7. Accept that there will be setbacks and bumps in the road, but also keep in mind that with the right tools, many symptoms are reversible. This too shall pass.
8. Remember that seeking help is empowerment, not weakness. Do not put off getting the mental health help you may need. Anxiety and depression are extremely common in chronic illness. They are not the cause, but they are a nearly universal outcome, and they need to be addressed to find full healing.
9. Stay in tune with your body and listen to those "gut" feelings. Honor your perspective and experiences. You know your body best!
10. Be compassionate toward yourself. Work on self-love. Believe that your healing is not a matter of if, but when.

What wisdom do you think is most relevant for your own situation? Create a list of important points and refer back to them often.

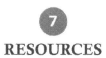

RESOURCES

Use this space to keep a list of books, documentaries/movies, podcasts,
websites, groups, community resources,
and other tools that you would like to tap into.

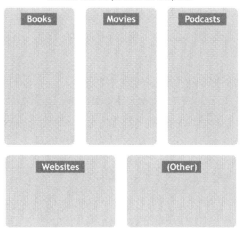

7: RESOURCES

The important information page in the U.S. passport also directs people to additional resources for how to register with the embassy and how dual citizenship works. In terms of chronic illness, I think it's important to direct patients to additional resources too.

Books

I encourage you to add the following books to your reading list, if you haven't already discovered them:

- Accessing the Healing Power of the Vagus Nerve - Stanley Rosenberg
- Break the Mold: 5 Tools to Conquer Mold and Take Back Your Health – Jill Crista

- Disjointed: Navigating the Diagnosis and Management of Hypermobile Ehlers-Danlos Syndrome and Hypermobility Spectrum Disorders - multiple authors; edited by Diana Jovin
- The Body Keeps the Score - Bessel Van Der Kolk
- The Driscoll Theory Newly Revised - Diana Driscoll
- The Toxin Solution - Joseph Pizzorno
- Through the Shadowlands: A Science Writer's Odyssey into an Illness Science Doesn't Understand - Julie Rehmeyer
- Toxic: Heal Your Body from Mold Toxicity, Lyme Disease, Multiple Chemical Sensitivities, and Chronic Environmental Illness - Neil Nathan

Movies

Below are some ideas for movies/documentaries/TV series that address issues commonly faced by individuals who have chronic conditions/disabilities. Keep in mind that some of these can be triggering or difficult to watch for some individuals; others find that these are helpful to show family members or friends.

- Brain on Fire (movie – anti-NMDA receptor encephalitis, an autoimmune condition)
- Heal (holistic wellness documentary)
- Moldy (documentary featuring Dave Asprey)
- Proven (holistic wellness documentary)
- The Fundamentals of Caring (movie – Duchenne muscular dystrophy)
- Unrest (documentary – myalgic encephalitis/chronic fatigue syndrome)
- We Are Visible (documentary – Ehlers-Danlos syndrome)

Podcasts

There are many excellent podcasts out there. These are some of my favorite ones for individuals who are interested in learning more about the trifecta and other empowering resources:

- Bendy Bodies with the Hypermobility MD – Dr. Linda Bluestein
- Beyond Your Diagnosis – Derek & Victoria
- Chronically Badass – Kris Grenier
- Hypermobility Happy Hour – Kerry Gabrielson
- Invisible Not Broken – Monica Michelle
- Just a Spoonful – Kaitlyn Blythe
- Made Visible – Harper Spero
- Move Daily Health Podcast – Freyja Spence & Dain Wallis
- The POTScast with The Dysautonomia Project – Jillian & Rylee
- The Rest Room – Natasha Lipman
- Thriving with Stripes – Dr. Patricia Stott & Thomas Stott

You can locate these podcasts through websites and smart phone apps such as Apple Podcasts or Google Podcasts. Keep in mind that opinions offered in podcast commentary should not be considered medical advice, and similar to what you may find on the internet, conflicting or misguided information can be shared on these types of resources.

Websites

Below are a handful of the many websites that offer may helpful information about the trifecta conditions.

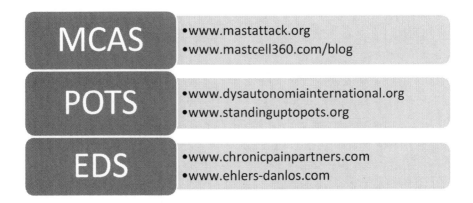

MCAS	•www.mastattack.org •www.mastcell360.com/blog
POTS	•www.dysautonomiainternational.org •www.standinguptopots.org
EDS	•www.chronicpainpartners.com •www.ehlers-danlos.com

Other

You can also use this section to reflect on the resources available to you in your personal circle and local community. Whether it be the presence of helpful or compassionate friends and family, local organizations, or support groups, brainstorm any other resources that you can tap into throughout your healing journey.

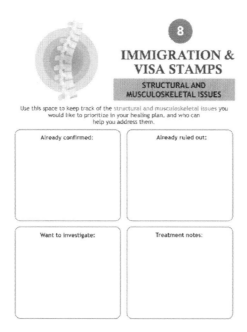

8: IMMIGRATION & VISA STAMPS

"This is a new nation, based on a mighty continent, of boundless possibilities."

- Theodore Roosevelt, page 16 of the U.S. passport

These pages make up some of the most coveted aspects of the passport: the immigration and visa stamps from travel. However, it's not always about where you've been or how many you possess... everyone's stamps look different. You may have to table some dream locations for a while due to financial or health reasons, or accept a drought where few may be experienced at all, but it's important to lay down your intentions and to specify which resources are in your holistic wellness toolbox for further exploration.

As you continue along in this book, fill in these passport pages according to your experiences: the treatments you have tried that were helpful, the treatments that you have tried that were not so helpful, and the things that you would like to experiment with. Note that this section is organized by category, with separate pages outlining what I consider to be each of seven keys to successful healing from chronic illness, which will make up the remaining chapters of this book. Addressing internal/external health stressors, the nervous system, nutrition, structural and musculoskeletal issues, movement/exercise, detoxification, and emotional trauma are essential foundational aspects to healing from chronic conditions.

Have you ever noticed that the passport has quotes at the top of the immigration pages? I encourage patients to add their own quotes as their journey unfolds. I tend to be an overachiever with a never-ending to do list, so I've written down Bible verses on the importance of rest in my own wellness passport. Some patients find it helpful to utilize one new quote each week to help boost their healing mindset.

With a vision and ideas in place, you can then move forward to address the variables and factors in the coming chapters with ease, periodically reflecting back to make sure that you are on track and utilizing resources as you are able.

The idea of a holistic healing passport may be a little bit cheesy, but I truly believe that there is great power in writing down our intentions, reminding ourselves of our identity, and staying organized in terms of where we've been and where we'd like to go. Take advantage of this tool as a way to bring further direction and clarity to your healing plan. Print it out or journal on these components, and as you go through the rest of this book, jot down notes or ideas that you can come back to and try later.

BEST-CASE SCENARIOS

Some of the topics that we are about to discuss can be overwhelming, particularly if you're faced with financial constraints when it comes to your healthcare (or the healthcare of your family). The purpose of the Trifecta

Passport exercise is to map out the *best-case scenario*, even if it's not all a possibility right now. Fill up the pages with ideas, even if you know you'll have to put many of them on the backburner for a while. Attempting to try every avenue at once is not only financially challenging but can also put extra strain on the entire physiological system as it's trying to heal, so it's useful to have an overview of the resources you'd like to experience over time.

One of my biggest frustrations with functional medicine is that it's not a resource that's currently universally available to all. (I am hoping that this changes as our medical system and insurance reimbursement standards evolve.) Functional medicine providers tend to work with a certain demographic of individuals who pay for out of pocket expenses. (Of course, there are always exceptions to this, and some functional medicine doctors do work with insurance plans.)

My frustration is not directed at individual providers—who are often paving the way with innovation, passion, and high standards for excellence—but rather at the system at large. There's certainly the argument where investing in your health for out of pocket medical expenses can save money and improve quality of life in the long run. However, we need to recognize that our medical culture is embedded with subconscious and conscious systemic racial/socioeconomic disparities at play.

One solution suggests including insurance-covered group functional medicine care to help make sure that marginalized communities have access to this option, while at the same time appropriately reimbursing our pioneering functional medicine providers for their important work. Many clinics around the country are already utilizing this approach, and it may be worth looking into for your own care. Another approach is to pursue care with a primary care provider or integrative doctor in a traditional insurance-covered medical setting who may utilize aspects of natural and functional medicine. Some functional medicine providers also offer discounts or sliding scale fee plans for certain scenarios.

When it comes to the topics ahead (especially the content in Chapters 5 and 6), many patients get discouraged if they don't have the means to investigate those types of issues on a customized basis. Don't lose heart if this applies to you. There's no perfect blueprint for healing, and those who find success each tell a different story. Health stressors investigated by functional medicine or naturopathic approaches can be very helpful for some, but there are plenty of other ways to creatively approach your healing if this isn't accessible to you. For now, grab a pen and start jotting down some best-case scenario ideas for your own care as you read along.

HOUSE CLEANING

Before we dive into the fun stuff, the tools for healing, I'd like to share one last little practical bit of information: remove the clutter. I'm not necessarily talking about feng shui-ing your living space—although, on second thought, that can also be really healing. I'm talking about taking the physical and literal baggage you carry from provider to provider down a notch.

Many patients arrive at my office with a binder of information that contains their medical history, labs and test results, prior procedures, doctors' notes and anything else that they can think of. Unfortunately, there can be a stigma with patients who cart around massive binders, and in reality, the medical staff rarely have time to look at all of it.

The first thing that I suggest is that you come up with a concise, one-page summary of your past medical history, known conditions, medications/supplements, etc., that you can carry to your appointments. It's also helpful to write out the top three goals or focus areas that you would like to address with the provider you are about to visit, so that you don't get sidetracked or go blank during your appointment.

I also recommend that patients put all their lab and test results into an Excel spreadsheet that they can print or bring on a USB drive to the appointment. Having these two concise references helps a provider to understand the full picture without being overwhelmed in the (usually short) amount of time you have together. It can also ease any anxiety that you may feel as a patient, especially when seeing a new provider for the first time.

So, take the time to get organized. And while you're at it, consider cleaning out your home of clutter and reassess any relationships that deplete you. There is great power in make life simpler, creating a comfortable space for healing, setting healthy boundaries, and honoring who you are and where you want to go.

WELLNESS PASSPORT: TAKE-HOME MESSAGES

- It's helpful to have a healing roadmap with clearly defined objectives, goals, and treatment ideas. Staying organized in the process is very empowering. You can download a Trifecta Passport worksheet to help organize your customized plan at: www.originwellnesscolorado.com/passport.
- Reflect on your identity and vision. Who are you? What makes you unique? What are you passionate about? What brings you joy? What would you like to do when you experience better health?
- Review your "demographic" information for chronic illness. What does your stable baseline look like today? What medications, supplements and other treatments have you found helpful to manage symptoms up to this point? Document your starting point with a photograph.
- Summarize your "dream team" for your medical care. Who are the providers currently on your team, and what other types of providers would you like to tap into?
- Use a subjective numeric scale to track progress. Reflect on how you would rate your current stress level, overall feeling of wellness, physical health, mental/emotional health and energy level. Every few months, rate these areas (without looking back at what you put last time before you rate your current status). Healing can be a slow process with many highs and lows, so this exercise can help show you that you are making progress in certain

areas, and it can also help you hone in on the areas that may be neglected in your treatment plan.

- Create an emergency plan with the help of your care team. Determine actions to be taken in the event of an emergency room visit or hospitalization as well as what to do for an at-home flare-up of symptoms.
- Reflect on wisdom that can help guide you through the healing process, such as the importance of listening to your body and being compassionate toward yourself.
- Create an ongoing list of resources that you can utilize in the future. Websites, podcasts, online and support groups, movies, community resources and books can help shed light on the healing process.
- Keep track of the internal health stressors (such as viral and bacterial infections, gastrointestinal issues, hormonal imbalances, etc.) that you've investigated, been diagnosed with and had ruled out. Describe the treatment responses you've had for internal health stressors.
- Keep track of the external health stressors (such as exposure to mold, heavy metals, electromagnetic radiation, etc.) that you've investigated, been diagnosed with and had ruled out. Describe the treatment responses you've had for external health stressors.
- Retraining the nervous system is a foundation for healing from persistent illness. Document what nervous system programs and approaches you've tried, and what you'd like to try in the future.
- Keep track of the nutritional approaches you've tried. Which ones have been helpful, and which ones have not been helpful? Are there any dietary strategies you'd like to try in the future?
- Orthopedic concerns (such as structural and musculoskeletal issues) can have a big impact on our quality of life, nervous system state and overall healing. What issues do you currently have that

you would like to address, and what types of providers can help you with that?

- Exercise is a very important part of a healing plan. What types of movement do you enjoy? Create short- and long-term goals for physical activity and describe the resources that can help you get there.
- Focusing on detoxification is integral for healing from chronic conditions. Evaluate strategies that can assist with both physical and mental detoxification.
- The concepts in this chapter will make more sense as you continue to read the rest of the book. The following chapters will offer ideas to help you fill in the Trifecta Passport workbook as you go.

Chapter 5:
INTERNAL HEALTH STRESSORS

O ut of all the areas to address with patients suffering from chronic illness, the concept of health stressors is probably one that I am most passionate about—and one that appears to be frequently overlooked. If the body is dealing with a lot of unidentified health stressors, patients may find themselves facing an uphill battle with more of a *Band-Aid approach of masking symptoms* as opposed to helping the immune system recognize and remove the underlying root problems.

Internal vs. External Health Stressors

Because the term "health stressors" encompasses so many areas, I've separated the concept into "internal" and "external" health stressors in Chapters 5 and 6, respectively. Internal health stressors include things that you may be exposed to in isolation, including imbalances in the form of bacterial infections, viral infections, hormonal and adrenal abnormalities, allergies and gastrointestinal issues. Examples of external health stressors include exposure to extraneous factors that may have a broader impact on the general community, including toxic heavy metals and chemicals, biotoxins from substances like mold, and the effects of radiation and electric and magnetic fields (EMFs). What all of these health stressors have in common is that they are considerably prevalent, and while some individuals may be exposed to them and have proper immune and detoxification responses that eliminate them easily, patients who are chronically ill are more susceptible to struggle with clearing them naturally.

From a clinician perspective, I've worked with patients with severely disabling cases of dysautonomia who, after addressing the presence of mold illness or Epstein-Barr virus—in the *absence* of any POTS-specific treatment—have had a complete and sustained remission of their POTS symptoms. I've worked with patients with severe subluxations and dislocations from EDS who, by strictly focusing on gastrointestinal health and reduction in exposure to toxins, have experienced a dramatic reduction in their orthopedic pain and dysfunction. I've also watched patients with MCAS go from a state of perpetual reactivity to going off their mast cell medications after working with a provider to uncover and address these root issues.

In terms of the trifecta wellness passport model, these internal health stressor areas are the first chart in the "Immigration" section for a reason: they should not be overlooked. Diving into treatments like exercise programs and lymphatic support without first addressing the underlying health stressors is like plunging to the bottom of the ocean with a bowling ball stuck to your leg, and then being thrown two children's floaties as an afterthought. Do not skip this step! Even if it takes multiple providers or spans the course of several years, do yourself a favor and investigate these health stressors to see if they are big players in the root issues behind your health concerns.

Bacterial Infections

Bacteria are single-celled organisms that have the ability to reproduce on their own. Most bacteria in the human body are harmless or even beneficial, and it's been estimated that fewer than 1% of all bacteria cause disease in humans.[1] However, infectious bacteria can reproduce quickly in the body, and many give off chemical toxins that can be damaging to our tissues. Unhealthy bacteria trigger mast cells to launch into response mode, which can trigger chronic inflammation if the source persists; this scenario tends to go hand in hand with autonomic dysregulation and tissue-level inflammation that could exacerbate POTS and EDS.

Examples of common bacterial infections include:

- *Streptococcus* ("strep")
- *Staphylococcus* ("staph")
- *Mycoplasma pneumoniae*
- *Borrelia burgdorferi* ("Lyme disease")
- Other vector-borne bacterial issues, some of which are also considered intracellular parasites (bartonellosis, babesiosis, anaplasmosis, ehrlichiosis, etc.)
- Gastrointestinal: *Clostridium difficile* ("*C. diff*"), *Escherichia coli* ("*E. coli*"), *Salmonella, Helicobacter pylori* ("*H. pylori*"), *Shigella*
- Sexually transmitted infections: gonorrhea, chlamydia, syphilis
- Less common infections: meningitis, encephalitis, tuberculosis, cholera, tetanus, anthrax, botulism
- Also notable: alpha gal transmission (sugar molecule transmitted by a tick, technically not "bacteria" but often transmitted alongside other tick-borne bacteria)

There are many risk factors for developing bacterial infections. The presence of other medical conditions and the associated medications used for those conditions are consistently recognized to impact the immune system's ability to ward off infections. For example, long-term use of certain medications like proton pump inhibitors appear to pose risk factors for bacterial infections in several different patient populations.[2-4]

It's been well established that gut bacteria direct innate immune cell development that protects us from harmful infections.[5] However, the vast majority of patients with the trifecta have some degree of leaky gut and intestinal dysbiosis that contribute to symptoms as well as susceptibility to infection. Leaky gut will be further discussed in the gastrointestinal issues section of this chapter.

Poor nutrition, lack of sleep and stress can also impact the immune system's ability to fight infections. Many patients with chronic illness find that they get sick frequently and that it takes their body longer to recover from infections. A small subgroup of patients falls on the opposite end of the spectrum, where the immune system is overactive and they rarely get sick, and these patients will commonly note high levels of systemic inflammation. Regardless of whether the immune system appears to be on the immunosuppressed or overactive end of the spectrum, it's important to evaluate for and treat the presence of harmful bacterial infections.

Many of these infections start out as acute issues but turn into bigger players as chronic and debilitating health stressors; chronic Lyme disease and *Streptococcus* infections are a great example of infections that can become a long-standing issue for many in the chronic illness patient population. Indeed, bacterial infections can trigger an increase in overall mast cell activation and/or an increase in dysautonomia, and many present as stealthy chronic infections that are undetected by conventional medical testing. It's very important to address any and all bacterial infections with the help of a functional medicine or naturopathic provider.

The testing for bacterial infections can be tricky and is not always covered by insurance. In the example of chronic cases of Lyme disease and its co-infections, many of the testing options are notoriously unreliable and, similar to the testing for MCAS, the process can yield frustrating results. For the sake of the scope of this book, I will not dive into details about the specifics of every single one of these bacterial infections, but I hope that they will be on your radar as potentially important areas to investigate, depending on your symptoms and health status.

Toolbox Tips: The bacterial infections that I note most often in my patients who present with chronic illness are presented in Table 10.

Table 10. Examples of Bacterial Infections Commonly Noted in Patients with Chronic Illness

CONDITION	SYMPTOMS	TESTING	TREATMENT
Clostridium difficile	Classic symptoms include abdominal cramping, diarrhea, fever, nausea, dehydration, and blood or pus in the stool in more severe cases. Kidney issues, sepsis, ileus, toxic megacolon and bowel perforation can result. Neuropsychological manifestations have been well researched and can include depression, psychosis, schizophrenia, Tourette's, tics, autism spectrum disorders, OCD and attention-deficit disorder/attention-deficit hyperactivity disorder (ADD/ADHD).	A comprehensive diagnostic stool analysis is the gold standard for detecting *C. diff.* Practitioners may also utilize organic acid and SIBO testing and investigate candida in order to have a more complete idea of gastrointestinal health.	Antibiotics are traditionally used for acute *C. diff* infections, but antibiotic resistance has been known to occur. Fecal microbiota transplantation is sometimes considered for advanced cases. Natural strategies including herbal extracts and essential oils are supported in the literature.[6]

131

CONDITION	SYMPTOMS	TESTING	TREATMENT
Chronic Streptococcus ("Post Streptococcal Disorder")	Acute rheumatic fever, choreas/movement disorders, muscle pain, kidney problems like glomerulonephritis, obsessive compulsive disorder (OCD) and neurological tics/myoclonic disorders have been noted. PANDAS (Pediatric Autoimmune Neuropsychiatric Disorders Associated with Streptococcus) manifests in children as OCD, motor and vocal tics, moodiness, irritability and anxiety attacks. More subtle chronic symptoms can include fatigue, rash and low-grade flu-like symptoms.	Anti-streptolysin O (ASO) titer is a blood test that detects antibodies 3–8 weeks post strep infection (and sometimes remains positive for several months). Streptozyme testing is another option. More specific tests evaluate for antihyaluronidase, antideoxyribo-nuclease B and antistreptokinase antibodies.	Conventional medicine uses antibiotics for the rapid stress test and ASO titers.

Natural medicine suggestions for chronic infection can include immune-boosting supplements, herbs, antimicrobial substances and essential oils. |

CONDITION	SYMPTOMS	TESTING	TREATMENT
Lyme Disease	Acute symptoms include bull's eye rash (not present in every case), headache, fever, joint pain, numbness and tingling. Post-Lyme syndrome symptoms include neck pain, stiffness, rash, chronic fever, brain fog, headaches, fatigue, gastrointestinal problems, muscle and joint inflammation, difficulties with vision and hearing, psychiatric conditions, facial nerve palsy and polyneuropathy. More severe neurological symptoms, heart problems, meningitis, encephalitis, seizures and other life-threatening complications can occur.	Standard testing is a two-tiered method (Lyme Screen Test and Western Blot Test) with notoriously poor sensitivity and specificity. IGeneX evaluates for tick-borne pathogens using immunoblot testing which has increased sensitivity compared to the two-tiered method. Functional medicine doctors often investigate immune markers, T and B cells, genetic testing, inflammatory markers and immunoglobulin levels. Co-infections commonly transmitted by ticks and alpha gal allergy may also be investigated.	Traditional treatment includes antibiotics when Lyme disease is caught early enough, and some doctors also utilize antibiotics with Post-Lyme syndrome. Natural methods to treat Post-Lyme syndrome often include ozone and IV therapies, chelation, hyperbaric oxygen therapy, infrared saunas, other electromagnetic treatments, colonics, essential oils and specific antimicrobial herbs, and much more.

Lyme Disease deserves a whole chapter (or book!) in itself, and there are many great resources out there that further outline natural treatment approaches.

CONDITION	SYMPTOMS	TESTING	TREATMENT
Mycoplasma Pneumoniae ("Walking Pneumonia")	Symptoms can include cough, fever, shortness of breath, fatigue, headache, sore throat, rash, chills, muscle pain, and gastrointestinal issues. Some patients are asymptomatic. Severe cases can lead to acute respiratory distress, thrombotic issues, cardiac problems, and neurological conditions.[7]	Antibody testing is the current gold standard for serology diagnosis.[7] X-rays don't always show infection but are sometimes used.	Antibiotics are used with the more severe infections. Steroids, plasmapheresis and intravenous immunoglobulin therapy are sometimes used in hospitalized patients but have mixed responses in the literature.[7] Natural treatment options typically focus on boosting the immune system with supplements, vitamins and herbal antimicrobials. Inhalation therapies are also sometimes utilized.

Natural Antibacterial Agents

Many foods and herbs have natural antibacterial effects, and this section is not intended to guide treatment nor provide a comprehensive list of options. Rather, the goal is to show a glimpse into some of the many options that can be further investigated for bacterial infections.

Garlic and ginger have a longstanding history of use for their antibacterial effects, and they are effective against various types of bacteria.[8,9] Some substances like echinacea have support for killing a wide variety of bacteria including Strep, while others like clove appear more effective for very specific singular strains like *E. Coli*.[8,10] Goldenseal is known for its effectiveness against resistant staph infection as well as urinary tract and gastrointestinal infections.[11] Neem oil, pau d'arco, St. John's wort, berberine, black walnut, silver and anise may also be good options for certain bacterial infections.[12,13]

Essential oils have increased in recent popularity as natural options against microbes. Oregano oil is highly touted as one of the more powerful oils to fight bacterial infections.[14,15] Thyme, basil and myrrh oils also show promising evidence in this area.[15-17]

Honey is also highly supported as an antimicrobial substance that's effective against several types of human bacterial pathogens.[18] Propolis is a resinous mixture of saliva and beeswax combined with exudate from botanical sources. Honeybees use it to seal unwanted open spaces in the hive. Propolis mixed with honey has tremendous health benefits and it is antihistaminic in addition to being antibacterial. Manuka honey is created by bees that pollinate a native New Zealand flower that blooms for a short time each year, and clinical studies show that it's also a powerful inhibitor of multiple drug-resistant pathogens.[19]

Probiotics can reduce risk of antibiotic-associated diarrhea that can occur during the treatment of bacterial infections. It continues to be best practice to take a probiotic following antibiotics, and additional benefits are likely with supplementation following herbal antimicrobials too.[20]

None of the treatment plans for these infections are black and white, nor are they simple. Rather, they ought to be integrated with the rest of the clinical picture in order to reduce the toxic/infectious burden and restore immune, detoxification organ, hormonal, neurological and gastrointestinal health simultaneously. Working with a functional medicine or naturopathic provider in this realm can also guide you to treatments that utilize natural antimicrobial substances (as opposed to prescription antibiotics) when appropriate and to address the ever-important work of restoring proper gut function and microbial balance.

Bacterial Infections & The Trifecta

Bacterial infections should be on the radar of patients with the trifecta. Many patients with chronic illness find themselves continually immunocompromised and more likely to suffer from persistent bacterial infections. Bacterial infections have the potential to induce mast cell activation, dysautonomia and tissue-level inflammation.

Mast cells produce cytokines and chemokines in response to bacterial exposure,[21] but it's unclear whether this patient population has any unique characteristics during the pathogenic response. Lyme disease is a frequently reported comorbidity with the trifecta conditions, and it's been known to trigger mast cell activation and cytokine release.[22] Certain toxins released by microbes have also been shown to affect the autonomic nervous system.[23] The bottom line: bacterial infections are likely potent triggers for increased inflammation and addressing them can have a profound impact on overall healing.

Viral Infections

Viral infections differ from bacterial infections in several ways. Viruses are smaller organisms that cannot survive without a host. They reproduce by attaching themselves to cells, and they are very specific about the cells they attack.

Examples of common viral infections include:

- Epstein-Barr virus (EBV)
- Varicella-zoster virus (cause of chickenpox and shingles)
- Cytomegalovirus (CMV)
- The common cold, influenza virus, coronavirus
- Human papilloma virus (HPV)
- Human herpes virus (HHV)
- Human immunodeficiency virus (HIV)
- Mosquito-borne viruses: dengue, yellow fever, West Nile
- Less common viruses: Powassan virus, viral hepatitis, viral meningitis, polio, measles, ebola, rabies

Epstein-Barr virus (EBV) is a common chronic viral infection that often occurs in patients who present with the trifecta. EBV is also known as human herpesvirus 4. EBV spreads through bodily fluids such as saliva and it's extremely prevalent, with most cases suspected to be transmitted before adulthood. It's estimated that at least 90% of the human population will experience EBV at some point in their lifetime.[24,25] When acute, EBV can cause infectious mononucleosis ("mono"). The virus often becomes chronic and can also lie dormant as a latent infection for years or even decades before some type of life event may trigger it to reactivate and become symptomatic.

Table 11. Epstein-Barr Virus Symptoms, Testing & Treatment

CONDITION	SYMPTOMS	TESTING	TREATMENT
Epstein-Barr virus	Initial symptoms often include swollen lymph nodes, fatigue, fever, sore throat, rash, enlarged spleen and swollen liver.[26] Chronic symptoms can include severe fatigue, persistently enlarged lymph nodes and spleen, recurrent fevers, headaches, rash, aching muscles and joints, depression, and hypersensitivity to mosquito bites.[26] Mucocutaneous disease, uveitis, encephalitis, vasculitis, myocarditis, hemophagocytosis and angioedema are also noted in the more serious chronic cases.[27]	Viral capsid antigen (VCA) EBV-VCA IgG (0–6 weeks of infection); EBV-VCA IgM (peaks at 2–4 weeks of infection, then declines slightly and persists for the rest of your life) Early antigen (EA) appears in early phases and usually falls to undetectable levels after 3–6 months; some people may test positive for antibodies for several years Epstein-Barr nuclear antigen antibodies (EBNA) Typically appears 2–4 months after onset of symptoms *	Prescription antivirals used in clinical trials have been largely ineffective for EBV.[29] Natural antiviral agents including herbs and supplements may be considered for some cases, in addition to other naturopathic and functional medicine treatments that support immune and organ health.

*EBV Antibody Profile Testing is offered by LabCorp, Mayo Clinic and other labs. Monospot testing is not recommended for general use by the CDC, as it's not accurate for EBV[28]

Natural Antiviral Agents

Antiviral activity against EBV has been noted with several plants and herbs, including andographis paniculate (green chireta), polygonum cuspidatum root (resveratrol), saururus chinensis (Asian lizard's tail), psoralea coryliforea (babchi) and Epigallocatechin-3-gallate (EGCG, the major green tea catechin).[30-35]

A number of additional herbal and natural substances are purported to have general antiviral properties and are sometimes utilized, such as echinacea, lemon balm, flavonoids like quercetin and luteolin, elderberry, stinging nettle, ginger, curcumin, vitamin D, vitamin C and monolaurin (a derivative of lauric acid found in coconut oil).[36-47]

Blood ozone treatment and IV therapies are sometimes used to help the body address chronic viral infections. Blood ozone is a treatment performed by a licensed practitioner where medical-grade ozone gas is mixed with some of your blood, which is then recirculated in order to purify the blood of viruses, bacteria and fungi.[48] Some patients better absorb nutrients like vitamin C intravenously as opposed to oral supplementation. While these approaches can be costly, certain patients respond very well to these treatment options.

Viruses do not have clear-cut treatments and addressing them properly entails supporting the entire system. Like the treatment of bacterial infections, viral infections ought to be addressed with the rest of the clinical picture in order to reduce the toxic/infectious burden and restore immune, detoxification organ, hormonal, neurological and gastrointestinal health simultaneously. Functional medicine and naturopathic providers typically address these conditions and organ systems. Chronic viral infections can wreak havoc on the entire system, and their detection and treatment should be a priority with your medical team.

Viruses & The Trifecta

Similar to the importance of addressing bacterial infections, viral infections are extremely important health stressors that can profoundly impact well-being for patients with the trifecta conditions and other types of chronic illness. A wide variety of viral infections have been shown to trigger dysfunction in the autonomic nervous system.[23] When exposed to viral particles, mast cells have similar cytokine and chemokine responses as they do to bacteria.[49] Viruses are also known to result in chronic joint inflammation, including arthritis as well as connective tissue conditions like tendonitis.[50-51] In addition to impacting tissues and systems on the cellular level, viral infections add to the burden of a (typically) already inflamed system, adding stress to the organs and increasing an already heightened immune response. Addressing potential viral infections is a key component of healing from chronic illness.

Fungal Infections

Fungi live in plants, soil, the air, water and the human body. Like bacterial microbes, there are good and bad types of fungi, and certain good types can become problematic when they are present in overly abundant quantities. Fungal infections often affect the skin, but they can also be problematic in the organs and particularly in the gut.

Examples of common fungal infections include:

- Athlete's foot, jock itch, intertrigo and ringworm
- *Candida albicans*
- Tinea versicolor
- Oral thrush

Candida albicans is a yeast that lives in the human digestive system including the mouth and intestinal tract. Friendly bacteria normally keep candida at low levels in the digestive tract, but many patients with chronic illness experience an overgrowth and imbalance of candida. Antibiotics, birth control pills containing estradiol, cortisone and chemotherapy are examples of medications that can contribute to candida overgrowth.[52,53] Diabetes, stress, immunosuppression, heavy metal/mercury exposure, ingestion of antibiotics from food sources, leaky gut, mold exposure and high intake of alcohol and sugar may also be contributing factors.[52,53]

Candida is the most common human fungal pathogen, and while it's a normal part of the gut flora, when in excess or in immunocompromised patients, candida can cause problems.[54] As the candida overgrows and takes over the digestive system, it can break through intestinal walls, allowing the yeast to travel to other areas of the body including the sinuses, throat, reproductive organs, lungs and skin. Candida is capable of producing over 100 symptoms, and its effects are not limited to the gastrointestinal tract. Symptoms tend to vary according to your diet. The yeast organisms feed on sugar, alcohol, fermented foods, sweets (and even fruit) and release more toxins with these foods, leading to increased symptoms. Exposure to excess amounts of the fungus elicits a response in mast cells similar to the studied response of mast cells to exposure to bacteria, viruses and parasites,[55] and candida may also contribute to leaky gut and food sensitivities.[56]

Table 12. *Candida Albicans* Symptoms, Testing & Treatment

CONDITION	SYMPTOMS	TESTING	TREATMENT
Candida albicans	Fatigue, gastrointestinal issues (constipation, diarrhea, bloating), cognitive symptoms (anxiety, depression, brain fog, irritability, mood swings), skin issues (eczema, rashes, psoriasis, hives), recurring urinary tract and yeast infections, nail infections, chronic sinus infections, joint pain, allergies/sensitivities, insomnia, food cravings, oral thrush, weight gain, hair loss, visual changes	A comprehensive stool analysis and organic acid testing are commonly used tests to detect candida with functional medicine providers. Some food allergy/sensitivity test panels will also test for candida. A candida antibodies blood test also exists, though it's unclear how accurate this is at detecting current vs. past infections.	Prescription antifungals are sometimes utilized, but resistance and allergies can result. Dietary modifications are key to reducing overgrowth of candida. Herbal antifungals also appear to play an important role in candida treatment.

Candida infections can be very stubborn, often requiring a multifaceted treatment approach to see progress. A diet change alone or one supplement alone is generally insufficient to reduce the impacts of *Candida albicans* overgrowth.

An anti-candida diet typically consists of food sources low in sugar, carbohydrates/starches and other sources that feed the yeast. These diets can be very restrictive and should not be followed long-term. The goal is to "starve" the candida for a few weeks, in conjunction with other treatments that will help kill/remove the yeast and its toxin by-products. This type of a cleanse is not appropriate for every patient. Consult your medical team if you think that candida may be an issue for you.

To complete a candida cleanse, patients typically *focus on* consumption of:

- Non-starchy vegetables and greens
- Lemons, limes
- Nuts and seeds (except for peanuts)
- Unsweetened nut/plant milks
- Herbal tea
- Gluten free oats, brown rice, and quinoa for grains
- Certain oils (such as coconut oil, avocado oil, olive oil and flaxseed oil)
- Organic chicken and turkey, cage-free eggs

Many sources recommend *avoiding* the following during treatment of candida:

- Alcoholic and caffeinated beverages
- All processed and packaged foods
- All sweeteners and sugar sources, except for stevia. Anything sweetened with sugar, cane juice, honey, molasses, maple syrup, rice syrup, maltodextrin, fructose, corn syrup, dextrose, etc., must be avoided
- Anything containing yeast
- Cereals, most grains
- Cheese and dairy products; non-dairy substitutes
- Fruit and fruit juices, including berries and dried/candied fruits
- Peanuts

- Smoked/processed meats, red meat
- Soy products
- Vegetables such as carrots, beets, nightshades, starchy vegetables like potatoes, winter squash
- Vinegar-containing foods

Following several weeks of a candida cleanse dietary approach, most patients begin to carefully reintegrate other food choices with the help of their medical team. A low-toxin dietary approach (see Chapter 8, "Nutrition") will reduce the likelihood that the candida overgrowth returns.

Candida robs the body of magnesium and zinc, so patients may want to consider supplementing with high quality sources of these nutrients for about three months. Fatigue and headaches are common side-effects of the treatment of candida. Attention to hydration, gastrointestinal motility (at least two bowel movements a day) and a daily probiotic are also important.

Natural Antifungal Options

The use of phenolic agents or caprylic acid from coconut oil may be an efficacious alternative option compared to antibiotics for the treatment of candida.[57] Substances like allicin (garlic), aloe vera, curcumin/turmeric, grapefruit seed extract, kombucha, pomegranate, undecylenic acid, uva ursi and xylitol have literature support for reducing candida growth and in some cases killing existing candida.[58-66] Berberine, black walnut, cloves, oregano and myrrh also show potent antifungal effects.[67-70]

Probiotics including *Lactobacillus* have also been researched with promising results.[71,72] Undecylenic acid, grapefruit seed extract and oregano oil also appear to disrupt the biofilm of candida; these substances may serve as powerful potential treatment approaches.[73-76] Certain essential oils may also be useful as natural antifungals.[77]

Some foods may also have antifungal effects. Cinnamon, fermented foods, ginger, olive oil, onion, radishes and rutabaga have demonstrated antifungal properties in the literature.[78-80] This section describes a small example of the multitude of natural options for fungal infections, but natural substances can present with potential side effects and drug interactions, so it's important to check in with your care team if you're considering natural treatment of candida or other fungal issues.

Fungal Infections & The Trifecta

Candida albicans has been shown to induce mast cell activation, and mast cells are believed to be part of the early induction of innate inflammation following the presence of candida overgrowth.[81] A fungal infection in the heart was described in a case report of a 24-year-old patient with the vascular type of EDS that was later associated with additional chronic complications, but literature is scarce regarding this topic in the hEDS population.[82] Specific literature regarding dysautonomia and fungal infections is also lacking, but it's clear that overgrowth of fungi can affect the body systemically. Because patients with the trifecta so frequently experience gastrointestinal issues, for most patients, it's important to rule out *Candida albicans* overgrowth with functional medicine testing.

Other Gastrointestinal Issues

We've already discussed several issues that can influence the gastrointestinal system, including bacterial infections like *C. difficile* and fungal infections like *Candida albicans*. I would be remiss to not also mention some other common culprits of gastrointestinal distress in patients with the trifecta conditions.

Examples of common gastrointestinal issues include:

- Parasitic and protozoal infections
- Dysbiosis and leaky gut
- Small intestinal bacterial overgrowth (SIBO)
- *C. difficile* (already discussed)
- *H. pylori* (already discussed)
- *Candida albicans* (already discussed)
- Digestive enzyme deficiency
- Celiac disease
- HCL (hydrochloric acid) deficiency
- GERD (gastroesophageal reflux disease)
- Gastric ulcers
- Eosinophilic esophagitis (EoE)

Gut health is tremendously important and is almost always a factor in the health of patients who are chronically ill. The gut has been called the "second brain" and many chronic conditions, including cognitive issues, are linked to gastrointestinal health.

"Leaky gut" or increased intestinal permeability has been a catchphrase in the past decade (plus), and it describes a process that occurs in the intestines and can lead to disease, though it is not considered a disease itself. In a nutshell, leaky gut describes the porous layers in the gastrointestinal tract remaining open for too long due to tight junction and intestinal barrier dysfunction. Intestinal permeability is regulated at the site of nutrient absorption called the brush border in the small intestine. When this occurs, food and toxin molecules are absorbed into the bloodstream, where they can affect other organs and areas like the liver, skin, brain and joints. Cancer, autism spectrum disorders and autoimmune conditions are among the dozens of health problems potentially connected to leaky gut.

Some theorize that this mechanism could be responsible for and/or worsened by the abundance of food allergies and spontaneous reactions that occur with ingestion of various foods, a phenomenon commonly noted within the chronic illness patient population. Stress, medications, the Western diet, alcohol consumption, low stomach acid, intestinal infections, high glucose levels, small intestinal bacterial overgrowth, and exposure to toxins and pollution in our environment are theorized factors contributing to leaky gut.

Zonulin is a biomarker that mediates leaky gut when it binds to receptors in the microvilli of the intestine, resulting in the opening of the tight junctions. Tight junctions play a major role in regulating what is absorbed and excreted.

Lipopolysaccharide (LPS) is a bacterial endotoxin that serves as a marker of transcellular leaky gut. Specifically, LPS molecules are present on certain bacteria, and they are naturally liberated into circulation when the bacteria die. These molecules are linked to significant increases in inflammation and are associated with cognitive dysfunction including anxiety and depression, cardiac disease, type II diabetes, Alzheimer's disease, reduced pain tolerance and damaging oxidative stress.[83-85] LPS activates the immune system, leading to inflammatory cytokines on a systemic level, alterations in neurotransmitter levels, blood brain barrier breakdown and changes in synaptic plasticity in the brain.[86] All of these changes contribute to a frustrating, vicious cycle.

Parasites are another important consideration, and most individuals in Westernized cultures are surprised to realize how common they are in the general population. A parasite is an organism that lives on or in a host organism. In humans, three main classes of parasites can cause disease: helminths, protozoa, and ectoparasites. Some parasites like malaria are associated with certain developing countries. In the United States, giardia infection (via contaminated water) and toxoplasmosis (infection spread by cats) are considered more common offenders.

147

However, roundworms, pinworms and tapeworms are also more common than you may realize.

Scientific case reports have noted a connection between small intestinal bacterial overgrowth (SIBO) and the trifecta. Under normal circumstances, the small intestine is devoid of bacteria when compared to the large intestine, which is rich in healthy bacteria. However, in the case of SIBO, an overgrowth of commensal bacteria occurs in the small intestine, and the root of the issue is all about *location*. When the small intestine does not move food along quickly enough, bacteria may grow and stick around, leading to dysfunction. The valve that connects the small and large intestine (ileocecal valve) may also be part of the issue, and when it's not working properly, a back flow can occur, which can also contribute to the bacterial overgrowth. Over time, this can lead to increasingly debilitating symptoms in the gut and beyond.

Gastroesophageal reflux disease (GERD) is a common condition that occurs when the sphincter between the esophagus and the stomach does not function properly. This can cause stomach contents to push up into the esophagus. Heartburn is the most common symptom of GERD, and when this occurs regularly, the esophageal tissue can be damaged. Late night meals or meals before exercise can worsen symptoms. Spicy foods, chocolate, acidic beverages, high fat foods, and peppermint or spearmint are notorious dietary culprits associated with increased GERD issues. Alcohol intake weakens the esophageal sphincter, and smoking may also contribute to developing the condition. Some experts also theorize that food allergies play a role in GERD. A poorly functioning diaphragm muscle or a hiatal hernia may also contribute to symptoms by impacting the tone and pressure of sphincter.

Eosinophilic esophagitis (EoE) is a chronic inflammatory immune condition that has identical symptoms to GERD, but its mechanism occurs due to white blood cell buildup in the esophagus between the mouth and stomach. Esophageal strictures can occur where the passageway between your throat and your stomach is narrowed. Most often, EoE presents as difficulty swallowing, and food impaction can also occur. White blood cells are not normally present in the esophagus, and diagnosis requires an endoscopy with biopsies as well as to rule out other conditions. Elimination of allergens from the diet may help reduce symptoms of EoE, and some theorize that functional medicine treatment of causes of global inflammation can aid in reducing the esophageal dysfunction seen in EoE.

Celiac disease is an autoimmune disease that leads to damage of the small intestinal villi from the consumption of gluten, a protein found in wheat, barley and rye. Many patients with the trifecta have been diagnosed with celiac disease or find themselves gluten sensitive but note that removal of gluten from the diet alone is not usually sufficient to restore proper gastrointestinal function, though it can help dramatically in some individuals.

Table 13. Common Additional Sources of Gastrointestinal Distress

CONDITION	SYMPTOMS	TESTING	TREATMENT
GERD (gastro-esophageal reflux disease)	Heartburn, persistent sore throat, hoarseness, chronic cough, frequent throat clearing, difficult or painful swallowing, asthma, unexplained chest pain, bad breath, erosion of enamel on teeth, a feeling of a lump in the throat and an uncomfortable feeling of fullness after meals are commonly experienced with GERD. Barrett's esophagitis and esophageal cancer can occur with untreated and persistent GERD.	GERD diagnostic testing usually consists of an upper endoscopy, X-rays with barium, ambulatory acid (pH) testing and esophageal manometry.	GERD is traditionally managed by either proton pump inhibitor (PPI) or histamine-2 receptor antagonist medications. Some research indicates that long-term use of PPI medications carries potentially serious risks.[87,88] Over-the-counter antacid use is also common. Surgical procedures are reserved as a last resort for severe cases. Certain natural substances can reduce inflammation and heal the lining of the GI tract. *

*Natural substances sometimes used for GERD include zinc carnosine, d-limonene, aloe vera extract, glutamine, glycine, n-acetyl glucosamine, and gamma oryzanol. Slippery elm and deglycyrrhizinated (DGL) licorice root may also provide symptom relief. Other supplements such as pancreatic enzymes, Betaine HCl, phosphatidylcholine, and Huperzine A are sometimes utilized, depending on the patient. Adjuncts such as acupuncture and dietary/lifestyle modifications are also important aspects of care to consider.

ISSUE	SYMPTOMS	TESTING	TREATMENT
Increased Intestinal Permeability ("leaky gut")	Chronic diarrhea or constipation, bloating, fatigue, headaches, cognitive difficulties, joint pain, skin problems, nutritional deficiencies and food sensitivities are often attributed to leaky gut. Vague symptoms are often linked to leaky gut, but it's important to dig deeper to investigate whether other gastrointestinal factors may be present.	Testing of leaky gut is somewhat controversial, and though some companies advertise and manufacture "leaky gut" tests, many providers assume leaky gut is inherently at play in certain patients who are sensitive to foods or experience chronic conditions and consider it more of a clinical diagnosis. **	Restoring proper intestinal permeability is usually a multifactorial and multistep process that involves removing offenders, restoring proper transit time, re-inoculating the environment with friendly bacteria and repairing damaged intestinal mucosa. ***

**Technically, leaky gut is not truly a "diagnosis" but more of a common finding or physiological phenomenon. Lactulose/mannitol tests have historically been used to identify intestinal permeability in patients with other conditions like inflammatory bowel disease, but they do not appear to particularly accurate/useful. Some providers will utilize blood tests that look at zonulin and antibodies to specific markers like LPS.[89] Functional medicine testing can shed some light into the intestinal lining function as well as other important gastrointestinal factors like microbial balance, pathogens, etc. Some providers find organic acid testing, a comprehensive stool analysis, food allergy testing and microbiology testing useful, though these tests are not specific to intestinal permeability.

***For treatment, many practitioners utilize some version of the "8 R" approach, which also includes attention to things like mindful eating, lifestyle modifications, reducing flare-ups, replacing digestive and pancreatic enzymes, adding supplements specific to healing the gut lining, and restoring a diverse diet. Working with an integrative provider to determine the causal factors related to leaky gut is key. Often, dietary changes to reduce exposure to food-based toxins is advised, in addition to investigation into unwanted pathogens.

CONDITION	SYMPTOMS	TESTING	TREATMENT
Parasitic Infection	Symptoms depend on the type of the parasite. Many gastrointestinal forms involve nausea, diarrhea, constipation, abdominal pain, cramping and bloating, weight loss and fatigue. Other systemic symptoms are common and can include things like food cravings, itching or crawling sensation under the skin, insomnia and fevers. Serious consequences including sepsis, liver damage, gastrointestinal obstruction, vision loss and other issues can occur, depending on the type of parasite.[90]	Comprehensive stool testing identifies some parasites that are present in the intestines. Blood tests can help to identify specific systemic infections (like Chagas).	Medications such as antihelminthics are often utilized as the first approach within conventional medicine. Some courses need to be repeated in order to be effective for different phases of eggs and worms. Many natural substances and foods are used to help the body kill and remove parasitic infection; working with a well-versed integrative professional is key in this process. ****

****With parasite treatment, addressing other factors that influence gut health (such as microbial balance and intestinal permeability) is also important to enhance effectiveness of treatment and reduce likelihood of relapse.

CONDITION	SYMPTOMS	TESTING	TREATMENT
Small Intestinal Bacterial Overgrowth (SIBO)	Bloating, abdominal pain, diarrhea, constipation, loss of appetite, early fullness, nausea, flatulence, unintentional weight loss, brain fog and fatigue are most common. Some associate restless leg syndrome, interstitial cystitis, muscle pain, bad breath and rosacea with SIBO. Complications including vitamin deficiencies, osteoporosis, kidney stones, and protein or carbohydrate malabsorption are also reported. *****	The lactulose breath test is the gold standard for detecting SIBO. In this test, a non-absorbable sugar is swallowed and gases (which arise from bacterial fermentation as the solution passes through the intestines) are measured in the breath over the next several hours.	The treatment depends on which type(s) of gases are measured abnormally in the test. Methane-dominant SIBO is typically treated with allicin (herbal antibiotic) or rifaxamin plus metronidazole or neomycin. Hydrogen-dominant SIBO is typically treated with herbal options including berberine, oregano, neem and/or cinnamon. The prescription alternative of rifaximin is also used to treat hydrogen dominant SIBO. Mixed SIBO typically utilizes allicin and berberine, or a combination of the prescription medications listed above. ******

*****Symptoms can vary depending on whether the patient experiences methane-dominant or hydrogen-dominant SIBO (or a combination of the two). Methane-dominant cases tend to fall on the constipation end of the spectrum, whereas hydrogen-dominant SIBO is characterized by diarrhea.

******Dietary changes (such as the GAPS, SCD, Low FODMAP, Siebecker food guide or elemental diet) are consider a key part of treatment.
Prokinetics such as erythromycin, low dose naltrexone, or prucalopride are recommended to maximize the migrating motor complex and reduce the likelihood of recurrence; alternately, natural prokinetics such as Iberogast, MotilPro, and ginger may be used. Pancreatic enzymes, digestive bitters, Betaine HCl and probiotics are sometimes used after treatment. Visceral manipulation can assist with ileocecal valve dysfunction, and manual therapy to the cervical and lumbar spine can also be useful for patients with SIBO.

Natural Treatment Approaches for Gut Issues

Natural approaches to removing parasites sometimes includes focusing on certain foods (like garlic, papaya, nuts, beets, pomegranate, pumpkin seeds and carrots) as well as supplements that may assist (like mimosa pudica, turmeric, wormwood, cinnamon oil and berberine, to name a few) and adequate hydration. Natural approaches vary widely based on the type of parasite; more serious infections may need to be addressed in a more aggressive (drug-based) manner.

Herbal antibiotics may be as effective as prescription drugs in the treatment of SIBO,[91-92] and the currently recommended natural treatment options for SIBO are listed above in Table 13. Supplements that may be useful for the treatment of GERD are also listed in the above table, though this listing is not all-inclusive. Celiac disease offers perhaps the most straightforward treatment—elimination of all gluten from the diet—

although many patients find that this alone does not resolve symptoms, so a more in-depth functional workup may be warranted.

Many natural approaches are out there for other GI issues, like eosinophilic esophagitis and gastric ulcers, but there's no silver bullet for finding healing, and each patient presents with a unique picture of contributing factors. It's essential to work closely with a medical provider to address any gastrointestinal concerns. Functional medicine/ naturopathic providers can be another great resource to help identify gastrointestinal issues and restore proper microbiome function across a whole host of different gut problems.

Gut Issues & The Trifecta

The gastrointestinal system has been discussed at length in its regards to mast cell activation and cellular-level mast cell characteristics. Gastrointestinal issues are frequently reported in the MCAS patient population, with self-reports of abdominal pain and gut symptoms ranging from 68% to 94% of MCAD patients surveyed or evaluated across multiple studies.[93-95]

Gastrointestinal mast cells engage in crosstalk with the enteric nervous system, regulate gut endothelial and epithelial functions, and contribute to host defense against viral, bacterial and parasitic invaders.[96] Gut-level mast cell hyperplasia and activity has been associated with many conditions, including celiac disease, food allergies, irritable bowel syndrome and inflammatory bowel disease.[96]

Research from 2019 evaluating 139 subjects with MCAS and 30 controls found that 30.9% of patients with MCAS had SIBO, and of those who tested positive, 67.6% had marked improvement with antibiotic treatment.[97] The authors theorized that MCAS could cause SIBO by mechanisms of altered GI function or altered GI motility related to mast cell mediator release.[97]

According to one comprehensive study of 20 years of Mayo Clinic patients, 56% percent of patients with EDS (various subtypes) were reported to have gastrointestinal issues.[98] When viewed from the opposite angle, other research indicates that 40%–50% of patients with irritable bowel syndrome and functional dyspepsia, respectively, appear to have joint hypermobility syndrome (JHS) or hEDS.[99]

A 2010 study found that 86% of patients with JHS/hEDS had gastrointestinal symptoms, with indigestion, GERD, abdominal pain, constipation and diarrhea comprising the most prevalent types of issues in this patient population[100]. Interestingly, preliminary research also indicates that prevalence of celiac disease may be higher in JHS/hEDS patients (16% compared to 1% in the general population).[101] It appears that postprandial distress syndrome (a type of dyspepsia characterized by bloating and fullness after eating) could be strongly correlated with JHS/hEDS.[102] Initial research also found that 59% of patients with JHS/hEDS had problems with esophageal motility.[103]

While it's tempting to assume that altered motility and biomechanic-related gastrointestinal issues in patients with hEDS are inherently collagen- and connective tissue-based, the exact nature of this relationship has not been confirmed.[99] More research is needed on the mechanisms between hEDS and gastrointestinal function, but it does offer an interesting theoretical perspective.

POTS also boasts an abundance of literature documenting concurrent gastrointestinal symptoms. Research indicates that gastric emptying abnormalities are present in about two-thirds of patients with POTS.[104] One study found that 87% of children with orthostatic intolerance also experienced gastrointestinal symptoms for more than one year, and the majority of these (78% of patients) had symptoms resolve when the orthostatic intolerance was treated.[105]

Additional research indicates that the prevalence of gastrointestinal issues with POTS may be as high as 91%, with nausea, abdominal pain, constipation and dysphagia being the most common culprits.[106] Associations between eosinophilic gastrointestinal disorders (EGID) and POTS exist, with an estimated five- to ten-fold higher prevalence of POTS in patients with EGID compared to the general population, though mechanisms are not yet understood.[107]

In summary, various gastrointestinal conditions, including those listed in this chapter, have been adequately documented in patients with all conditions of the trifecta. It's clear that this area is not only extremely prevalent but also especially important to address as part of a comprehensive plan for healing.

HORMONAL IMBALANCES

Investigating hormones can sometimes feel like opening Pandora's Box. However, many patients with chronic illness have abnormalities in the hormone department, and it's important to have awareness of this and how it may relate to your own health.

Examples of common hormonal issues include:

General:
- Thyroid conditions (hypothyroidism, hyperthyroidism, Hashimoto's disease)
- Adrenal or cortisol abnormalities
- Hyperparathyroid-related hormone abnormalities (often apparent by elevated calcium in blood work)
- Infertility
- Insulin resistance and diabetes
- Estrogen dominance

In Women:

- Premenstrual dysphoric disorder (PMDD)
- Ovarian cysts and Polycystic Ovarian Syndrome (PCOS)
- Hirsutism (excessive hair growth in male patterns)
- Menorrhagia (abnormally heavy or prolonged periods)
- Endometriosis

In Men:

- Hypogonadism (decreased production of testosterone)

As you can see, the term "hormones" really does encompass many systems and potential conditions. There are over 50 different hormones in the human body, all with unique functions and interactions. This topic deserves a book of its own, but for the purpose of this chapter, I'll keep this as a simple reference and jumping-off point for further individualized research. The conditions that I see most often in patients who have the trifecta are general symptoms of estrogen dominance, polycystic ovarian syndrome (PCOS), and thyroid issues.

Table 14. Hormonal Issues Commonly Noted in Patients with MCAS, POTS and EDS

CONDITION	SYMPTOMS	TESTING	TREATMENT
Estrogen Dominance	In women: irregular menstrual periods, symptoms of PMS, mood swings, fibrocystic lumps and/or swelling/tenderness in breasts, abdominal bloating, anxiety, headaches, hair loss, weight gain, cold hands and feet, memory and cognitive problems, fatigue, insomnia In men: gynecomastia (breast tissue development), infertility, erectile dysfunction	Functional medicine hormonal testing gives the best picture of hormonal balances and shows patterns in relation to different phases of the menstrual cycle, which is important compared to a single blood draw or urine sample. The DUTCH (Dried Urine Test for Comprehensive Hormones) or a similar alternative is considered the gold standard for this type of testing. Comprehensive testing typically evaluates sex/adrenal hormones and their metabolites, diurnal cortisol/metabolites, melatonin and markers of oxidative stress.	Mainstream medicine sometimes utilizes aromatase inhibitor medications, which reduce the conversion of androgens into estrogen, but these should be considered with caution. Topical progesterone creams are also sometimes recommended. The use of supplements, addressing underlying root factors, dysbiosis and gut issues, dietary changes, modifying certain lifestyle factors and reducing exposure to toxins and exogenous estrogen sources can be helpful.

CONDITION	SYMPTOMS	TESTING	TREATMENT
Hypothyroidism	The thyroid gland is not producing enough thyroid hormone, resulting in symptoms such as fatigue, cold sensitivity and body temperature dysregulation, abnormal heart rate, constipation, slow metabolism and weight gain, dry skin, low libido, thinning of the outer (lateral) eyebrows, abnormal menstrual cycle, depression and hair loss.	The typical thyroid panel includes tests for thyroid stimulating hormone (TSH), free T3/T4, total T3/T4, thyroid antibodies. Iodine loading is also sometimes tested, and a goiter (enlarged thyroid) will be evaluated if present.	Conventional medicine often prescribes thyroid hormone replacement as a treatment.

Natural/functional alternatives include iodine and other supplements, addressing other systems such as gastrointestinal function, evaluating for nutrient deficiencies and toxins/heavy metals, adrenal support and diet/lifestyle modifications. |

CONDITION	SYMPTOMS	TESTING	TREATMENT
Polycystic Ovarian Syndrome (PCOS)	Female endocrine disorder where ovaries are enlarged with small cysts on the outer edges. Sometimes characterized by amenorrhea (no menstrual cycles) or oligomenorrhea (irregular menstrual cycles), acne, hair loss on the head, hirsutism (extra male-like hair growth on the face). May be associated with obesity, diabetes, sleep apnea, infertility, miscarriage and heart disease.	There's no definitive test to diagnose PCOS. Ovarian cysts are visualized with transvaginal ultrasound. Risk factors such as hormonal imbalance and abnormal insulin/glucose levels can be measured with lab tests. DHEA and testosterone are sometimes elevated in PCOS.	Address insulin resistance, inflammation, obesity and dietary factors. Some opt to regulate menstrual cycles with synthetic birth control. Medications and/or supplements are sometimes used to stimulate ovulation or address root issues. A thorough workup with a functional medicine or natural medicine provider is often very helpful to determine underlying factors with PCOS.

Natural Treatment Approaches for Hormonal Imbalances

Sleep hygiene and stress management are important factors in a comprehensive plan for hormonal imbalances, as are dietary modifications and removal of environmental toxins.

Synthetic hormone treatment options are widespread, but they often exacerbate symptoms, particularly in patients with MCAS. Bioidentical hormones derived from plants offer additional alternatives to consider. Many patients find that supplementation with substances that naturally help the body remove estrogen or support the adrenals or the thyroid are better-tolerated alternatives to help naturally restore hormonal balance. For example, Panax ginseng, licorice, ashwagandha and certain vitamins and minerals are often used to support the presence of abnormalities in the hypothalamic-pituitary-adrenal axis and low cortisol.[108] Selenium, iodine, zinc and other vitamins/minerals are often used to treat hypothyroidism and subclinical hypothyroidism naturally.[109] Supplements for estrogen dominance often include diindolylmethane (DIM), calcium-d-glucarate, saw palmetto, chaste tree berries and certain vitamins and minerals.[110,111] The herb chasteberry may also be useful for premenstrual issues.[112] N-acetyl L-cysteine (NAC), inositol and magnesium supplementation may be useful for certain conditions such as PCOS,[113-115] in addition to approaches that focus on any existing concurrent insulin resistance, methylation issues, thyroid problems, detoxification struggles and estrogen dominance.

These are a handful of examples of more natural substances that may be better tolerated by patients with chronic illness. Not to belabor the point, but working with a specialist who has a background in natural/functional medicine can make all of the difference in terms of identifying and managing hormonal issues, and in turn, calming this area can profoundly impact the quality of life for patients who have any of the trifecta conditions.

Hormonal Issues & The Trifecta

Mast cells are directly affected by hormones due to their receptor sites; for example, mast cells express receptors for progesterone and estrogen, the two hormones that regulate the menstrual cycle.[116] Estrogen and progesterone attract peripheral mast cells to the uterus and can directly cause degranulation. Many hormone experts recommend removing dairy from the diet due to the potential for exposure to hormones as well as inflammatory beta casein (milk protein). Beta casein stimulates a cascade of inflammatory release of mast cell mediators and cytokines that affect the uterine lining and menstrual period.[117]

Uterine mast cells release mediators like histamine and heparin, which can influence how heavy the period becomes. Histamine rises and falls with estrogen, so many patients find themselves experiencing more symptoms around ovulation and in the premenstrual window. Many patients note that antihistamines and natural antihistaminic substances help relieve symptoms of premenstrual syndrome (PMS) and premenstrual dysphoric disorder (PMDD). Prostaglandins also have a well-established role within the menstrual cycle and pregnancy.

Research from 2016 evaluated nearly 400 patients with hEDS and determined that the most common gynecological complaints included menorrhagia (heavy/prolonged bleeding) (75%), dysmenorrhea (menstrual cramping) (72%) and dyspareunia (pain with intercourse) (43%).[118] Surprisingly, endometriosis was not commonly reported. Hormonal fluctuations and flares in symptoms were noted prior to menstruation, during puberty, in the postpartum period and in patients taking oral contraception.[118] Premature births and cesarean section delivery rates were consistent with that of the general population, but the study did note a higher rate of spontaneous abortions in patients with hEDS (28%).[118]

A smaller study found that nearly 82% of patients with dysautonomia had premenstrual symptoms. Out of these, nearly a third of patients tended to experience dysautonomia-related crises in the time frame leading up to their period, leading researchers to conclude that hormonal fluctuations may disrupt autonomic nervous system homeostasis.[119] Given that neurohormonal imbalances have been connected to the etiology of certain types of POTS, this is not surprising. Subsequent research found that high levels of progesterone and estrogen in the midluteal phase of the menstrual cycle were associated with greater increases in renal-adrenal hormones, which resulted in more volume retention and improved standing tolerance in patients with POTS compared to the follicular phase (where rising estrogen leads to ovulation). Thus, it's possible that the menstrual cycle regulates the renin-angiotensin-aldosterone system to affect hemodynamics in female POTS patients, though caution is warranted in interpreting these results due to study methodology and small sample sizes.[120]

In conclusion, it appears that all three of the trifecta conditions have complex relationships with hormones, and hormonal investigation and intervention may be warranted as part of comprehensive care in certain patients.

Treatment Spotlight:
CranioBiotic Technique & Neuromodulation Technique

I utilize a form of assessment and treatment called CranioBiotic Technique (CBT) to help the body address certain issues in a natural manner. CBT is a technique devised by Dr. Tony Smith, and it utilizes muscle testing of neurovascular reflex points to help the body determine what to prioritize. Specifically, CBT targets infections and chronic illnesses through brain stimulation and simultaneous stimulation of organ and infection points on the body. The infection points correlate to certain health stressors, such as viral infections like Epstein-Barr virus; bacterial infections such as strep,

Candida and SIBO; and parasites, mycotoxins, protozoal infections and more.

There are various practitioners around the United States (and beyond) who have been trained in CranioBiotic Technique. Similarly, Lyme Stop is a natural technique specific to Lyme disease and co-infections like Bartonellosis, but it's only performed by a handful of doctors in the United States.

Similarly, Neuromodulation Technique (NT) is an approach that is sometimes used with patients who suffer from allergies, autoimmune conditions, bacterial and viral issues, gastrointestinal problems and more.[121] Neuromodulation Technique combines autonomic nervous system muscle testing with corrective commands or statements, spinal or cranial nerve stimulation, and breathing techniques.[121]

I cannot cite peer-reviewed research in support of these types of treatment for health stressors, but I can offer personal and clinical anecdotal opinions that these strategies can be tremendously helpful for reducing the impact of the cumulative burden on the system—and without the need for prescription medications or invasive treatments. However, every patient is unique and responds differently to different treatment approaches. Trial and error may come into play before finding the approach that best suits a patient's health stressor load.

Internal Health Stressor Conclusions

Unfortunately, we don't have a large-scale study investigating the prevalence of these health stressors in the MCAD population. Most patients with chronic illness experience a smattering of viral, bacterial and gastrointestinal issues in addition to potential hormonal or adrenal imbalances that need to be addressed with the help of a professional. For many patients, the full system cannot recover until every part is addressed in a specific fashion.

As you've probably noticed by now, I am a huge proponent of functional medicine doctors and/or naturopaths who can address "root issues" like viral and bacterial infections, gastrointestinal health and CIRS/biotoxin illness, as well as provide resources for detoxification strategies, nutrients via supplements or infusion, EMF reduction, etc. I think that this area is a crucial starting point for patients with MCAD; diving into treatment without addressing the health stressors first may hinder the body's ability to heal.

These areas need to be addressed carefully and with a customized, patient-specific plan in play, and it's not an overnight fix by any means. In the example of a patient beginning a treatment plan of binders to remove mycotoxins or heavy metals (discussed in the next chapter), if they have not addressed gut health/motility issues or the function of other detox organs, the treatment can actually be dangerous and toxins can be reabsorbed. Again, working with a reputable medical provider—and one who is well-versed in the trifecta—is essential. Patients with MCAD may not tolerate supplements (especially those with multiple ingredients), and there are many other reasons that this part of the process can be lengthy and require patience and trial and error.

One of the biggest things that I notice clinically is that patients tend to skip investigating health stressors altogether and want to jump right to mast cell-, EDS- or POTS-specific treatments. Of course, many patients do need to be on some combination of medications and/or supplements initially to help them stabilize, but the ultimate goal is to remove the source(s) of what's up-regulating the system so that the entire body is less taxed and better able to heal (while consequently needing to utilize fewer prescription/over-the-counter options). Some patients spend a lot of time and money focusing on treatment approaches for factors like diet and medications, but again, without *also* addressing the underlying health stressors that are triggering a chronic state of dysfunction and inflammation, it tends to be a frustrating uphill battle. Likewise, some patients do not find that they can reduce inflammation or reach food diversity until they've started a nervous system retraining program. The order that concerns are addressed is a complicated topic that you should discuss with your holistic care team if multiple health stressors are present.

It's important to note that this chapter did not address certain topics like allergies and nutritional deficiencies specifically. These areas are often strongly influenced by the presence of the health issues discussed in this chapter and Chapter 6, and it may be important to investigate nutrient levels and allergies specifically with your care team, particularly if they are not improving as you address other root issues.

INTERNAL HEALTH STRESSORS & THE TRIFECTA: TAKE-HOME MESSAGES

- Bacterial infections, in theory, can trigger chronic inflammation when left untreated. Mycoplasma pneumonia, streptococcus, Lyme disease, *C. difficile*, *H. pylori* and *Staphylococcus* are examples of some of the many bacterial infections that may need to be considered in patients with chronic illness.
- Viral infections can also influence patients with the trifecta on a chronic basis. Epstein-Barr virus is a notoriously stubborn infection that can occur, but there are many others that should be considered as part of a comprehensive evaluation of health stressors.
- *Candida albicans* is a commonly encountered chronic fungal infection, and its overgrowth can lead to over 100 different symptoms in the body.
- Many other chronic gastrointestinal problems appear to impact patients with the trifecta, including increased intestinal permeability, SIBO, parasitic infections, celiac disease, GERD, eosinophilic esophagitis and others.

- Hormonal imbalances and abnormalities related to the thyroid, insulin resistance and sex hormones should be on the radar of patients seeking a comprehensive evaluation of chronic illness.
- Patients with MCAS, POTS and EDS should prioritize addressing the possibility of internal health stressors early in their healing journey.
- Treatment strategies to address internal health stressors may include antimicrobial/antiviral/antifungal agents, nutritional and dietary changes, attention to hydration, supplements to reduce inflammation and support the body's ability to detoxify and restore proper hormonal imbalances, treatment to improve gastrointestinal digestion and elimination as well as leaky gut, movement/exercise, adequate sleep, stress reduction, treatment of structural or musculoskeletal issues, therapy for emotional healing, and nervous system retraining. A multifaceted approach is key, and these topics will be further discussed in the following chapters.
- Out of all the internal health stressors discussed in this chapter, which ones have you investigated or confirmed? What treatment approaches have you tried? Are there areas you still would like to investigate? Reflect on this topic in your Trifecta Passport worksheet.

Chapter 6:
EXTERNAL HEALTH STRESSORS

This chapter focuses on "external" health stressors that we may all be exposed to at some point in our lives. These include biotoxins from mold, heavy metals, additional environmental chemical-based toxins, and radiation and electromagnetic fields.

Biotoxin Illness & Mold

Mycotoxins are a type of biotoxin that is the by-product of fungi (mold). Harmful toxins are produced by these microbes, with the most common offenders coming from molds such as Alternaria, Aspergillus, Chaetomium, Fusarium, Penicillium, Stachybotrys and Wallemia.[1]

Mold is a difficult trigger to avoid. A nationwide study of 100 office buildings noted that 43% of buildings had current water damage and 85% had past water damage, a contributor to mold growth.[2] Other research showed a 50%–68% of prevalence of dampness or mold in residential homes.[3,4] Mold illness is believed to be much more prevalent than acknowledged by the medical system, and mycotoxins are a common problem reported among patients who also have the trifecta.

Not all individuals are equally susceptible to illness from mold. Human leukocyte antigens (HLAs) are found on the surface of nearly every cell in the human body. They help the immune system to differentiate between body tissue and foreign substances. There is an HLA-DR genetic makeup associated with mold toxicity risk, which impacts ~25% of the general population, explaining why most family members or coworkers can be in the same environment and have no health issues alongside someone who is really ill.[5]

HLA-DR/DQ (DRB1, DQB1, DRB3-5) gene carriers do not make the antibodies needed to deactivate and remove mold toxins. When they're not tagged and removed by the body, these toxins circulate freely. This creates a vicious cycle as the body recognizes foreign substances but is unable to effectively clear them, leading to immune system over activation.

Some experts also believe that under the right circumstances, individuals without this genetic variant can still become very sick from mold. For example, individuals without biotoxin-specific genetic variants may suffer from measured allergies to molds and exhibit severe reactions. Individuals who display neither the genetic variant nor the allergy are also documented to have serious health complications following toxic mold exposure.

Mold toxins are lipophilic, and their molecular structure consists of fatty acid molecules, so the toxins tend to migrate and deposit in the brain, which can lead to alterations in neurons and hormone production alongside neurological symptoms. Due to the fact that mycotoxins are stored in fat, women and individuals with a higher body fat percentage may be more at risk. This can create a vicious cycle problem as individuals who are sick from mold often also have difficulty losing weight. For many people who are doing the right things in terms of diet, lifestyle and exercise, mycotoxin exposure is the missing part of the puzzle.

There are many symptoms associated with Chronic Inflammatory Response Syndrome (CIRS) and biotoxins. Dr. Ritchie Shoemaker is one of the leading experts on the topic, and his website is a great resource (www.survivingmold.com).

Dr. Shoemaker's work delves into CIRS, described as an "acute and chronic systemic inflammatory response syndrome acquired following exposure to the interior environment of a water-damaged building with resident toxigenic organisms, including, but not limited to fungi, bacteria, actinomycetes and mycobacteria as well as inflammagens such as endotoxins, beta glucans, hemolysins, proteinases, mannans and possibly spirocyclic drimanes, as well as volatile organic compounds."[5]

Mold can grow within 24–48 hours of water damage occurring. Buildings that have humidity above 50% are at increased risk. Mold is not always visible in buildings until walls are taken down or other spaces are investigated. Inhaled mycotoxins are the most frequent way by which mold toxins enter the body through the lungs. They can also coat the throat and be swallowed into the gastrointestinal system where they break down the intestinal lining and subsequently impact our vital organs. Mold releases volatile organic compounds in addition to mycotoxins which is a double whammy!

Mold can also be ingested via foods. Peanuts and coffee are commonly contaminated with mold, and it can be present in other foods such as aged cheese, dried fruits, and alcoholic beverages.[1] Patulin is a type of mycotoxin most commonly present in apple juice and apple products such as jams and ciders. Mold is often present in animal feed and consumption of animal products is another potential route of human exposure. Farm animals and pets often develop tumors and other symptoms linked to mold in their food supply, with urine metabolite markers from the animals confirming suspicions of mold toxicity. Mycotoxins are especially common in the grains consumed by humans, too.

Common symptoms of mold illness include: fatigue, muscle weakness, headaches, severe anxiety and depression, brain fog, joint and muscle pain, dizziness, weight gain, chest tightness and pain, numbness and tingling, insomnia, visual abnormalities, menorrhagia (abnormally heavy or prolonged periods), body temperature dysregulation, mood swings, night sweats, frequent urination, excessive thirst, sensitivity to light/touch/noise, a metallic taste in the mouth, asthma, skin rashes, eczema, ringing in the ears, sinus issues and gastrointestinal problems. Alternating diarrhea and constipation are common. Many patients experience extreme food cravings, sensitivity to electric and magnetic fields, and odd reactions to medications and supplements (like insomnia from sleep aids). The impact of mold on anti-diuretic hormone in the kidneys can increase thirst and urination and may also be connected to secondary POTS symptoms.

Out of all the clinical symptoms described by experts, brain fog appears to be one of the most common and most severe issues. Patient reports of feeling overwhelmed with extreme bouts of anxiety and a feeling of doom are also nearly universal, in my clinical experience.

Some patients experience seizure-like events, fractures that won't heal, or strange tics or spasms. Dr. Neil Nathan, another prominent biotoxin expert, notes that hallmark symptoms connected to mold can include the tendency to have frequent electric shocks, vibrating or pulsing sensations in the spine, and ice pick-like pains, though not all patients experience these symptoms.[1] Mold symptoms may be worse with barometric pressure changes, rain and snow storms, and following snow melt in the spring.

Connections between mycotoxins and conditions such as Alzheimer's disease, Parkinson's disease and amyotrophic lateral sclerosis are well documented. Mycotoxins also tend to make other underlying health problems much more pronounced. Lyme disease shares many symptoms and biotoxin pathways with mold and sometimes it's difficult to determine what to address first in patients who test positive for both issues. Mold tends to be accompanied by more respiratory issues and greater environmental patterns, whereas a hallmark of Lyme is migrating/wandering symptoms. That being said, many people do present with both problems, and an integrative provider can help determine what to address first.

Mold in Buildings

While many patients find themselves impacted by known historic exposures to mold, it's also important to determine whether the current home and office environments contain mold spores. The ERMI (Environmental Relative Moldiness Index) is considered the more accurate test across the board for investigating a room for the presence of mold. The ERMI uses the analysis of settled dust in homes and offices to determine the concentrations of the DNA of 36 different species of molds. The HERTSMI (Health Effects Roster of Type-Specific formers of Mycotoxins and Inflammagens) is a less comprehensive and more affordable alternative to the ERMI that analyzes five different species of mold. The ERMI and the HERTSMI offer a comprehensive scoring system with clear-cut recommendations for patients with CIRS based on numeric cut-offs, making it easier to determine whether to remediate a space.

The gold standard dust testing can cost upward of $300 (HERTSMI) to $500 (ERMI) per room when using a testing company, compared to other dust sample testing brands that have significantly lower pricing (typically under $160 per sample) but different reliability, technology, and less user-friendly scoring to help guide decisions. For this reason, some patients opt to complete the gold standard testing in the room that they suspect is affected by mold and use more affordable testing for other parts of the house when faced with financial limitations.

Companies such as Immunolytics offer mold plate testing in rooms at a significantly more affordable price point but with higher rates of false negatives. Air sampling kits that capture indoor and outdoor spore counts are generally believed to be significantly less reliable than dust sampling, while many "experts" in the industry will swear by them.

The testing can be completed by a professional company or by individual homeowners. Certain mold testing companies are more well-versed in this area than others, and it's best to work with a company that's familiar with the health impacts of CIRS and knowledgeable in dust sample testing. If a company is not open to performing the more reliable testing methods or if they don't seem well educated on how mycotoxins can impact health, you may want to search for another business. When these companies come in, they should also perform a thorough inspection, assess dampness with meters, and ensure that the source of the leak or water damage has been completely uncovered and fixed prior to remediation.

Any company can put a "mold certification" badge on their website, but it's up to you to screen them first. In my experience, the vast majority of companies do not handle mold properly. Unfortunately, the industry can be corrupt; some companies provide false information, belittle patients, contaminate other spaces with mold when completing their work, and offer unsound remediation advice such as "just open the windows and it will be fine." Just as trifecta patients must shop around for doctors, the same is true when facing companies that offer mold testing and remediation.

Remediation of mold is a complex topic. Some experts recommend relocating, particularly for severe patient illness cases. If you do choose to remediate, many companies use toxic chemicals in the process, which can spell disaster for patients with the trifecta conditions and can actually make the mold problem worse. The rare companies using "eco-friendly" options for remediation may be better in theory but are not guaranteed to provide sound remediation tactics. You must be your own advocate and oversee the details of the process when working with outside companies.

If the mold is isolated to one part of the building, it's important to have a physical barrier and negative air pressure containment vented outside of the building before any building materials start coming down to reduce contamination to other rooms and air ducts. (Even with these

176

precautions, the whole house can be impacted.) It's important that contaminated belongings such as mattresses, bedding, pillows, clothing, books/papers and other permeable items are disposed of. Other practices such as stand-alone air scrubbers (used without creating negative air pressure, vented into the home, and often left there for days) and fog machines are controversial.

Individuals with CIRS should not remain in the building while the remediation is taking place. I typically recommend that my patients remove themselves from the area for at least one week following remediation. After remediation, it's important to re-test the area, keeping in mind that it can take 4–6 weeks for dust to build up again before the dust sample testing will be accurate. Some people also find that replacing furnace filters and having their air ducts professionally cleaned can help.

Basic Tips for Remediation:
- Do it yourself testing kits may only catch about 10% of indoor molds. Do yourself a favor and invest in the reputable types of testing and if needed screen for professionals who know what they are doing.
- Find someone with several mold inspection credentials, and then call to see if they are familiar with terms like CIRS and what type of dust sample testing they utilize. If they only do air samples, keep looking!
- Avoid conflict of interest by having separate companies for testing and remediation.
- Ask detailed questions to understand every step of the testing and remediation process, and don't be afraid to speak up if you want something done differently. Don't hesitate to fire companies that are not respecting your needs and wishes. If a company tells you to just open the windows or use fans to clean the air, run the other way!

- If possible, have mold testing done several times: before any building materials come down (to determine the impact on your belongings in different spaces), following removal of building materials and 4-6 weeks following the final remediation.
- Make sure a containment barrier is set up with negative air pressure (vented outdoors) before any building material starts coming down. Avoid cross contamination of other spaces by making sure all involved parties wear proper protective gear that does not come into other areas.
- Do not accept companies that want to spray something over mold. This "solution" is simply a stain remover that can make spaces more toxic and can increase the mycotoxin concentration/growth. Do not allow for the use of seals and special paints; mold seeps through products like Kilz ®. Bleach can also make matters worse.
- Mold should always be removed completely, and best practice is to remove two additional feet of building material in each direction beyond the growth found. This is one of the biggest reasons why people end up needing to have remediation done a second time.
- Following removal of all moldy materials, a wipe-down of the space from ceiling to floor should occur. Some experts suggest using a simple solution of dish soap and water and changing towels after each pass. Botanical solutions and fogging chemicals are recommended by some companies, but the efficacy is unclear and it's unknown how these options impact individuals with CIRS.

Prevention of mold growth is key. Individuals looking to buy or rent a home often find the process frustrating and stressful. New homes are not immune and often carry the added burden of off gassing of volatile organic compounds from building materials, which can also make people sick. Paper building materials in newer buildings are the perfect breeding spot for mold. At a bare minimum, it's important to avoid places with finished basements, flat roofs, poor ventilation and skylights.

However, historic buildings and buildings more than a few decades old certainly carry increased risk from more years of wear and tear. Some people hire mold-sniffing dogs or use professional mold testing before buying or renting homes. Some states have laws that will help protect renters if mold is discovered. It's always wise to try and prevent the scenario from day one by evaluating for different factors.

Factors that Increase Building Mold Risk:
- Does the land slope toward the building, resulting in pooled water?
- Does the roof have damaged/missing shingles?
- Do you see moss or vines growing on the outside of the building?
- Does the interior pass the sniff test? Do you sense any musty odors? Are air fresheners or candles covering up unwanted odors?
- Does the building have a finished basement or a basement with carpet?
- Do windows and doors show any signs of mold or water issues?
- Does the building have a flat roof?
- Does the building have skylights?
- Do attics or crawlspaces show any unusual signs or discoloration?
- Do bathrooms have any evidence of mold growth around the tub, on grout and caulking, on tiles, or in the area above the tub/shower?
- Are signs of water damage present in cabinets under the kitchen and bathroom plumbing? Around the toilet or tub?
- Do kitchen appliances (dishwasher, fridge, freezer) have odors or signs of water damage around them?
- Do closets have signs of water damage?
- Do the washing machine/dryer and their connections show any signs of water issues?

These suggestions aren't perfect for eliminating mold risk, but they can help reduce the odds that you face a major issue later.

Testing for Mold

Physiological testing to determine the presence of mold toxins is a tricky subject. A simple and quick at-home measure called Visual Contrast Sensitivity (VCS) testing is available online, and positive tests are reportedly 92% specific for CIRS.[6] Biotoxins affect the optic nerve and the VCS test measures your ability to see details at low contrast levels. The VCS is a useful screening tool to raise the index of suspicion of biotoxin illness, but other conditions can cause abnormal results in retinal function.

VCStest.com offers an affordable ($10) test that takes about 15 minutes to perform with the use of a home computer, and the results generate a helpful PDF that contains information that you can take to your healthcare provider. These results are certainly not diagnostic on their own but provide a simple and affordable tool as an adjunct to the other tests, and this can also serve as a simple test to revisit following treatment to determine whether systemic inflammation may have calmed down.

Blood tests are also not diagnostic in themselves but can indicate whether certain aspects of the biotoxin pathway are impaired or struggling. Low levels of MSH, VIP and VEGF and high levels of C4a, TGF-beta-1, leptins and MMP-9 are suggestive of persistent inflammation noted with biotoxin issues, but other conditions such as Lyme disease and its co-infections will have a similar (abnormal) result with blood tests.[1]

Some providers will order blood draws for mold allergy testing such as mold IgE antibodies, which may indicate whether someone is hypersensitive to mold, but this testing is not as useful in terms of determining which type of mold is creating toxicity issues and what treatment options are best suited for the particular mycotoxin at play.

At present, there are two main "gold standard" tests that evaluate levels of specific mycotoxins in the urine:

- Real Time Laboratories Mycotoxin Test
    - This test evaluates for 15 of the more common mycotoxins that cause illness via ELISA technology.
    - Limitation: Cost (about $100 more than the other urine test); false positives are possible.
- Great Plains Laboratory MycoTOX Profile
    - Liquid chromatography and mass spectrometry are used to determine the presence of 11 common mycotoxins from 40 different species of mold.
    - Limitation: Turnaround to get test results can take longer (~2–3 weeks compared to the Real Time test of 1 week).
    - Note: False negatives are possible if the patient is taking glutathione or n-acetyl cysteine prior to this test, because these substances influence the mass of the toxin so that it becomes undetectable through the mass spectrometry testing technology. This company recommends that patients send in an "unprovoked" urine sample since the reference range is based on a regular sample.

Unfortunately, these tests revolve around the ability to capture actively circulating mold toxins. The sickest patients sometimes test negative with urine testing because their bodies are unable to remove toxins on their own. For this reason, some doctors advocate taking oral glutathione (500 mg) twice a day in the week prior to the urine collection to aid the body in detoxifying bioaccumulated substances.[1] However, as mentioned above, depending on the laboratory technology, glutathione may need to be avoided prior to testing for mycotoxins. The urine collection should be done first thing in the morning and fasting for 12 hours beforehand may increase the excretion of mycotoxins.[1] It may also be helpful to sit in a sauna for 10–30 minutes prior to the urine collection.[1]

Glutathione and sauna strategies may improve the test accuracy for certain laboratories, but they can also provide a big flare-up of symptoms because they are mobilizing toxins faster than the body can unload them. Individuals with certain genetic predispositions such as sulfite sensitivities may find glutathione supplementation particularly problematic. This could also be due to a buildup of oxidized glutathione and a lack of the cofactors that help recycle it back to its reduced form. Dr. Nathan suggests that patients whose symptoms are exacerbated while taking glutathione should stop taking it and send out their urine sample immediately.[1] Binders such as activated charcoal and bentonite clay need to be avoided for 72 hours–1 week prior to the urine sample, and the urine sample should be frozen before shipping to improve testing accuracy.

The tests are not perfect, and they can still be negative even with the above steps and a confirmed history of exposure to mold. The urine tests are more useful for confirming that mold toxins are present at baseline and are less useful to track progress or quantities over time. This is because the values depend not just on the toxic burden, but on the patient's ability to detoxify. Often, as a patient's health improves and their ability to detoxify is enhanced with a lower systemic inflammatory burden, more mycotoxins can be measured in the urine over time.[1] Numbers going up may also indicate continued exposure to mold, or excess treatment with binders and antifungal therapy.[1]

Additional functional medicine testing such as an organic acids test (OAT) can be helpful for patients who suspect that mold is an issue. Organic acids testing functions like a vehicle emissions test for the body and (depending on the laboratory) evaluates over 75 metabolite markers found in the urine. These metabolites can help to indicate the status of candida/fungal issues, bacterial issues (such as an absence of good bacteria or presence of problematic types of clostridia), nutritional and antioxidant deficiencies, fatty acid metabolism, aspergillus mold metabolites, oxalate levels, neurotransmitter levels, and mitochondrial marker abnormalities. Patients with illness from mold exposure often present with issues with stubborn candida overgrowth, high oxalates, poor detoxification capacity, and dopamine issues that are evident on the OAT.

Table 15. Summary of Mold-Related Illness

CONDITION	SYMPTOMS	TESTING	TREATMENT
Mold Illness	Most common symptoms include: fatigue, muscle weakness, headaches, severe anxiety and depression, brain fog, joint & muscle pain, dizziness, weight gain, chest tightness and pain, numbness and tingling, insomnia, visual abnormalities, menorrhagia, body temperature dysregulation, mood swings, night sweats, frequent urination, excessive thirst, sensitivity to light/touch/noise, a metallic taste in the mouth, asthma, skin rashes, sinus issues and gastrointestinal problems. Some patients experience frequent electric shocks, seizures and severe neurocognitive issues.	Environmental mycotoxins: ERMI, HERTSMI Patient mycotoxin levels and types: Urinary Mycotoxin Panel from Great Plains Lab or Real Time Lab Organic acids testing and blood tests of inflammatory markers and the biotoxin pathway can also be useful but are not diagnostic in themselves. Visual Contrast Sensitivity is sometimes used as a screening tool for CIRS but is not diagnostic in itself.	Removal of environmental trigger(s). Toxin binders specific to strains of mold present. Immune, mitochondria and detoxification support. Some patients may also require intranasal treatment of mold colonies and biofilm targeting substances for full recovery. Treatments to improve gastrointestinal motility, organ health, and nervous system regulation should be integrated for best results. Adequate attention to hydration, sleep, exercise and other lifestyle factors is essential.

Treatment Considerations for Mold Illness

Once it's been identified that you are suffering from biotoxin illness or CIRS, there are several steps and treatments necessary to help remove the toxin buildup, restore proper organ and immune system function, replenish depleted nutrients, and eliminate re-exposure. This treatment should be guided carefully with the help of a medical professional who is well-versed in an integrative approach to the treatment of mold.

The general process for addressing mold typically entails the following approaches:

- Ensure proper remediation (or relocate). Get rid of belongings and prevent continued mold exposure following remediation.
- Verify that the air you are breathing is clean. Air filtration down to the mycotoxin level of 0.01 microns is important. IQ Air and Pure Air Doctor are some brands that may assist with this. (However, make sure that the place is free of mycotoxins before using filtration machines, and do not recycle them to new locations.)
- Ensure that you are not ingesting mycotoxins. Many experts recommend avoiding foods like baked goods, cantaloupe, cheese, corn, dates, figs and other dried fruits, grains, grapes, mushrooms, peanuts, pickled foods, potatoes, soy sauce, sweets, vinegar, and yeast. Patients who also have candida issues may need to follow a more exhaustive list. Wine and other alcoholic beverages, kombucha/fermented beverages, apple cider, fruit juices, coffee, black and oolong tea, and sweetened beverages may also need to be avoided.
- Ensure that you are not getting exposed from supplements and medications. Medicinal mushrooms, the probiotic *S. boulardii* (controversial; some experts still recommend it for mold toxin binding), and certain brands of bee propolis can make mold

185

problems worse. Certain medications and supplements (including some B vitamin brands) are activated by aspergillus and need to be avoided.

- Ensure that you are having one to three bowel movements per day while undergoing a mold detoxification program. Hydration, fiber intake, exercise, dietary or herbal bitters, and bile support may help with gastrointestinal motility.

- Ensure that you have adequate detoxification support that factors in both phases of detoxification (further explained in Chapter 11). If you can't tolerate supplements for liver support, there are other lifestyle practices that can help.

- Fill your diet with organic foods that support detoxification and herbs/spices that boost the immune system and have antifungal properties. Examples of these dietary approaches will be discussed in further chapters.

- Determine which types of mycotoxins are an issue for your body and pair that information with an appropriate plan to bind them in the gut. A push-catch system that times liver/gallbladder/bile support prior to toxin binding may enhance the efficacy of the treatment when done properly, but sensitive patients may not tolerate this approach, especially early on. When approached correctly, symptoms should not occur with binders, and trial and error is necessary to find the right dose and frequency of use.

- Integrate holistic tools to maximize the benefits. Address mental toxins. Include nervous system retraining, adequate attention to self-care, breath work, gentle physical exercise, ample sleep and sweating. Gentle movement in fresh outdoor air is foundational to healing from mold. Some experts recommend peloid therapy (mud baths), infrared saunas and castor oil packs. Some patients also benefit from body work, lymphatic drainage and addressing structural/musculoskeletal issues at the same time.

- Whole-body and nasal mold colonies may need attention in the early, middle or latter stages of mold treatment. The experts differ in their opinions on the timing of these treatments and adding them in too soon can cause big flareups in symptoms.
- Systemic antifungals are recommended in many cases, and there are prescription and natural supplement options. Your doctor may guide you to herbal antifungals like holy basil, olive leaf extract, berberine, thyme, oil of oregano, pau d'arco, and others.
- Some experts claim that nasal colony mold issues need to be investigated to find full recovery, particularly if you are still experiencing issues after a toxin binding program. Both herbal and prescription nasal sprays are also available as antifungals. Colloidal silver and xylitol are some of the more natural options. Some people also tolerate essential oils (vaporized in the air) for nasal treatment of mycotoxin-induced illness.
- Enzymes and biofilm busting substances are often used in the very last phase of mold treatment.
- Candida, oral thrush, vaginal yeast infections, and topical fungal issues often go hand-in-hand with mold; it's important to address these areas and particularly gastrointestinal health as part of a mold treatment plan.

As part of the process, it may be wise to think outside of the box and revisit your hobbies and the physical environments outside of your home and workplace. Some experts assert that mold-sick individuals are attracted to "moldy hobbies" that feed mold because when they remove the hobbies, the existing mold in their system dies and releases more toxins, making them feel worse. It's possible that there's a fascinating subconscious biological influence at play here. Cabin lovers, mushroom foragers and swimmers may certainly fall into this category!

There are some discrepancies between expert opinion on the order of how mold should be addressed. Removal from ongoing exposure is a clear first step for everyone. Some experts suggest a stepwise approach to CIRS (like the Shoemaker protocol) that begins with toxin binders and then focuses on treating different biomarkers, one step at a time. Others feel strongly that oral and/or nasal antifungal treatment should be concurrent with the first or second phase of toxin binding.

Regardless of which approach you take, it's essential to remove yourself from continued mold exposure. Most experts assert that it is necessary to get rid of all permeable belongings (like clothing, bedding, furniture, papers, books, etc.) in the contaminated home or workspace. Couches are one of the most common hiding places for mold spores. Air purification systems that have been exposed to mold need to be replaced so that they don't recirculate the spores in the new location; simply changing the filter is not enough. Micro Balance Health Products makes laundry detergents and cleaning solutions that can help reduce re-exposure to mold spores, and some patients make their own formulas for cleaning purposes.

Binding agents are necessary to help the body remove mycotoxins via the stool. Certain binding agents are more effective for certain toxins. In some cases, prescription and natural approaches are both available. Toxin binder decisions often come down to personal tolerance, cost, access, and the specific type of mold present in the urine. With all toxin binders, care must be taken in terms of dosing as well as timing, as taking them too close to meals or other medications/supplements can reduce their efficacy and potentially impact medication absorption and nutrient factors. It's generally advised that you should time a medication at least 30 minutes before a toxin binder and leave at least 60–90 minutes after a toxin binder before consuming anything or taking other medications and supplements, though it's always good to research instructions for a specific type of binder before you begin taking it.

It's important to go slowly. Patients who are both toxic and sensitive often react to supplements or toxin binders and require special considerations for dosing and frequency that are often a small fraction (for example, 1/16th of a dose) of what the recommendations may say. When biotoxins congregate in the liver, they are bound to the bile and sent to the gastrointestinal tract to be eliminated via the stool. However, enterohepatic circulation recycles the bile when it reaches the small intestine in order to conserve bile, which means that toxins can recirculate, particularly when gastrointestinal transit is delayed or when high levels of toxins are bound. Going slow is the name of the game. Some patients may also find that they need to reduce the frequency of toxin binders from daily to every other day or even one to two times per week. Pushing through increased symptoms while focusing on detoxification is not the way to go; a gentle approach can help reduce the potential for flareups.

Prescription binders for mold include cholestyramine (Questran) and colesevelam hydrochloride (Welchol). Cholestyramine must be ordered from a compounding pharmacy in order to be effective at eliminating mold. These medications are traditionally used for high cholesterol, and they are helpful for mold because they bind the toxin more strongly than the toxin binds to bile, reducing the issue of the toxin recirculating from the small intestine.

Nonprescription binders include activated charcoal, bentonite clay, chlorella, chlorophyllin, the probiotic *Saccharomyces boulardii*, glucomannan, propolmannan, zeolite, and n-acetyl cysteine. Quicksilver Scientific makes a product called Ultra Binder (sensitive formula is also available) that contains zeolite, bentonite clay, gum arabic, activated charcoal, chitosan and aloe leaf for broad-spectrum binding of mold and heavy metals. OptiFiber Lean or GI Detox Plus are other toxin binding options for sensitive patients. These toxin binders are available in powder (mix with water) forms, capsules and liquid formulations. It's important to note that some sources of chlorella or zeolite may be contaminated with heavy metals, and not all products are created equal.

According to Dr. Nathan, certain mycotoxins are better bound by certain products. Based on your individual urine test results, you can then make educated decisions about the best course of action. Consult your care team and reference his book for more information on dosing and treatment parameters.[1]

A common side effect of toxin binders is constipation, so it's important to work with your care team to ensue regular bowel movement to help remove the toxins. Deficiencies in certain nutrients and immune function are also important to address while undergoing toxin binding treatment.

While many patients respond to toxin binders and removing themselves from a moldy environment, commensurable bacteria growing in the sinus area may prevent a full recovery in some patients and can be measured with a nasal swab test. Treatment for mold colonies in nasal passages is complex and requires close work with a medical doctor. This step may be necessary for some patients to experience full relief.

Factors that support the system through a mold detox can include a variety of supplements and food choices that specifically support the different phases and pathways of detoxification. While some mycotoxin types rely on glutathione for detoxification pathways, other species rely more heavily on a process called glucuronidation for their removal.[7] Some individuals have more susceptibility to difficulty with certain phases and pathways of detoxification, so genetic testing can help guide mold treatment and customize nutrient and supplement choices; see Chapter 11 for more information.

Adjuncts to treatment are important and can include nervous system retraining programs, meditation, craniosacral therapy or osteopathic cranial manipulation, sound therapy, frequency specific microcurrent, homeopathic remedies, hyperbaric oxygen therapy, low dose immunotherapy, ozone, lymphatic drainage, visceral manipulation, acupuncture, massage and other modalities. Some patients may also be appropriate for intravenous infusion of phosphatidylcholine or other substances.

As patients begin mold treatment programs, they often see a shift in symptoms from central (struggling organ function, neurological deficits) to more superficial (skin-related) manifestations. Expert theorize that this is a sign that the body is pushing mycotoxins to the outermost layer of the body to get rid of them. The bigger gauge of progress lies in whether, over time, the basic bodily functions are trending toward improvement.

It's also important to note that it can take many months, or even a year, for patients to see the results of these efforts, though most patients notice some type of improvement in certain types of symptoms with a few weeks to months of starting. Healing from mold is not linear, but it is very probable with the right approach.

Mold & The Trifecta

While peer-reviewed research has yet to examine the prevalence of mold illness in patients with MCAS, POTS and EDS, most clinician experts note that CIRS seems to go hand-in-hand with these conditions.

Patients who are sick from mold frequently experience dysautonomia.[8] One study found that 93% of patients with chronic fatigue syndrome had evidence of at least one elevated mycotoxin in the urine, and many of these patients also exhibited orthostatic intolerance and POTS.[9] A recent review highlighted the importance of looking into damp and mold hypersensitivity syndrome (DMHS) as an underlying cause of autonomic system dysregulation. The same authors also noted connections between myalgic encephalitis/chronic fatigue syndrome (ME/CFS) with joint hypermobility and Ehlers-Danlos syndrome after exposure to damp microbiota.[10] These associations are fascinating and it's clear that more research is needed to further investigate potential mechanisms between mold, POTS and EDS.

Mold activates mast cells directly as part of an innate immune response that results in the release of chemical mediators, including prostaglandins, histamine, and tryptase, as well as pro-inflammatory cytokines.[11] In his book "Toxic," Dr. Neil Nathan describes how mast cell activation is often triggered by mold toxicity, and how patients need to reduce carbohydrates (particularly simple sugars) in order to avoid feeding mold issues and candida.[1] He also notes that addressing mast cell activation early in the treatment process can help reduce reactivity so that patients may better tolerate treatment specific to mold.[1]

Recent research suggests that mold may be linked to the pathogenesis of autism spectrum disorders via mechanisms related to the mast cell immune response.[12] Mold ingested in pancake mix has been described to cause fatal anaphylaxis in a patient who presented with signs of MCAS.[13] It's undeniable that this type of toxin can be a trigger for this patient population.

Clinically, the treatment of mold via toxin binders can sometimes reverse symptoms of POTS, musculoskeletal pain/connective tissue inflammation and mast cell sensitivity. Patients with *and without* a known exposure to mold should both consider working with an integrative provider to rule out this potent health stressor.

Environmental Toxins

The current industrialized world sets the stage for human exposure to numerous hidden environmental toxins on a daily basis. Addressing toxins should be one of the biggest priorities for patients with MCAS, POTS, EDS and other chronic illnesses. Failing to address this area means that a patient will fail to unlock a dramatic gold mine of healing potential.

Toxicant-induced loss of tolerance (TILT) describes either a series of low-level exposures or a one-time major exposure to toxins that is followed by a loss of tolerance to foods, drugs and chemicals that previously did not bother the patient.[14] This phenomenon does not describe the mechanism behind every illness, but it may explain why certain symptoms occur at the same time as other health problems. For example, TILT is a theory that could explain why many patients with MCAS and other chronic disease, though typically presenting with a long-standing history of chronic ailments, also will report a point in time when they suddenly found themselves unable to tolerate everyday substances and foods. It could also be connected to the abrupt onset of dysautonomia symptoms experienced by some patients.[14]

The human body has mechanisms in place to clear out toxins. Why does it seem that the younger generations are struggling so greatly to "detoxify?" One theory is that younger generations are experiencing these types of symptoms earlier and earlier in life due to an exponentially higher rate of exposure to toxins coupled with decreased efficiency in the body's ability to process them. The baby boomer generation began to show symptoms around the age of retirement and menopause. The current 20- and 30-somethings are now alarmingly symptomatic, and their kids are often severely symptomatic starting at infancy. In addition to increased exposure throughout life, it appears that each generation is passing potent health stressors like heavy metals, bacteria, and viruses from the parent to the fetus, which only compounds the issue of individuals arriving into this world predisposed to a greater toxic buildup.

Fifty years ago, air quality and soil quality were different, and the body was less burdened with filtering out all the noise from the environment. However, today the body is faced with a higher toxic load burden, and for most people the amount of exposure exceeds the body's processing ability. When the body is not able to break toxins down, it's forced to sequester them in the bloodstream or tissues somehow until it has an efficient way to remove them.[15] In the cases of certain heavy metals, like lead, the body will store them in the bones until the bones begin to break down (such as during hormonal changes like menopause) when they may be released again. Toxins not only contribute to different symptoms and disease but can also serve as catastrophic catalysts that may magnify the disruption caused by other factors when combined with the right conditions.[14,15]

In addition to exposure over our lifetime, humans can be exposed to harmful toxins prenatally. It appears that each generation is more and more likely to start life as a newborn with a higher toxic burden than their parents' generation, simply from the higher level of toxins that are passed from the mother to the growing fetus.

The Environmental Working Group (EWG) conducted an eye-opening study in 2005 that examined the umbilical cord blood of 10 newborns.[16] They detected 287 chemicals, of which 208 cause birth defects, 217 are toxic to the brain and nervous system, and 180 are linked to cancer.[16] Flame-retardants, pesticides, gasoline, consumer product ingredients, and waste from burning coal and garbage were some of the sources associated with the measured toxins.[16]

Toxins themselves have been linked to numerous diseases and symptoms, but public knowledge may only encompass a superficial understanding of this. The movie-famous Erin Brockovich helped fight for the residents of Hinkley, California, after they were exposed to drinking water contaminated with hexavalent chromium—but tainted water is just one obvious source of toxins.

The reality is, regular daily effects of hidden toxins are commonly found to be slow, stealthy and less obvious. Environmental toxins can cause more gradual and silent chronic ailments that go undetected. Over time, neurotoxicity can lead to memory and cognitive decline, headaches, or motor and sensory difficulties associated with brain atrophy, edema, changes in blood flow, alterations to nerve myelin, and influences on receptors and metabolism.[17] Endocrine toxicity can impair metabolic function and is connected to libido and reproductive issues.[18]

Immunotoxicity appears connected to everything from asthma and allergies to chronic disease and cancer.[19] Different types of toxins can also act in a detrimentally synergistic manner. For example, aluminum and pesticides create more cell damage when they are both present than when either is alone.[15]

It seems that much of conventional medicine has been turning a blind eye to the research that confirms the dangers of an increasing toxic burden. In some cases, there appears to be a disconnect between medical provider acknowledgment of the presence of everyday toxins and how these toxins may translate to symptom and pathology development in chronically ill patients. Clinically, one major challenge is the lack of priority given for toxin testing and treatment options. Poor insurance coverage and limited reliability for the more affordable mainstream tests further complicates matters.

Regulatory agencies are in place to protect consumers, but allowed chemicals vary across different countries. There are some alarming statistics out there about the United States' toxin regulations (or lack thereof). According to the Natural Resource Defense Council, there are 80,000 synthetic chemicals out there, most of which have not undergone full testing.[20] Only 11 chemicals are banned in the U.S., compared to over 650 in Canada and over 1,300 in Europe.[20]

In the U.S., the cosmetic industry's panel has only evaluated a small portion (about 11%) of the cosmetic ingredients recognized by the FDA.[20] Perfumes in particular are worrisome, as the word "parfum" is not regulated and could potentially mean a cocktail of harmful chemicals.[20] In fact, due to the concept of "trade secrets," fragrance houses are protected from disclosing their ingredients to the public. Perhaps more shocking is the fact there are no laws in place to regulate the words "natural" and "organic" on personal care products.[20]

Common Toxin Sources

Regularly encountered toxin sources may include poor air quality, chemicals in drinking water and food sources, additional types of heavy metal exposure and exposure to other environmental possibilities such as mycotoxins that come from water-damaged buildings (previously discussed). Toxins can enter the human bloodstream simply by breathing or by skin contact/absorption. Toxins are present in nail salons and electronic products and are the by-products of living in an increasingly industrialized world. However, there are many other toxins that humans are exposed to on a regular basis that need to be examined.

There are agricultural and industrial toxins, such as pesticides, hormones, herbicides, pollution and radiation.[21] Household and workplace toxins may circulate from building materials, rugs, paint, cleaning supplies and the presence of dangerous materials like asbestos.[21] Toxins are in personal care products, including health and beauty aids, perfumes and cosmetics.[21] Toxins can impact residents who live near fracking wells, power plants and sources of coal burning.[21] When seeking a safe location for childcare, the Agency for Toxic Substances and Disease Registry recommends that parents consider the former use of the site, nearby sites/activities, naturally occurring contamination and the safety of drinking water.[22]

Food toxins—including genetically modified organisms (GMOs), food coloring, artificial flavors, preservatives and artificial sweeteners—are becoming increasingly embedded in the food supply.[21] Even organic food sources from grocery stores may not be immune to certain toxins. Short of a home-grown garden, it's difficult to know for certain what exactly the crops have been exposed to. In addition, herbal and other over-the-counter supplements may be toxin contaminated.[23]

The danger of phthalates is becoming better known in the consumer world, where they can be present in everything from children's toys and makeup to plastic containers.[20] According to the Natural Resources Defense Council, "Phthalates can seep into food through equipment used in processing plants such as tubing, gloves, conveyor belts, lids, adhesives and plastic wraps."[20] Vinyl items in the home such as blinds, flooring and shower curtains most likely contain phthalates.[20] Air fresheners contain phthalates, even those labeled as "natural" or "unscented."[20]

Everyday items in the kitchen are hidden toxin sources. Plastic from water bottles, milk jugs and food storage containers leach into food and beverages.[20] Pizza boxes and popcorn bags aren't safe either! Pizza boxes tend to be treated with per- and polyfluoroalkyl substances (PFAs) which increase water and grease stain resistance.[20] Nonstick cookware, stain resistant fabric/carpet and Goretex clothing are other common sources of PFAs,[20] and the toxin is associated with liver, pancreas, thyroid and hormone abnormalities.[24]

It's becoming more common knowledge that seafood such as canned tuna, marlin and sea bass have higher mercury levels. Silver dental amalgams for fillings are also high-risk factors for release of mercury in the body. Certain jewelry and household products like broken thermometers, thermostats and switches may be other sources of mercury exposure.

Bleaching creams, antiseptics, disinfectants, preservatives in cosmetics, toothpastes, lens solutions, vaccines, contraceptives, immunotherapy solutions, fungicides and herbicides are also known to be contaminated with mercury.[25] There's great debate about vaccinations, but it's important to note that mercury is present in many other everyday products than you may realize.

Additional concerning substances include benzene found in soda and cigarettes, chloroform (by-product of chlorine) found in water, vinyl chloride found in dry-cleaning chemicals and cigarettes, polychlorinated biphenyls found in non–wild-caught fish ("farmed fish") and certain plastic products, and polycyclic aromatic hydrocarbons produced from asphalt, burning coal, cigarettes and charred meats.[26]

Tattoos have been associated with chemical toxicity and the masking of cutaneous disease and malignancy.[27,28] Polycyclic aromatic hydrocarbons and phenols are present in black tattoo ink, and it appears that tattoo ink is unregulated and often used for other tasks like printing and painting cars.[29] In addition to the ink-associated risks, tattoo complications can include bacterial and viral infections, localized and generalized inflammatory problems, hepatitis and infectious endocarditis.[30]

The dangers may not be isolated to permanent tattoos. Paraphenylenediamine is a chemical in temporary henna tattoos that has been associated with severe reactions and even fatalities.[31] Tattoo removal procedures may also pose hazards; a case report noted cardiotoxicity and death in one patient.[32]

There are enough reputable sources on everyday toxins to make your mind spin! And if you're exposed to these toxins regularly, it's easy to imagine how after a few decades, and certainly by middle age, this could very well trigger a number of symptoms and health conditions, particularly if your body has an inefficient or "clogged" toxin elimination system.

The liver, kidneys, skin and gastrointestinal tract are some of the body's most important detoxification passageways. Sluggish and dysfunctional livers are more common than you would think. The typical blood tests may only pick up abnormalities with end-stage organ issues, so blood work alone is not ideal for determining if the liver is *thriving* or simply *surviving*. Dietary fiber and gastrointestinal motility also play a role in detoxification, and when the gastrointestinal system is sluggish, the body may reabsorb toxins when it cannot eliminate them efficiently.

The ability to remove toxins is also influenced by mitochondrial function, exercise, glutathione, nutrients and thyroid function.[15] When the system has chronic disease processes occurring on top of a toxic load exposure (which is presumably the case for the majority of people reading this book and a large percentage of people in Westernized cultures), the toxins and by-products of other issues can fuel each other. It also appears that bacteria may "feed off" heavy metals and toxic chemicals present in the body.[33] Thus, it's not a stretch to imagine that toxin exposure on a regular, chronic basis can easily be tied to inflammation "storms" and flare-ups as well as residual, systemwide issues.

Heavy Metals

It's been well established that exposure to heavy metals can translate to severe health problems. Heavy metals are important for certain biologic processes, but they can be harmful in excess. Out of all sources, 35 metals are of the greatest concern due to residential, dietary and occupational exposure. Out of these, the following heavy metals are of the greatest concern to humans: aluminum, antimony, arsenic, bismuth, cerium, cadmium, chromium, cobalt, copper, gallium, gold, iron, lead, manganese, mercury, nickel, platinum, silver, tellurium, thallium, tin, uranium, vanadium and zinc.[34] Five of these are ranked as "priority" metals due to their high degree of toxicity and public health concern: arsenic, cadmium, chromium, lead and mercury.

Sources of heavy metals come from the atmosphere, soil, water, foods and industrial processes.[34] Sewage discharge, urban runoff, mining, erosion of soil, natural weathering of the earth's crust, industrial effluents and insect/disease-controlling agents applied to crops have all been implicated in the increased human exposure to heavy metals.[35] Arsenic, cadmium, chromium, copper, lead, nickel and zinc are commonly found in wastewater, creating a risk for the general population.[36] Very few metals (like aluminum) can be removed with elimination activities; the majority of metals accumulate in the body and food chain, resulting in the potential for chronic health consequences.[34]

Heavy metals accumulate in soft tissues when they are not metabolized. The simplified explanation for their effects on the body boils down to an increase in oxidative stress on the cellular level.[34] Heavy metals attach to protein sites and displace cellular reactions from occurring at their natural binding docks, which results in the malfunctioning of the cells and subsequent toxicity.[34]

Toxicity depends on the dose, route of exposure, duration of exposure and unique individual factors (like genetics, age, sex and nutritional status), though severe health consequences—including multiple organ damage—have been noted from minor exposures of the "priority" metals.[34] Heavy metals can have destructive consequences to the blood composition, brain, kidney, liver, lungs and other organs. Progressive muscular and neurological degenerative conditions including multiple sclerosis, Alzheimer's disease, muscular dystrophy and Parkinson's disease have been associated with heavy metal toxicity.[34] Over 100 hazardous effects of heavy metal exposure have been noted, including allergic, carcinogenic, circulatory, central and peripheral nervous system problems.

Table 16. Common Sources of Heavy Metal Toxicity

HEAVY METAL	SOURCE	SYMPTOMS
Aluminum	Food, water, air and soil Certain vaccinations[37] Deodorant and other cosmetic products Aluminum cans, foil, pots and pans Antacids, buffered aspirin, astringents Baking powder and baking mixes Food additives: anticaking agents, coloring agents[38] Siding and roofing material Kidney dialysis may pose a risk factor due to contaminated dialysates and phosphate binders.[34]	Nausea, vomiting, mouth ulcers, skin ulcers, rashes, diarrhea and arthritic pain Nervous system issues, bone issues, kidney problems, loss of balance and coordination, and memory problems are also possible, with some indicators that aluminum may be connected to Alzheimer's disease[38]
Arsenic	Drinking water Rice, chicken, seafood Soil, ground water runoff and air from smelting Cigarettes Soaps, dyes, paints, metals, semiconductors, drugs Certain fertilizers, pesticides, animal feeding operations[39]	Low levels: Nausea, vomiting, hand/leg pricking sensation, blood cell abnormalities, blood vessel damage, heartbeat abnormalities Long-term exposure: neurological problems, skin lesions, peripheral vascular disease, hypertension, cardiovascular disease, diabetes, pulmonary disease, cancers (particularly bladder, liver, lung and skin cancer)[40,41]

Cadmium	Rechargeable batteries Tobacco smoke Food sources from soil contamination Plastics, pigments, metal coatings	Kidney damage and kidney stones are common consequences. Lung issues, gastrointestinal problems and fragile bones are also noted
Chromium	Soil, water, air and food source contamination Fertilizers, sewage Burning of oil and coal; emissions from chemical plants Petroleum Pigments, industrial metals Tattoos Antifreeze, cement, wood preservatives[42]	Gastrointestinal symptoms (nausea, vomiting, ulcers, epigastric pain, diarrhea) are frequently reported. Ulcers on the nasal septum are common with occupational exposure. Vertigo, fever, muscle cramps, sinus issues, lung problems, kidney and liver damage, organ failure and death have also been noted
Lead	Plumbing pipes Food, tea leaves Drinking water (from older pipes) Ammunition Children's toys Cosmetics Fertilizers and pesticides Smelting of ores Factory chimneys Additives in gasoline Pigment in house paint Exhaust from automobiles Soil wastes Wastes from battery industries Metal planting and finishing operations[34,43]	Acute symptoms (typically from occupational exposure): abdominal pain, headache, kidney problems, fatigue, arthritis, loss of appetite, insomnia, hallucinations, vertigo Chronic exposure: psychosis, autism spectrum disorders, hyperactivity, dyslexia, allergies, paralysis, birth defects, mental retardation, weight loss, muscle weakness, kidney damage, brain damage, death[44]

| Mercury | Food sources, particularly fish (Consumption of aquatic animals by humans is the major route of human exposure.)[45] Mercury amalgam fillings (Dental preparations are the other common source of human toxicity.) Certain vaccinations Agriculture, mining, pharmaceuticals, municipal/industrial wastewater, incineration, and products such as thermometers and fluorescent lamps are other sources | The nervous system and brain are big targets of mercury toxicity, which can result in memory problems, tremors, irritability, alterations in hearing and vision, psychiatric illness, brain fog, autism spectrum disorders and depression[46] Damage to the lungs, diarrhea, nausea, vomiting, skin rashes, hypertension, headache, hair loss and fatigue are also commonly noted |

Heavy Metal Testing

Functional medicine testing of heavy metals is typically a blood metals panel or hair test. Nonmetal toxin urine testing is also available. Porphyrins profile testing can also be helpful. Companies including Quicksilver Scientific, Great Plains Laboratory, Genova Diagnostics and many others offer this type of laboratory analysis.

Heavy Metal Treatment

Chelation therapy has traditionally been used to help the body remove certain heavy metals through the kidneys and urine, but it's a controversial treatment option, and serious adverse effects can occur.

Certain toxin binders may help patients remove heavy metals in the stool. Examples of metal-specific toxin binders include activated charcoal, apple pectin, bentonite clays, chlorella, cilantro, diatomaceous earth, zeolite, and others. Over time these may help reduce the presence of heavy metals and other potential mast cell triggers, which can result in a reduction in symptoms.

As mentioned in the mold section, toxin binders are tricky in that they must be carefully spaced away from other medications and supplements and sometimes even foods. And just like anything else, they do have the potential to trigger anaphylactoid reactions in patients with mast cell activation issues. Working closely with a specialist is crucial when using these compounds. Like the concept of removing mold toxins, if the body's detoxification pathways are not working efficiently or the patient is not having regular bowel movements, these products can rerelease heavy metal toxins back into the tissues, causing major problems. They may also pose a risk of malnutrition if they are not timed and spaced appropriately.

Certain supplements and herbs may help to remove heavy metals and support detoxification organs in the process. As a potent antioxidant and chelator of heavy metals, alpha lipoic acid (ALA) appears to reduce the cognitive impairments associated with aluminum heavy metal toxicity.[47] Recent reviews support the use of natural heavy metal chelators such as cilantro, garlic, gingko, green algae, milk thistle, phytochelatins, triphala and turmeric.[48,49] Sulfur-rich foods including shallots and onions may help remove lead from the body.[50] Selenium from Brazil nuts aids in detoxification and actively binds methylmercury in the body.[51] Other foods/beverages that may bind heavy metals include Atlantic dulse, barley grass juice powder, blueberries, chlorella, curry, green tea, lemon water, spirulina and tomatoes.[52]

Strategies to reduce sources of air toxins can include increasing house plants and use of HEPA air purifiers as well as careful consideration of the materials present in the home. Newer home air filtration systems can measure the amount of circulating volatile organic compounds (VOCs), which can be very helpful. Food sources, health and beauty aids, household products and workplace exposures should be evaluated carefully.

Additional methods to support detoxification are shared in Chapter 11, "Detoxification."

It's very important that the patient addresses their concerns carefully with their healthcare team instead of attempting to detox without medical advice. Again, if a patient does not control or manage their detoxification carefully, and repair the necessary organs (particularly the gut, liver and kidneys) in a particular sequence, more toxins can be unleashed than the body can safely process, and toxins may recirculate.[15]

Similar to removing mold toxins, adequate attention to organ and immune system support, gastrointestinal motility, hydration, sleep, and other factors are key to helping the patient recover from heavy metal and other toxin exposure. Vitamin deficiencies are associated with poorer responses to heavy metals and need to be addressed. Removing existing continued sources and prevention of further exposure is also very important.

Prevention
Tips to reduce exposure to heavy metals:

- Remove your shoes and limit dust in the home, since metals may be present in dust and dirt.
- Consider reducing fish dietary intake.
- Avoid peeling paint, imported toys, and imported candies.
- Consider showering and changing clothes at work before coming home if you work with metals. Also prioritize proper ventilation in your workspace.
- Avoid living near industrial factories, if possible.
- If you have older plumbing or use well water in your home, consider having the water tested for heavy metals. Utilize filtered water for drinking and bathing.

- Address mercury amalgam fillings with the help of a reputable biologic dentist.
- Read labels and utilize clean cosmetic/beauty products.
- Eat organic foods and be cautious with sources of rice and meat.
- Avoid being present when pesticides or herbicides are sprayed around the house and ensure use of a good air filtration system in the home.
- Use a mask/sit inside when pumping gasoline for your vehicle. Avoid secondhand car exhaust.

Environmental Toxins & The Trifecta

How do heavy metals and other toxins relate to the trifecta? Toxic substances may have a direct effect on the heart and autonomic nervous system, mast cells, joint inflammation and tissue collagen properties. The cumulative load of heavy metals (in isolation or when combined with other types of toxic burden) can put tremendous strain on the immune system and our organs of detoxification.

Many patients with MCAS have some type of low-level liver abnormality on testing, and a poorly functioning liver can negatively impact the body's ability to clear or render inactive certain mast cell mediators, leading to a vicious cycle scenario.[15] Logically, if a patient has a sluggish liver, a high toxic burden, and MCAS, it's like a triple whammy.

Toxins can also damage DNA, alter gene expression and cause damage on the cellular level.[53] It's plausible that toxins could be connected to some of the epigenetic changes noted in current generations of patients presenting with chronic conditions like MCAS.

Many types of heavy metal exposure are triggers for mast cell activation.[17-19] Mast cell degranulation has also been noted to increase by 72% after high-dose short-term exposure to diesel exhaust fumes.[54] These are a few examples of the hundreds of studies available on the subject of the influence of toxins on the immune system response. Whether inhaled, ingested or absorbed through the skin, toxins have a profound impact on the immune system and mast cell activation, and their influence on specific organs like the gastrointestinal system only compounds existing inflammatory matters.

By-products of toxic chemicals in the gastrointestinal system called gut endotoxin metabolites contribute to histamine levels and symptoms like hives.[15] Toxic substances contribute to an increase in intestinal permeability or "leaky gut" (discussed in Chapter 5), which can trigger system-wide inflammatory reactions.[55]

Potential connections between dysautonomia or Ehlers-Danlos syndrome and toxins are less investigated in the literature, but many speculate that toxins also influence these conditions. One case report described autonomic dysfunction as a predominant symptom of botulinum toxin poisoning.[56]

The presence of heavy metals may block the actions of acetylcholine, an important neurotransmitter than impacts vagus nerve function.[57,58] As you will see in the next chapter, the vagus nerve has profound impacts on the entire system and our ability to heal. The added impact of heavy metals and toxins on the cellular level can have a tremendous effect on an already overburdened system.

Radiation and Electromagnetic Fields (EMFs)

In addition to the exposure to toxins that are ingested or absorbed through the skin in everyday life, the last few decades of increasing access to technological advancements also put human bodies at more risk for invisible harm. Many patients report that getting off the grid can work wonders for their symptoms. There are certainly some theorists who link viral pandemics to the effects of cell phone tower radiation. The intent of this section is not to propagate paranoia, but it *is* important to recognize that this factor can influence our patient population, a population that tends to already be inflamed and hypersensitive to other environmental factors.

According to the National Cancer Institute in America, "Electric and magnetic fields are invisible areas of energy (also called radiation) that are produced by electricity, which is the movement of electrons, or current, through a wire."[59] Electric fields occur regardless of whether a device is turned on, whereas magnetic fields occur only when current is flowing.[59]

Electromagnetic field (EMF) radiation exposure is vastly more common than we realize. Coffee makers, dishwashers, electric blankets, electric wiring, hair dryers, lamps, power lines, shavers and vacuum cleaners are examples of common everyday "extremely low frequency EMFs," although some experts claim that this name is misleading because these still can cause harmful effects.

The more concerning radiofrequency radiation sources include many of our everyday devices: cell phones, e-readers, tablets, laptops and smart watches. These are often claimed to be "non-ionizing" sources of radiation, though this is a controversial point. Standing near household electrical motors and digital components in appliances like the refrigerator, using a clock radio, and sleeping near the wall of the house's main power meter may also be EMF sources to consider avoiding. Highest sources of (potentially) everyday EMF frequencies include full body scanners and direct broadcast satellites. Cellular phones, microwave ovens, radars, radios and wireless networks make up the second-highest category in terms of frequency of EMF output.

EMFs have been long associated with problematic health effects in anecdotal claims, but it's another area where the medical system seems to be skeptical to the growing risks and negative health implications. The National Cancer Institute (America) maintains that "no consistent evidence for an association between any source of non-ionizing EMF and cancer has been found."[59] They note that while studies have looked for associations between prenatal or preconception exposure via the parents, the results have been inconclusive in this area as well.[59]

Many experts appear to have a healthy dose of skepticism for the National Cancer Institute's stance as well as what they constitute as "non-ionizing radiation." The National Cancer Institute failed to acknowledge studies that, from a research standpoint, provided ample evidence of the harmful effects of EMFs. Furthermore, plenty of evidence exists to show that EMFs are harmful in some physiological way or another, even outside of cancer. This topic is highly controversial and EMF exposure is becoming increasingly difficult to avoid in Westernized cultures.

Researchers first noted skin-specific reactions (flushing, itching, pain, papules, pustules, redness) and heart and central nervous system symptoms in patients who were exposed to electronic screens and mobile phones in studies conducted back in the 1980s.[60,61] Further research in the early 2000s on electro-sensitivity noted headaches in about 85% of cell phone users, and a significant number of subjects also reported burning, cognitive symptoms, dizziness, fatigue, itching, nausea and redness.[62]

Additional research has shown that overnight EMF exposure negatively impacts soundness of sleep and well-being in the morning.[63] Interestingly, the same study also found that patients tended to shift to the side of the bed that was furthest from the source of radiation during the night.[63] Mobile phone emissions have been shown to alter brain waves and human lymphocyte function for up to 72 hours after exposure.[64,65]

Multiple scientific review articles assert that using a cell phone for 30 minutes a day over several years or decades increases the risk of developing a brain tumor, in some estimates up to 40%–50%.[66,67] Cell phone radiation has been connected to all sorts of diseases, including cardiovascular symptoms, childhood leukemia and other types of cancer, immune system issues, infertility, neurodegenerative diseases, and allergic and inflammatory responses.[66,67]

In the past decade, electric companies began installing new smart meters (digital gas and electric meters) that track when someone is home. While at first glance they seem like a good idea for energy efficiency and use of resources, some voice concern that the EMF grid radiated from smart meters could cause health problems. Following the mandate for smart meters in Victoria, Australia, a 2014 case series noted that subjects most frequently reported insomnia, headaches, tinnitus (ringing in the ears), fatigue, cognitive disturbances, dysesthesias (abnormal sensations) and dizziness.[68] While the average radiofrequency emitted by smart meters is no greater than holding a cell phone to the head, it's possible that smart meters emit "brief and very intense radiofrequency pulses" that may have a detrimental effect on health in susceptible individuals.[69-71]

Table 17. Electromagnetic Field Sensitivity Symptoms, Testing and Treatment

CONDITION	SYMPTOMS	TESTING	TREATMENT
EMF sensitivity	Headaches, skin issues/rashes, fatigue, ringing in the ears, brain fog, memory issues, insomnia, dizziness/vertigo, gastrointestinal issues, depression, dysesthesia, heart rate irregularities, restless leg syndrome, visual issues, muscle pain, chest pain, and nerve inflammation are reported in studies.	To date, there are no official testing methods to determine how much an individual is impacted physiologically by EMFs. Handheld EMF meter devices can be purchased for home testing of electric and magnetic fields and radiofrequency radiation.*	Many patients find that turning off the wireless internet at night or getting rid of smart meters significantly reduces their symptoms and insomnia. Avoidance of Bluetooth devices, cell phones, televisions, home appliances and computer screen time may also help.

*Better (more sensitive) EMF meter devices show down to 0.1 milligauss or 0.01 microtesla levels, which may aid the patient who is hypersensitive. These devices are useful for assessing various areas of the living space where you spend the most time. Don't forget to test your car and different Bluetooth devices, too! Readings at different times of day and at different air temperatures will vary. Budget and cell phone versions of these devices are often unreliable.

Various products exist (such as jewelry, gemstones, cell phone and laptop EMF blockers, etc.) that claim to mitigate the harmful effects of radiation, and they are a useful idea, but there's little science backing some of these claims. Patients with severe sensitivity may want to consider living and spending time away from power lines, satellites and radio towers when possible.

EMFs & The Trifecta

How does this relate to the trifecta? Some research exists supporting links between exposure to EMF radiation and mast cell activation. Sweden-based researcher Olle Johannson has conducted several studies evaluating the influence of EMFs on mast cells. His research has concluded that EMFs may increase the quantity of mast cells, their migration/infiltration, and rate of degranulation in patients with electro-hypersensitivity.[72]

Low level EMFs are capable of stimulating autonomic nervous system activity and have been investigated in their potential to induce cardiac changes like atrial fibrillation.[73] Evidently, there's less speculation of connections between EMFs and Ehlers-Danlos syndrome and a scarcity of research is present on this topic regarding dysautonomia. However, the consensus is that patients with some or all conditions in the trifecta often find themselves extra sensitive to EMF sources and also find that removing them can help dramatically with certain symptoms. This may be one small piece of the puzzle, but it's something to consider for all patients who have chronic conditions.

WIDESPREAD TRIGGER ELIMINATION

Below is a room-by-room checklist to use when assessing for sources of common toxins, mold and EMFs in everyday life. For those concerned about additional everyday chemical/toxin exposure, a more thorough screening tool, such as the Environmental Influences Questionnaire, may be more appropriate. Various occupational screening tools are also available online.

OVERALL ASSESSMENT

1. Is there mold or water damage? If found, relocate or *carefully* remediate with professional help.
2. Are pesticides, insecticides or herbicides used around the exterior of the home? Vacate the premises if this is scheduled, or better yet, reconsider these treatments and investigate more natural options, if possible.
3. Is the building near high-voltage wires or transformers or near an electric distribution station?
4. Do you use a smart meter for utilities? Consider opting out if possible.
5. Is wireless internet turned on at night? Consider using a router on a timer.
6. Do you live on or near a golf course? Pesticides and runoff can influence drinking water, and chemicals sprayed on the course can enter homes.
7. Does the home have a hot tub?
8. Do you live close to a high-traffic road?
9. Do you make pottery, paint, refurbish furniture, work in a photography darkroom or engage in other forms of art? Toxins alone may not be reason to leave these hobbies, but it's important to be aware of methods to reduce your exposure (such as wearing a mask and gloves, selecting materials carefully, ensuring proper ventilation, etc.)
10. Is the environment cluttered, dark or aesthetically unpleasing? Living spaces can influence the human body. When clutter is reduced from the home or work environment and when the space

213

is a place that generates peace, some believe that the body may also be better able to detoxify and heal.

ALL ROOMS: GENERAL ASSESSMENT

1. Are candles, air fresheners, or other synthetic scented products present?
2. If the home is newer, is off gassing of carpets/flooring and furniture an issue?
3. Do the carpets, furniture or curtains contain flame or stain repellants?
4. Do you have PVC-containing mini-blinds? If they are from Mexico or Asia, they may contain lead.
5. Does the house have vinyl flooring? Wooden, bamboo, marble or ceramic may be better alternatives.
6. Do flooring finishes contain formaldehyde?
7. Do you use a humidifier in the home? If so, try to keep humidity levels below 50% to reduce mold growth and dust mites.
8. Do you use natural cleaners? Consider replacing any chemical-based cleaners with something like lemon juice, probiotic solutions or distilled white vinegar. Microfiber cloths and water can also be considered for sensitive patients.
9. Do you use gloves when you clean? Seek hypoallergenic, latex-free gloves and a facial mask for cleaning to minimize contact of irritants with skin pores and the respiratory system.
10. Do you have someone dust often? This can help reduce exposure to chemicals and mold particles that settle in dust.

KITCHEN ENVIRONMENT

1. Is the tap water filtered? A reverse osmosis or carbon filter may be advised to reduce exposure to heavy metals, volatile organic

compounds, water treatment additives, bacteria/viruses and other potential water contaminants.

2. Is there a designated allergen-friendly space for food preparation? Do you have a designated allergen-free section of the fridge/freezer? Use color coding for cutting boards, knives and cooking materials that are specific for the individual with allergies, if needed. Make sure there's a designated separate sponge as well.

3. Do you have adequate ventilation in the kitchen (fans, windows)?

4. Do you use aluminum or nonstick cookware? Glass, ceramic and stainless-steel cookware are better options. Non-chlorinated wax paper and non-treated parchment paper may also introduce less toxins with baking.

5. Do you use your own plastic food storage containers, aluminum foil, or plastic wrap? Consider the use of glass containers for food leftover storage. Be sure to avoid heating plastic kitchen components in the dishwasher or microwave.

6. Are there plastic containers (or packaging) from the grocery store holding food or beverages? Mesh bags are a good alternative to plastic storage of produce, and glass bottles and containers should replace any plastic kitchenware. Do you have plastic cutting boards? Consider wooden or glass alternatives. Beware of "BPA-free" marketing, as those products typically utilize other equally harmful toxins.

7. Are groceries organic and free of additives, preservatives and chemicals?

8. Are the bags in the trash can odorless?

9. If applicable, are baby bottles labeled with the #7 (polycarbonate plastic)? Are latex rubber nipples used? If so, consider alternatives.

BATHROOM

1. Is hand soap laden with chemicals? Does your deodorant contain aluminum/other chemicals? Do you use triclosan-containing toothpaste, toothbrushes or mouthwash?
2. Does your shaving cream contain parabens or other chemicals?
3. Do you use hair dye or nail polish?
4. Are additional shower, makeup and skin beauty products appropriate? Get out every single product used and do some research, aiming to eliminate and reduce the majority that are synthetic/chemical based. There are apps (such as Think Dirty, GoodGuide, Detox Me, and EWG's Healthy Living) that may help with this step.
5. Are feminine hygiene products free of chlorine, dyes, pesticides and other chemicals?
6. Is shower water filtered? A filter to remove chlorine and other chemicals may be helpful.
7. Are the bathtub or fixtures made out of porcelain? If so, they may contain lead.
8. Are adequate ventilation and cleaning techniques used in the bathroom to prevent mold/mildew growth?
9. Do you use vinyl-based shower curtain linings? Consider alternatives that are made with hemp, linen, beeswax coatings, or cotton.
10. If you deal with regular constipation, is a toilet footstool ready for action? If gastrointestinal issues are present, elevating the knees above the hips (on a Squatty Potty type step) can be a tremendous aid for facilitating easier bowel movements, which in turn can help with detoxification.

BEDROOM

1. Are electronics that emit EMFs (including alarm clocks and cell phones) near the bed? Are laptops or TVs used in bed? Create a sanctuary for sleeping in bed and base electronic use elsewhere. Consider a battery-operated clock near the bed. Avoid extension cords and power strips near the bed.
2. Is dirty laundry stored in a separate area from the bedroom? This may reduce reactivity.
3. Do clothes contain fabrics pretreated with anything? Waterproofing materials (like Gore-Tex) and clothes exposed to bug treatments should be avoided.
4. Is your bedding hypoallergenic? Also, consider the use of hypoallergenic pillow covers and a hypoallergenic mattress encasement.
5. Are the sheets made with pesticide-treated cotton or "wrinkle-free" (formaldehyde-treated) fabric?
6. Is anything made out of memory foam? Memory foam and other special bedding/pillow material may possibly emit toxins.
7. Is the mattress new? It's likely been treated with a chemical to retard flames and may experience some off gassing.
8. Are pillows hypoallergenic and replaced regularly? Dust mites or contaminants may influence patient tolerance to bedding and subsequent sleep quality.
9. Do you utilize an electric blanket? Overnight electric blankets have been shown to increase total exposure to EMF's by two- to four-fold, and they represent a substantial source of whole-body exposure.[74]
10. Is the bed close to the main source of electrical current?

LAUNDRY ROOM

1. Remove dryer sheets and scented detergents/fabric softeners/bleach from use. Distilled white vinegar is a chemical-less alternative to traditional laundry detergent. Wool balls for the dryer may be considered as an alternative to dryer sheets and fabric softeners.
2. Is the dryer filter checked regularly?
3. Do you take clothing to the dry cleaners? Machine washing and washing by hand are preferred to reduce toxin exposure.

LIVING AREAS

1. Are pets allowed on furniture (or in bed)? This can increase cross-contamination of triggers.
2. Are houseplants present? Certain houseplants are known for their ability to contribute to cleaner air, though this alone is typically not sufficient to counteract poor air quality.

VEHICLE

1. Is the vehicle new? Does it have off gassing issues or seat covers that were chemically treated?
2. Is the vehicle old? Does it potentially have invisible water damage?
3. Do you drive with the windows down? In some instances, this can be helpful to reduce exposure to inhaled irritants within the vehicle, but in other instances this can increase your exposure to car exhaust, cigarette smoke and other environmental pollutants.
4. Do you pump your own gas? Avoid inhaling fumes when pumping gas. Consider delegating the task or using a mask and waiting inside the vehicle while gas is pumping.

5. Do you use a Bluetooth device while driving? Aim to minimize the use of your phone for calls, music and apps while driving. Dust off those old CDs!

WORKPLACE

1. Assess lighting and ventilation factors.
2. Is the location close to a wireless internet router or other EMF sources?
3. Assess postural ergonomic factors.
4. Do you use a computer more than six hours per day or a cell phone more than two hours per day?
5. Have your computer and other electronics been treated with brominated flame retardants (PBDEs)?

OTHER TIPS FOR TRIGGER ELIMINATION

1. Remove shoes before entering the home to reduce cross contamination.
2. Invest in a HEPA-type air purifier with a carbon filter (or several, depending on the room/living area size). Do not relocate these from previously contaminated environments. Replace the filter regularly. (Don't clean it!)
3. Change the house furnace filter quarterly.
4. Ensure clean water adherence when out of the home. Use glass containers and avoid bottled water/beverages from plastic bottles.
5. Avoid exposure to paint, and if the house needs to be painted, ensure that low- or no-VOC paint is used.
6. Consider naturally treated hardwoods floors and rugs as opposed to carpet.
7. Vacuum often and consider delegating this task to other family members. Delegate additional house-cleaning tasks and leave the

house when they are being done, if possible. Try not to do all the house cleaning at once and make sure to open windows/increase ventilation with fans.

EXTERNAL HEALTH STRESSORS & THE TRIFECTA: TAKE-HOME MESSAGES

- Mycotoxins are a very prevalent type of biotoxin, and past or current exposure to mycotoxins can have a powerful impact on health for individuals who are genetically susceptible.
- Symptoms of mold illness are widespread and often carry heavy neurological and cognitive symptoms. Strange symptoms including electric shocks, seizure-like events, unusual tics or spasms, a metallic taste in the mouth, and vibrating or pulse-like sensations are often reported, in addition to other symptoms common among individuals with chronic mysterious illness.
- The Environmental Relative Mold Index (ERMI) utilizes dust samples and is the gold standard for evaluating whether a building may have a mold problem.
- Patient testing for biotoxin illness typically involves a urine test to determine specific mycotoxin types. Visual contrast sensitivity screening and blood markers of inflammation may provide useful information but are not diagnostic in nature. Nasal swab testing may also assist in diagnosis and treatment of persistent mold-related issues.

- Environmental toxins are widespread and can have a profound impact on health, especially in individuals who are already immunocompromised or are struggling with chronic conditions.

- Heavy metals come from the atmosphere, soil, water, foods, household products and industrial processes and have well-documented evidence as contributing factors to human disease.

- Treatment of illness from toxins such as mold or heavy metals should be guided with the help of an integrative provider who is knowledgeable in the delicate process of binding toxins and removing them from the system. Adequate attention to organ and immune system support, gastrointestinal motility, hydration, sleep, vitamin deficiencies and other factors is key.

- Nervous system retraining programs, meditation, craniosacral therapy or osteopathic cranial manipulation, sound therapy, frequency specific microcurrent, homeopathic remedies, low dose immunotherapy, ozone and IV therapies, lymphatic drainage, visceral manipulation, acupuncture and other modalities are often utilized as part of a comprehensive healing plan for patients recovering from toxin-related illness.

- Reducing exposure to electromagnetic fields (EMFs) may be another important factor to address for patients who are sensitive to their environments.

- The removal of existing continued sources of toxins and prevention of further exposure is also very important for patients with chronic illness. Comprehensive assessments for the home and workplace are available online.

- Out of all the external health stressors discussed in this chapter, which ones have you investigated or confirmed? What treatment approaches have you tried? Are there areas you would like to investigate? Reflect on this topic in your Trifecta Passport worksheet.

Chapter 7:
RETRAINING THE
NERVOUS SYSTEM

When it comes to holistic healing from chronic illness, many patients check off most of the right boxes. They evaluate for and address root issues like the health stressors already discussed. They remove triggers like mold, dietary additives and pesticides, and chemical-laden beauty and household products. They invest in fancy machines to purify their air and water sources. They come up with an exercise routine and focus on detoxification and the lymphatic system. They reduce exposure to EMFs. They work hard on a healing diet and the right approach with supplements.

However, many patients still report a persistent feeling of anxiety and/or depression that they just can't shake. Many find that despite all these measures, they are still sensitive to certain triggers. Many feel that they have healed partway but are still mysteriously lacking some important piece of the puzzle. In my clinical experience, the missing piece and final roadblock often relates to abnormal patterns in the nervous system function.

Functional Naturopath and MCAS specialist Beth O'Hara suggests that there are four key aspects of healing from MCAS and histamine intolerance: identifying and addressing root triggers, foods and supplements, environmental toxin reduction and nervous system balancing.[1] She believes that when it comes to chronic illness, doing two or three of the four steps doesn't really work if you've been ill for a long time.[1] The concept of nervous system balancing—supporting the parasympathetic nervous system—through the rest, heal, digest and restore approach is key to finding lasting healing.[1] Beth O'Hara believes that parasympathetic nervous system support accounts for 33%–50% of the healing process in these patients.[1]

This component is so incredibly important that I've decided to devote an entire chapter to the topic. Counseling and psychotherapy are important modalities for patients with chronic illness and talk therapy can provide very useful insight into past and current sources of stress. However, one limitation to talk therapy is that it can perpetuate embedded and programmed subconscious responses of the nervous system as you relive the trauma. The goal of addressing the nervous system in this chapter is to teach you the resources available to bypass habitual neural circuitry (often malfunctioning from a history of trauma, big or minor/unrecognized) so that proper restoration of a relaxed and socially engaged state is possible.

The Autonomic Nervous System

The autonomic nervous system (ANS) is comprised of the brainstem, some of the cranial nerves, certain organs, and certain parts of some spinal nerves from levels T1 through L2 (thoracic spine and part of the lumbar spine) of the sympathetic chain. The ANS regulates the function of organs like the heart, lungs, liver, gallbladder, intestines, kidneys, stomach and sexual organs.

When I was in physical therapy school, I learned about the autonomic nervous system as a yin and yang concept of balance between two opposing systems. The parasympathetic nervous system (PSNS) is responsible for "rest and digest" moments, whereas the sympathetic nervous system (SNS) is known for the "fight or flight" adrenaline response. As part of this simplified explanation, the ANS is the body's system for determining when there's a threat (and the need to flee or freeze up/play dead) vs. the state where the body can focus on rest and digestion.

It's now believed that the ANS is comprised of three main subsystems: the PSNS, the SNS and the enteric nervous system of the gastrointestinal tract. The enteric nervous system communicates with the other two systems and is involved with regulation of digestive enzymes, gastrointestinal motility and gut immune defense responses. Autonomic nervous system issues are generally discussed as being either the result of an underactive PSNS or a compensatory overactive SNS (sympathetic overdrive).[2]

A cranial nerve called the vagus nerve (cranial nerve 10, "CN X") is at the forefront of the traditional conversation of ANS regulation. As part of the "rest and digest" system, the vagus nerve is a large structure that runs from the medulla oblongata at the base of the head to the transverse colon in the abdomen and plays an important role in a plethora of systemwide functions. The vagus nerve and its branches innervate the face, head and several organs. The vagus nerve has a direct influence on the heart, abdominal viscera, larynx, pharynx, bronchi and more. The nerve influences motor functions, PSNS functions like digestion, sensory functions that relay communications to the central nervous system, and even taste.

The vagus nerve has a powerful role in the messaging system between the gastrointestinal system and the brain. The vagus nerve is 80% afferent, detecting and relaying information from the organs to the central nervous system regarding physiological aspects like hunger and fullness, energy metabolism and inflammation.[3] The remaining 20% of its function is efferent, directing aspects of gut health like gastric capacity, digestive enzymes and gastric acid.[3] Bacteria in the gastrointestinal biome communicate by sending information to the brain via the vagus nerve. The vagus nerve appears to help mediate the gut epithelial cells and leaky gut as well as blood-brain permeability and what substances affect the brain.[3]

The vagus nerve has three primary functions:

1. Parasympathetic functions – The nerve is responsible for metabolic processes, heart rate, digestion, urination, sexual arousal, the pH of the gastrointestinal tract and salivation—our main bodily functions that occur while resting/feeling safe.
2. Sensory functions – The nerve processes sensory information from the heart, lungs, throat and abdomen, and has special functions related to taste behind the tongue.
3. Motor functions – The nerve provides movement to the neck muscles responsible for swallowing and speech.

When this nerve is not functioning properly, patients may find themselves more in sympathetic-dominant neural regulatory states, which can lead to increased fight or flight reactions, often to benign stimuli. Or, the body can also present in a "freeze" state as discussed in the next section. Factors commonly noted in the hEDS population such as Chiari malformation, intracranial pressure issues and upper cervical instability (discussed in Chapters 3 and 9) can lead to direct pressure on the vagus nerve and subsequent inappropriate nerve signals leading to dysautonomia. Because the vagus nerve relies on the neurotransmitter acetylcholine in its communications with organs, it's also theorized that impaired production or release of acetylcholine may be connected to dysautonomia.

Experts describe three categories of scenarios that could lead to a dysfunctional vagus nerve: top-down assault, bottom-up assault or full-body assault.[2] Top-down mechanisms refer to vagus nerve or brainstem trauma from concussion, craniocervical instability (CCI), cervicomedullary syndrome, Chiari malformation, low or high intracranial pressure, and extracellular fluid leaks.[2] Bottom-up assault refers to forms of vagus *sensory* neuritis, which could occur from leaky gut, MCAS and gastrointestinal autoimmune disease.[2] The full-body assault causes of vagus *motor* neuritis could include neurotoxins, heavy metals, autoimmune issues and certain conditions like Lyme disease or Rickettsial diseases.[2] In theory, any given patient could have multiple types of vagus nerve assault occurring at once.

The endocrine system also plays an important role in nervous system mechanisms. Endocrine organs and glands sense various processes of the body and secrete hormones (chemical messengers) that bind to cell receptors to trigger responses in the body. One of these organs, the hypothalamus, is considered the "master switchboard" that connects the endocrine system to the nervous system. Specifically, the hypothalamus scans our internal and external environments and tells the pituitary gland and adrenals to start or stop making the hormones that regulate our autonomic nervous system responses. This interconnectedness between the endocrine system and the nervous system is known as the hypothalamic-pituitary-adrenal (HPA) axis, and dysfunction in this area can have a major impact on our health. Cognitive perception of stressors in the environment can have a powerful influence on the physiological cascade that occurs and the level of inflammation that results, and the hormones released can alter short- and long-term physiological processes.

Emotional factors including history of trauma and post-traumatic stress disorder (PTSD) are closely connected to a dysfunctional nervous system status that is sympathetic-dominant. When you are spending more time in SNS activation, the body prioritizes the functions that would be more necessary for fleeing for your life (even if the trigger is something that logically does not require such a response). The PSNS functions that occur in safety, such as digesting that meal you just ate, are therefore less prioritized, and when this occurs on a chronic basis, numerous systems of the body can be affected. Some theorize that the vagus nerve oscillation between states of relaxation and stress is the common link between gastrointestinal issues, heart rate changes, respiratory abnormalities and other symptoms noted in patients with MCAS, POTS and EDS.

The Polyvagal Theory

It appears that the autonomic nervous system is more complicated than a simple teeter-totter fluctuation of neural impulses between fight or flight and rest and digest. In more recent years, there's been an expanded understanding of the vagus nerve and other cranial nerves and how they influence our ANS. Dr. Stephen Porges is the author of the Polyvagal Theory, which offers an expanded idea of the mechanisms behind our nervous system's resting state regulation.

The previously accepted yin and yang concept assumed that there was only one vagus nerve pathway, but the Polyvagal Theory notes that there are several distinct anatomical entities at play, including the dorsal branch and ventral branch of the vagus nerve. Each of these branches travels through its own path in the body. The ventral branch is myelinated, while the dorsal branch is not.[4] The ventral branch functions in conjunction with four other cranial nerves that all originate in the brainstem (CN V, VII, IX, XI).[4]

Further, it's believed that a third component that influences the ANS is SNS activity from the spinal chain. Specifically, spinal nerves go to the muscles and some of the organs, enabling a quick shift into fight or flight mode when necessary. These three components (dorsal branch, ventral branch and sympathetic chain) are the anatomic factors that influence which state our ANS finds itself in at rest and with activity, with "poly" referring to the many aspects of the vagus nerve.

From an evolutionary perspective, there are three neural circuits that form a response hierarchy. The newer circuit is social and reflects a well-regulated state that supports visceral organ homeostasis, as evidenced by good eye contact, relaxed facial expression and prosody of voice (proper intonation and rhythm). Individuals relying on this newer circuit respond well to human communication and can block out background noise to focus. The older circuits are associated with the flee (fight or flight) response or the freeze (shut down/collapse/pass out) response. Individuals relying on these circuits are more in-tune with lower frequency sounds (like background noise, which historically was desirable in order to hear predators) and tend to be programmed to prioritize detecting danger from their environment.[5]

Some bodies react to a history of trauma by going into a perpetual state of fight or flight, while others respond with a dissociative freeze response, where they are numb.[5] Others oscillate between the two states. These responses are how the body helped them to survive historically, but they are no longer necessary or useful once the person is removed from the situation and in a safe place. Over time, either one of these dysfunctional states, while never a conscious choice, can contribute to chronic system-wide health issues.

Dr. Porges discusses a term he calls "neuroception" or how our neural circuits determine whether a situation is safe or dangerous.[5] Various factors can influence our perception of situations; for example, if we are currently in pain, sleep deprived, hungry or suffering from a chronic condition that depletes the body's resources, we may respond differently to the same stimulus when compared to our neighbor.[4]

When we find ourselves in the desirable ventral vagal state, we are relaxed and feel safe. We may feel joy, love and satisfaction. The ventral vagal state is typically accompanied by a sense of relaxation, presence in the moment and the desire to build relationships with others socially. We are engaged with those around us with good eye contact and body language.[4,5] This is the state that is most conducive to healing.

When we find ourselves in a dorsal vagal state, we are often depressed and withdrawn. This is often referred to as "shut down" or "immobilize" or "freeze." We may feel sadness, anger, grief, apathy, hopelessness or lethargy. Some individuals report feeling paralyzed or dissociated when experiencing a dorsal vagal state. Our face loses its color, our voice becomes monotonous and lacks prosody, and our facial expression is often stone-faced. From an evolutionary perspective, freezing up to fake death was one of our strategies for survival. However, this type of a physiologic response becomes problematic when the system becomes stuck in this state on a chronic basis.[4,5]

When we find ourselves in a sympathetic chain dominant state, we are experiencing stress and are preparing ourselves for survival, known as "mobilization" or "fight or flight." As the spinal branch of the vagus nerve is activated, our muscles tense up and prepare for action. We may feel defensive or anxious and may notice an urge to flee. Our blood pressure rises, and our blood is shunted away from our abdomen and toward our extremities. Our pupils dilate, salivation is inhibited, the airways relax and our heart rate increases.[4,5]

In the animal world, after fleeing from a predator (mediated by a sympathetic response), the animal will stop and shake for a short time in order to dissipate the nervous system tension. However, humans lack this mechanism and often hold on to sympathetic energy physiologically and mentally, which is why certain treatment approaches like Tension & Trauma Releasing Exercises aim to help the body let go of this aspect of nervous system tone. The sympathetic nervous system should be activated 1%–3% of the time, but in our modern world it's common for individuals to be in this state much more than that.

Table 18. Components of the Polyvagal Theory of ANS Regulation[4]

Component of ANS	Associated with:
Ventral branch of vagus nerve	Social engagement and relaxation. Feelings of joy, satisfaction and love. Voice contains prosody. Bronchioles relax, allowing for adequate air flow to lungs. Good ventral vagal tone is associated with high heart rate variability and overall systemic stability.
Dorsal branch of vagus nerve	Depressive behavior and shutdown. Often accompanied by low blood pressure, syncope (fainting) or near-fainting, low levels of muscle tone, POTS symptoms, and less blood flow to the frontal lobes resulting in cognitive symptoms. Sweating, nausea, anxiety, dissociation, anger, sadness, hopelessness, fatigue, and fibromyalgia are commonly reported. Social isolation may be preferred when chronically in this state. Facial expression is usually dull. Bronchioles constrict, resulting in breathing abnormalities; possible connections to chronic obstructive pulmonary disease (COPD).
Sympathetic activity from the spinal chain	Stress and the body's response to mobilize/move for survival. Blood pressure rises and muscles tense (and sometimes shake) in preparation for fight or flight. Heart rate and respiratory rate rise. Pupils dilate and peripheral vision increases, blood flow increases to large muscles, the skin may be pale or flushed, blood thickens which increases clotting factors, hearing sharpens.

It appears that there are also two physiological "hybrid states" that can occur when different aspects of these systems engage together. Friendly competition (such as sports) can involve simultaneous activation of spinal sympathetic chain (mobilization) and the ventral vagus (social engagement) systems.[4] Similarly, sexual intimacy in a state of relaxation involves simultaneous immobilization (dorsal vagus) and feeling safe (ventral vagus) influences.[4]

Some theorize that autism spectrum disorders can be explained by an oscillation between a dorsal vagal state and sympathetic chain activity.[4] Another theory is that the reason that exercise works for some people to manage depression is because vigorous exercise essentially moves us from a dorsal vagal state into a sympathetic dominant state, temporarily alleviating shutdown symptoms.[4]

The ventral branch of the vagus nerve innervates the upper one-third of the esophagus, while the dorsal branch innervates the lower two-thirds of the esophagus. The vagus nerve and its impact on acetylcholine have been implicated to play a role in the unchecked inflammatory responses seen in eosinophilic esophagitis (EoE), a chronic allergic inflammatory condition of the passageway between the mouth and the stomach.[6] Depression, autism spectrum disorders and EoE are examples of the many chronic conditions that may be triggered or exacerbated by a poorly functioning vagus nerve.

When it comes to being able to engage with others socially in a ventral vagal state, it's much more complex than the vagus nerve itself. Five cranial nerves influence our level of social engagement.

Cranial nerve V, the trigeminal nerve, is responsible for chewing, swallowing and hearing. This nerve innervates a muscle called the tensor tympani which is responsible for adjusting tension on the eardrum to block out the sound of our own chewing so that we can hear others around us.

Patients with dysfunction in this nerve often suffer from hyperacusis or being extra sensitive to sounds around them.

Cranial nerve VII, the facial nerve, is responsible for chewing, hearing, and some facial muscle and saliva functions. This nerve innervates a muscle called the stapedius which regulates our sensitivity to certain frequencies of sounds. High frequency sounds such as our mother's voice are normally prioritized by the nervous system, but dysfunction in this nerve can result in individuals being more in-tune with low-frequency background noise, creating difficulty in hearing and comprehending human speech. This could present as something as simple as having an issue with hearing a conversation in a busy room or startling easy from background sounds that normally should not elicit such a reaction.

The glossopharyngeal nerve (cranial nerve IX) is responsible for swallowing and is necessary for normal feeding motor behaviors. The vagus nerve (cranial nerve X) was discussed above. Rounding out the group of five cranial nerves responsible for social engagement is cranial nerve XI, the spinal accessory nerve. This nerve innervates two neck muscles responsible for turning the head and expanding the visual field, the upper trapezius and the sternocleidomastoid.

These final three—cranial nerves IX, X, and XI—pass through the jugular foramen at the base of the skull, and some experts assert that we should treat them as one nerve, because parts of their fibers weave together.[4] Thus, our cervical spine (neck), swallowing and vagus nerve functions are closely connected. Factors like forward head position and low back posture, our diaphragm muscle/rib excursion/breathing pattern, pelvic floor muscle tone, and the alignment of the cranial bones and upper cervical spine are extremely important to address as they relate to our resting vagal state and blood flow to the brain. These topics will be described at length in Chapter 9, "Structural and Musculoskeletal Issues." Strategies addressing these five cranial nerves are extremely important in healing from chronic illness.

Virtually every patient I've met who has suffered from chronic illness presents with some aspect of neurological dysfunction related to the regulation of the autonomic nervous system (ANS). In my opinion, neurological programs that only focus on *conscious* strategies for calming and soothing the system, while valuable, fail to help reset and restore the complex relationships between the nervous system and our anatomy. We can listen to guided meditations until we are blue in the face, but if that approach is not accompanied by a method to increase awareness and bring us back into a ventral vagal state (particularly when we have gone about our day and are no longer listening to the meditation), we will find ourselves feeling "stuck" from the physiological influences that are outside of our conscious control.

Also, programs that *just* focus on the vagus nerve may miss the mark for certain patients, particularly those who suffer from:

- ADD and ADHD
- Anxiety and depression
- Auditory hypersensitivities
- Auditory processing disorders
- Autism spectrum disorders
- Chiari malformation, intracranial pressure issues, and cerebrospinal fluid leaks
- Craniocervical instability (CCI), which is commonly associated with EDS
- Dysautonomia/POTS
- Emotional regulation difficulties
- Hypothalamic-pituitary-adrenal (HPA) axis dysfunction
- ME/CFS (myalgic encephalitis/chronic fatigue syndrome)
- Misophonia (a strong reaction to certain sounds, such as dripping water, chewing, tapping)

- Mood dysregulation
- Motion sickness
- Multiple chemical sensitivity
- PTSD, trauma history
- Sensory processing disorders

These patients may need a specialized program that also addresses dysfunction in the nerves that innervate the middle ear muscles and cranial nerves V and VII.

Finally, programs that lack a focus on the cervical spine and other orthopedic biomechanics may fall short because the patient may continually fall back into a dorsal vagal state with the slightest perturbation. These patients would benefit from an approach that addresses all five of the social engagement cranial nerves in order to maximize their healing potential. It's important to be aware that proper nervous system retraining can require educating the patient to recognize when they are in a dorsal vagal state and specific home exercises that, over time, restore proper ANS regulation again. The end of this chapter discusses different types of strategies to help retrain the nervous system, and Chapter 9 discusses orthopedic considerations to maximize success.

The Enteric Nervous System

The enteric nervous system (ENS) is the biggest accumulation of nerve cells in the body and it's gained more attention in recent years as a major player in what is described as the gut-brain axis. It's comprised of an intricate network of more than 500 million neurons and glia found in the bowel walls.[7] The ENS has bidirectional communication between both the central nervous system and the autonomic nervous system.[7] Almost every cell of the bowel wall has close interactions with the ENS.[7] The ENS plays a role in bowel motility, epithelial secretion, blood flow, epithelial proliferation and repair, intestinal immune system modulation and other functions.[7] The motor part of the vagus nerve helps assist the enteric nervous system with rhythmic peristaltic contractions as part of digestion.[2]

The enteric nervous system may be a big player in terms of different types of disease etiology. Research supports that the ENS may directly affect conditions like Parkinson's disease through mechanisms of toxin/pesticide ingestion that impact genetic expression. By-products of protein misfolding from these triggers may then travel to the central nervous system via the vagus nerve and may be responsible for Lewy body pathology noted in Parkinson's disease.[7] Given the fact that so many chronic conditions stem from dysfunction in the gut, it's very plausible that the enteric nervous system plays a role in the propagation of inflammation leading to other types of disease.

While it's been well-established that vagus nerve function can influence our digestive health, it may also be important to consider that our own dietary factors could possibly impact what is getting transmitted to the brain via the enteric nervous system and the vagus nerve. It's clear that this large nerve has a powerful impact from both an efferent (motor impulses to our organs) and afferent (sensory information to our brain) perspective.

Vagus Nerve Support

Low vagal tone has been associated with a number of gastrointestinal conditions including irritable bowel syndrome (IBS) and inflammatory bowel disease (IBD). Damage to the endothelial tight junctions, known as leaky gut, may be attenuated by vagal nerve stimulation.[8] Reduction in bile secretion, activity of parietal cells, secretion of hydrochloric acid and pancreatic enzymes are all associated with low vagal tone.[9] These gut-specific factors are important for patients facing chronic illness and should be addressed with a knowledgeable integrative provider.

The main neurotransmitter that affects the vagus nerve is acetylcholine, which attenuates the release of inflammatory cytokines (including TNF and interleukins) from mast cells and other cells.[10] Natural choline compounds including alpha-glycerylphosphorylcholine (alpha-GPC) may provide support to the vagus nerve pathways, though research is currently lacking in terms of investigating their therapeutic use specifically for the vagus nerve.

Several products currently exist that are marketed to support the vagus nerve. They often contain a combination of substances like acetyl l-carnitine, alpha lipoic acid, B vitamins, devil's claw, Huperzia serrata extract, passionflower, skullcap, spirulina and turmeric. Huperzia serrata appears to improve deficient cholinergic nervous function[11] and acetyl l-carnitine may improve heart rate variability in patients with dysautonomia,[12] but more research is needed to investigate these combination products and their impact on ANS regulation.

Short chain fatty acids (particularly butyric acid), omega 3 fatty acids, l-citrulline, vagally mediated probiotics (such as *lactobacillus rhamnosus*) and zinc have ample literature backing and appear to support the vagus nerve from a nutritional perspective.[13-17] Ginger may also be useful for the vagus nerve, particularly for patients with gastrointestinal issues such as nausea.[18] Factors including adequate sleep and time-restricted eating (intermittent fasting) also appear to support the function of the vagus nerve.[19]

Vagus nerve activation (through an immune system response to inflammation or endotoxins) induces stimulation of the HPA axis and adrenals, which modulates inflammation in the body.[10] Stimulation of the vagus nerve has been found to reduce epileptic seizures[20-22] and reduce inflammatory cytokine synthesis and release.[10] Vagus nerve stimulation may also decrease cerebral edema and inflammation, reduce breakdown of the blood brain barrier, enhance both motor and cognitive recovery, provide neuroprotective effects and enhance synaptic plasticity.[9] Devices to stimulate the vagus nerve are discussed at the end of this chapter.

Chanting, gargling, humming and singing are theorized to stimulate the vagus nerve; these activities are encouraged in the process of resetting the nervous system. Drinking cold water, taking cold showers or splashing cold water on the face may also positively impact the vagus nerve. Positive effects of cold water have been shown in animal studies, and habituation to cold climates appears to enhance parasympathetic nervous system balance in humans, based on one small study.[23,24]

Activating the salivary glands is another method that, in theory, may positively impact vagal tone. To do this, you can imagine a juicy citrus fruit and fill your mouth with saliva, submerging your tongue for a short time in order to experience a hyper-relaxing response. Meaningful conversation, extended hugs/embraces and other types of social connections are also supported mechanisms to improve vagal tone.[25]

A combination of gentle abdominal self-massage and reclined spinal twists can help stimulate the vagus nerve. Acupuncture is another great option that appears to directly impact the vagus nerve and parasympathetic nervous system.[26,27] Yoga breathing techniques and breathing that utilizes the diaphragm muscle also increase vagal tone.

Journaling, reading, mindfulness, prayer, tai chi, massage, singing, laughter, coloring, playing with kinetic sand, doing a puzzle and other calming activities are also strongly encouraged and may positively impact heart rate variability and vagus nerve function.[28-31] Meditation is another important strategy to assist in changing the nervous system resting tone; various forms will be discussed later in this book. Slowing down is key!

Nervous System Retraining Approaches

This section discusses some of the options available for patients to help retrain (or rebalance) the nervous system.

It's very important to note that nervous system retraining has a complex relationship with trauma, and there are several key guidelines to utilizing the rest of the information in this chapter:

1. Every single individual who has experienced trauma should begin nervous system retraining approaches with the guidance of a trained professional.

2. Virtually every patient with chronic illness contains an aspect of trauma from singular or multiple events in their past. Trauma may be from early childhood, witnessing something that triggers strong emotions, prior experiences within the medical system, surgeries, physical or mental abuse situations, accidents, the loss of a loved one or pet and so much more.

3. Even seemingly "minor" traumas can be a big deal for the nervous system and can impact us physiologically (even decades later) without an overt awareness of them. Do not downplay what you have been through. Consider yourself to have experienced some type of trauma and make sure that you begin this work with a well-trained professional.

4. Sometimes less is more. Smaller than recommended doses are often helpful, particularly at the beginning of a new approach, until you can determine what type of an impact the approach may have on your system. While some of these programs give specific recommendations for the number of minutes per day, there is no "one dosage fits all" approach. This is one reason why it's helpful to work with a practitioner who can help you determine what type of a schedule is best for your specific system and baseline.

5. Embrace a long-term mindset when doing this type of work. Expect a comprehensive nervous system retraining program to take six months to one year to complete. There are no shortcuts here, and change is not overnight!

6. Paradoxical reactions to nervous system retraining can occur. For example, an auditory therapy may help give the nervous system the signals that it is safe and permissible to relax again as it starts to help restore ventral vagal tone. However, with a history of trauma, the signals of safety can actually be a trigger for the nervous system, because the brain may subconsciously say "I let my guard down before and look what happened to me! No, I'm not going there again." By working with a professional trained in these disciplines, you can learn how to interpret signals coming from your body, and in some cases, these signals will dictate your dosage and frequency of the approach. A paradoxical reaction does not indicate that the approach is a bad fit; rather it indicates that a slower pace is needed with extra attention to detail of the program parameters for that individual.

7. Trained professionals can also help you learn how to self-soothe and self-regulate the nervous system when unpleasant reactions do occur.

8. Some of these approaches (particularly the auditory therapies) may be contraindicated in patients who have uncontrolled epilepsy. You will also want to avoid these exercises when you are performing certain activities like driving or operating machinery since they can have a calmative effect.

Nervous System Baseline Assessment

In healthcare, we like to have concrete data to help determine the baseline status as well as whether our treatments are creating meaningful change. There are some formal and informal tests and questionnaires that I utilize before treatment, during treatment, and after treatment—repeatable measures that I consider my "asterisk signs" to determine whether we are on the right track when it comes to nervous system retraining.

These include:

- Physical exam characteristics such as breathing pattern, diaphragm activation, facial expression, respiratory rate and heart rate changes when going from sitting to standing, rib excursion, spine motion, and neck muscle tension.
- An evaluation of cranial nerve function, with special attention to the cranial nerves involved with social engagement (CN V, VII, IX, X, XI). These tests involve looking at face sensation, the corneal reflex, facial muscle motor function, the tongue and the response of the uvula with the "ah" test. Eye pupil size and reaction can also be affected with dysautonomia, and sometimes differences are noted in size between sides. These tests can provide valuable information. For example, when the uvula deviates to one side or the soft palate fails to lift, this is indicative of dysfunction in the vagus/hypoglossal nerves. If the uvula is asymmetrical with the "ah" test, it will deviate away from the affected side. This test in particular is a quick way to check for overall nervous system status, and at the end of the treatment session it's helpful to recheck if this response has normalized.
- A questionnaire called the BBC Sensory Scales, which assesses subjective information from 50 questions about auditory processing, visual processing, tactile processing, and digestion.
- Measurement of heart rate variability, equipment-permitting.

Heart Rate Variability (HRV)

Heart rate variability is the *variance in time between each heartbeat.* This is different from the heart rate itself. Individuals who have an imbalanced nervous system will have a measurably low HRV, whereas individuals in good health tend to have a higher HRV and better adaptability and responses to external influences. High HRV correlates with improvements

241

in parasympathetic (rest and digest) nervous system tone and in particular the desired ventral vagal tone.[4]

Interestingly, one clinician has noted that some POTS patients interpret variability in heart rate as palpitations when wearing heart monitors, and while increased HRV is generally considered a good thing, in some cases patients with dysautonomia may also show too much heart rate variability.[2] While more HRV is generally considered better in a healthy population, it's possible that there's a "sweet spot" for heart rate variability when it comes to patients with POTS, though research is needed to confirm this observation.

A number of different companies make devices that measure your heart rate variability; these devices can be used in conjunction with a separate treatment approach (such as breathing exercises, sound therapy, nervous system retraining programs, yoga and other therapies) to receive biofeedback on your overall progress over time. Elite HRV, Whoop and Oura are some popular brands. Some of these devices also have connected phone apps to track progress. HRV is usually measured first thing in the morning to determine your baseline "morning readiness score," and for athletes, the information can also be used to determine how hard to push the current day's physical activity. For patients with chronic illness, this information can also be useful in terms of pacing and planning activities.

Daily HRV baselines measurements are a handy way to assess progress across time, and additional sessions tracking HRV with activities like breathing exercises can provide unique biofeedback. I like that it provides objective data that can be tracked to help motivate patients to create new lifestyle habits for nervous system retraining. The downside is that it requires an initial purchase and sometimes has a monthly fee; also, not everyone prefers to have daily feedback on biometric analyses. However, it can be a useful clinical and home tool as an adjunct to the questionnaire and physical examination.

In addition to having an impact on the regulation of time between heartbeats, our emotions and our nervous system state are also reflective of our heart rhythm patterns. Chaotic patterns emerge when we are stressed, compared to a smooth pattern when we are in a ventral vagal state and experiencing gratitude, love and appreciation. Additional tools like the HeartMath device aim to analyze heart rhythm and use real-time biofeedback to help you regulate your heart rhythm and emotions and to track your progress over time.

Nervous System Retraining Toolbox

The great news is, we can reverse and reset these neural pathways, even when they've been dysfunctional for decades. There are several programs and treatment interventions available to patients—even beyond the heart rate and rhythm strategies discussed above—to assist in enhancing a predominantly ventral vagal state. Of course, these programs and approaches do not represent overnight/immediate fixes.

When it comes to switching between the dorsal vagal, ventral vagal and sympathetic chain states of freeze (immobilization), a relaxed social engagement, and fight or fight (mobilization with fear), it appears that we can easily be triggered into a less desirable state initially/early on in the process. When we learn tools to help us hit the "reset" button, we can transition back into the ventral vagal state of calmness. However, experts assert that even something as simple as a negative thought can switch us back over to the other two less desirable states.[4]

Thus, the key to success is repetition and empowerment. Persistence in exercises and strategies to shift the patient back into the ventral vagal state is key so that, over time, the system will be more stable, less easily perturbed and better equipped to handle future physical or emotional stressors. Empowerment lies in helping the patient to become more in-tune with their body and to understand and employ strategies that they can do on their own at home to bring them back into a ventral vagal state.

For patients with the trifecta, I recommend a minimum of the following:

- Daily breathing exercises
- Daily tapping exercises (also known as Emotional Freedom Technique)
- Daily mindfulness and/or meditation exercises
- Training on interpreting different physiological cues in order to help move yourself out of the sympathetic or dorsal vagal states
- Integrating one of the nervous system retraining programs or approaches into your treatment plan (see Table 19)
- Participating in an auditory therapy approach for nervous system retraining (see Table 20)
- Addressing structural and musculoskeletal factors with the help of a trained professional (physical therapist, osteopath, etc.) (see Chapter 9 for more information)

In some cases, it may also be important to address the presence of trauma with a mental health professional as an adjunct to addressing the nervous system in other ways.

Breathing Exercises

The diaphragm is a dome-shaped muscle connected to the lower part of the ribs. The diaphragm is the primary muscle that helps with breathing. As previously mentioned, the vagus nerve runs from the brain through the face to the thorax and abdomen. At the bottom of the rib cage, the nerve runs through the esophageal hiatus of the diaphragm. Movement of the

244

diaphragm around the vagus nerve helps stimulate parasympathetic nervous system tone. More movement of the diaphragm means more relaxation and less of a stressful physiological state. For this reason, exercises that help retrain the breathing pattern and use of the diaphragm can have a profound impact on the nervous system default regulatory state.

Breathing exercises should incorporate a longer exhale than inhale time, because inhaling increases sympathetic nervous system stimulation, and exhaling increases parasympathetic nervous system tone.

Three Daily Breathing Exercises
Inhale Positivity/Exhale Negativity

Find a quiet space to relax while sitting or lying down. Identify what "lies" or harmful thought patterns you tell yourself. Figure out a statement that contradicts those lies, sometimes referred to as a reversal statement. For example, if you find yourself thinking "I am too sick to work as much as I want to," instead use the reversal phrase "I contribute to society in meaningful ways."

Take a deep belly breath while inhaling through the nose, playing the reversal statement (the positive thought) in your head. Exhale the negative emotions associated with the lie statement and visualize the lie being released from your body. Continue to breathe and focus on increasing the positive thought and releasing the negative thought with each breath. Aim to spend more time exhaling than inhaling. Our nervous system is greatly in-tune with our thoughts, so what we tell ourselves really does matter!

4-6-8 Breath

Find a quiet space to relax while sitting or lying down.

- Inhale for a count of 4 seconds with a deep belly breath, keeping the neck and shoulders relaxed.
- Hold your breath for a count of 6 seconds (as tolerated; this should not be stressful).
- Exhale slowly and steadily for 8 seconds.

You can also modify this exercise by pursing the lips as you exhale to affect the pressure receptors on the arteries. The heart rate increases on inhalation due to the sympathetic nervous system response, and likewise the exhalation slows the heart rate, which can also offer a beneficial impact for patients experiencing dysautonomia.

This exercise is modified slightly from the traditional 4-7-8 exercise. This breath work focuses on greater time spent on the exhale, which can have a profoundly calming effect by decreasing sympathetic nervous system tone. This is a great exercise to perform when feeling flared, but make sure you are not exercising at the same time. It should be performed at rest. If you use biofeedback you will likely notice that your heart rate variability improves (gets higher) as you perform this exercise.

Variations of this exercise such as box breathing may also be helpful. Box breathing focuses on 4 phases of the breath in one breathing cycle: the inhale, breath hold, exhale and (second) breath hold. Most of the time the ratio for each phase of box breathing is 1:1:1:1, but you can modify it to have a longer exhale time.

Other breathing exercises that may be useful include alternate nostril breathing, diaphragmatic breathing with tactile (sensory) cues, a yoga practice called humming bee breathing and coherent breathing.

Twist and Breathe

While sitting in a chair or on the floor, or lying on your back, perform a gentle spinal twist stretch. Breathe deeply into the pose and feel the body release the tension with each exhale. Make sure that your breathing is deep and initiated by the diaphragm as opposed to shallow with upper rib and neck tension. You can also combine this with the "Inhale Positivity/Exhale Negativity" exercise from above!

Twist and Breathe Position Options

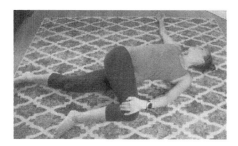 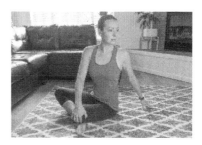

Create a routine for these exercises. Some patients find it helpful to do breathing exercises right before each meal so that they have better digestion. Set a timer and work up to a goal time of 5–10 minutes per day for your breathing exercises. You can also spend a few minutes doing them reactively to help calm the nervous system if you are feeling triggered.

Daily Tapping Exercises

Emotional Freedom Technique (EFT), also called tapping or psychological acupressure, uses fingertips to stimulate energy points on the body. These energy points are on the face and chest. The tapping is gentle, easy to learn, and typically has an immediate calming effect on the body. EFT may also help reduce food cravings, lower pain and decrease negative emotions. The tapping is done in conjunction with a specific process of thinking about something that is stressful to you. This practice impacts ventral vagal tone as well as the limbic system.

For some individuals, this practice can be intense initially; participants occasionally report feeling strong emotions during and after tapping. It's advisable to learn how to perform EFT with a trained provider before trying it on your own. You can learn more about EFT here: www.eft.mercola.com.

Daily Mindfulness and Meditation Exercises

Information about these options will be covered in depth in Chapter 11, "Detoxification."

Polyvagal Awareness Training

One way to conceptualize the three different nervous system states is to think of a ladder, where the dorsal vagal state is at the bottom, the sympathetic state is in the middle, and the ventral vagal state is on top. This is our evolutionary hierarchy of nervous system activation based on the polyvagal theory. Ideally, we want to be at the top of the ladder as much as possible.

The first step to awareness is recognizing the signs of when you're bottoming out on the ground in an immobilized/collapsed dorsal vagal state. It's very possible that this is happening nearly constantly for some individuals, especially as they first begin to address their nervous system. The key is to catch it early and often. If you're starting to feel lethargic, depressed, anxious, frozen or collapsed, instead of suffering through it, make a small intentional change in your day, even if for a few moments.

When the system feels paralyzed or frozen, you can gently wake it up with movement and body awareness. Activities that can help you shift out of the dorsal vagal state include simple intentional activities like going outside, drinking water, taking a walk, practicing yoga or stretches, doing neck exercises, practicing tai chi, trying guided meditation and focusing on breath work coupled with body positions (such as a gentle spinal twist). You can also try some gentle rocking back and forth with your feet on the ground. These actions can help serve as a catalyst to move your system up the ladder to shift toward a more balanced nervous system state.

Awareness of a sympathetic-dominant nervous system state is generally more obvious in terms of symptoms. When you're noticing signs of fight or flight, you may feel agitated, fidgety, hyperactive, and anxious. You may notice physical symptoms like nausea, a pounding heart and sweating. In these moments, it can be helpful to shift the nervous system through calming self-soothing activities like using a stress ball, playing with clay, gentle and slow rhythmic pressure on your skin, listening to guided meditation, drinking water, practicing breathing exercises (with a focus on the exhale) and journaling. It's also important to practice some meal hygiene strategies in order to avoid eating when stressed or rushed. These activities can help shift the system up the ladder toward more ventral vagal nervous system tone.

Once you feel well balanced and like you're in a relaxed and safe ventral vagal state, additional factors like sunlight, hydration, clean eating, singing, yoga, social interactions, playing musical instruments, creating art, walking, hiking and other forms of nervous system support may help keep the system on the top of that ladder. It's normal to move up and down the ladder, depending on the day (and even within different moments of the day). The key is to turn up the lights on these subtle nervous system shifts and to gently reset them when the balance is off. Building certain activities into a routine is helpful, but it's also important to work on building self-awareness of these different states in each moment. By focusing on movement when stuck in a frozen state and focusing on self-soothing when in fight or flight, you can remind yourself that you have the tools it needs to help the system heal and restore balance. Over time, with increased polyvagal state awareness plus the other strategies mentioned in this chapter, it's possible to shift the nervous system baseline to a more consistent ventral vagal state, and this can have a profound impact on the body's ability to heal in other ways.

Integrating a Nervous System Retraining Program into Your Treatment Plan

The following table is not all-inclusive, but it contains a summary of some of the options out there available to patients to help rebalance the nervous system. I have not tried all of these personally and cannot attest to most of the claims made about any of these programs. There is no "right approach," and many patients find that trial and error is necessary until they find a program that best suits them. Some patients prefer the self-guided video approach, while others appreciate a more tangible or tactile experience.

Table 19. Nervous System-Focused Treatment Programs

APPROACH	DESCRIPTION	RESOURCES
Dynamic Neural Retraining System (DNRS)	Annie Hopper's limbic system-focused home program with DVDs. Neuroplasticity seminars also available. Patients report improvements in systemic symptoms, nervous system issues as well as chemical sensitivities with this approach, also noting that it can be time-intensive (one hour a day for six months, or less time for longer duration).	www.retrainingthebrain.com

Gupta Program Brain Retraining	Program includes video sessions, audio exercises, meditations, coaching webinars, Facebook group and other online resources. A free 28-day trial is available to test the program out. Anxiety, depression, functional impairments, health related quality of life and pain responses all appear to be positively impacted by this program.	www.guptaprogram.com
Tension & Trauma Releasing Exercise (TRE)	TRE is an innovative series of physical exercises that activate a natural shaking reflex which helps dissipate sympathetic nervous system tone. This approach does not address trauma history consciously; patients learn how to do it on their own at home, but initial session(s) need to be with trained practitioner.	https://traumaprevention.com/
Wim Hoff Method	The 3 pillars of this approach include breathing, focus and controlled exposure to cold. Online videos with a 10-week program. Some patients are unable to tolerate cold showers or find this approach too intense initially; complex patients may need additional approaches.	www.wimhofmethod.com

Some individuals also find handheld vagus nerve stimulators to be helpful. GammaCore is a handheld device that offers gentle electrical stimulation to the neck area. This particular device is FDA-approved for migraines and cluster headaches. Many other medical devices are available by prescription only and may be specific for conditions like epilepsy.

In addition to one or several of the approaches in Table 19, I encourage patients (particularly those with sensory sensitivities or longstanding illness) to also consider auditory therapy to help retrain the social engagement system.

Table 20. Auditory Therapy to Help Retrain the Nervous System

APPROACH	DESCRIPTION	RESOURCES
BrainTap (auditory device and audio bundles)	BrainTap utilizes neuro-algorithms to help the brain experience several different types of brainwave patterns. We often experience alpha wavelengths with meditation, but BrainTap offers alpha, beta, delta, gamma and theta waves for a full spectrum experience. BrainTap Headset also delivers light pulses. This is a unique approach combining binaural beats, guided visualization, isochronic tones and 360-degree sound environment.	www.braintap.com

Neuvana Xen (auditory device)	Neuvana Xen is a vagus nerve stimulation headphone device created by a surgeon. This is a portable and self-guided program. Vagus nerve stimulation accompanies music from your own music library and streaming platforms.	www.Neuvanalife.com
Parasym (external stimulation device)	Parasym is a vagus nerve stimulation machine that delivers customized input via an ear clip on the tragus of the left ear (which is innervated by the auricular branch of the vagus nerve). This approach offers different frequency programming depending on your own needs/focus. Sessions are typically one hour per day for a minimum of 8-12 weeks.	http://www.parasym.co

Safe & Sound Protocol (SSP) (five hours of auditory therapy)	The SSP is a type of auditory therapy that strengthens middle ear muscles to improve parasympathetic state, social engagement, sensitivities, etc. The SSP is a shorter duration for the initial treatment (5 hours total over 1-3 weeks). This approach must be utilized with a trained practitioner but can completed via telehealth and the use of an app in most cases.	www.integratedlistening.com

It's important that listening/auditory programs are begun with the guidance of a professional, as the process of retraining muscles in the middle ear can sometimes elicit symptoms that require modifications or adjustments. While auditory devices may be more easily integrated for a general population, patients with a history of chronic illness and/or trauma need to be carefully monitored and trained in terms of interpreting responses to treatment.

It's also important to evaluate for exposure to electromagnetic fields (EMFs) when using these devices regularly. Certain shielding products can be worn to aim to minimize any impacts of EMF exposure during these therapies. Grounding (earthing) practices may also help reduce this potential.

As a practitioner, I work with clients and guide them through the Safe & Sound Protocol (SSP) and have witnessed profound changes within the treatment window, as well as in the months that follow. The SSP is specific in that it targets the middle ear muscles and helps strengthen them by exposing them to specific frequencies of sound paired to music. As discussed at the beginning of this chapter, when the middle ear muscles are inactive, lower frequency sounds like background noise are perceived as much stronger than the human voice.

Clinically, I note that patients are often easily startled and sensitive to background noise while having difficulty engaging in conversations, making eye contact, hearing people when there is background noise or understanding the entire meaning behind certain phrases. The middle ear muscles are primarily fast-twitch and they fatigue easily. Illness, fever and aging also reduce the function of the middle ear muscles. When the middle ear muscles do finally contract properly, the background noise can be dampened, the nervous system is less aroused or waiting to go into fight or flight/freeze mode, and the listener is better able to focus and perceive human speech (higher frequency sounds) properly.

Other potential benefits of the SSP include improvements in heart rate and blood pressure regulation, sweating, digestive function, facial expression, eye contact, voice intonations, memory and concentration, adrenaline rushes and adrenal dysfunction, understanding of human language and body language, ability to express oneself verbally or physically, insomnia, anxiety and depression, sensory stimulation to touch/sound/sight/taste, diversity of food choices, breathing and much more.

The SSP has been shown in peer-reviewed research to significantly increase vagal regulation of the heart—a vital component of ANS regulation.[32] Thus, I find it particularly useful for patients who have a combination of dysautonomia and exaggerated physiological response to external triggers. When auditory therapy targeting the middle ear is combined with a more global nervous system retraining program plus attention to the breath and biomechanical factors that influence our cranial nerves, greater (and more long-standing) improvements may be noted by the patient and reflected in follow-up testing.

There are many additional nervous system retraining approaches out there. Brainspotting (BSP) refers to a treatment technique focused on the idea that where you look with your eyes determines how you feel. Based on activity in the subcortical brain, practitioners utilize pointer devices to determine individualized associations between positive and negative emotions at different places in the visual field. BSP is used for those who have experienced trauma as well as those looking to tap more into their creative side.

Activities that combine coordination of the eyes, mind, body and breath, such as the Asian practices of tai chi and qi gong or rhythmical drumming practices in certain African cultures, may also help restore more beneficial nervous system tone.[33] Martial arts such as tae kwon do, aikido, jujitsu, judo, capoeira and kendo also involve coordination between breathing, movement and meditation, which can have a powerful effect on the nervous system.[33] Additional strategies such as biofeedback and other approaches to address mental health, discussed in Chapter 11, are also helpful treatment options.

As I mentioned, there is no silver bullet for retraining the nervous system successfully. It requires time and patience, but it can have a profound impact on the quality of life for patients with chronic illness. Most of these programs lack peer-reviewed research and it's difficult to compare them to each other in terms of efficacy. Alone, these programs may offer some change, but when a comprehensive and integrative nervous system approach is utilized, the impacts may be more profound and far-reaching.

RETRAINING THE NERVOUS SYSTEM: TAKE-HOME MESSAGES

- The autonomic nervous system is comprised of parasympathetic ("rest and digest") and sympathetic ("fight or flight" or "freeze") functions.
- The polyvagal theory (by Dr. Stephen Porges) proposes that humans fluctuate between three different neural states: ventral vagal-, dorsal vagal-, and sympathetic chain-dominant nervous system tone.
- The ventral vagal state is the desired mode of relaxation, safety and social engagement. We may feel joy, love and satisfaction. We are engaged with those around us with good eye contact and body language. The ventral branch functions in conjunction with four other cranial nerves that all originate in the brainstem (CN V, VII, IX, XI).
- The dorsal vagal state is often referred to as "shut down," "immobilize" or "freeze." This state is associated with depression, sadness, anger, apathy, grief and lethargy. Changes in the form of reduced facial expression and voice intonation are common. From an evolutionary perspective, freezing up to fake death was one of our strategies for survival. However, this type of a physiologic response becomes problematic when the system becomes stuck in this state on chronic basis.

- The sympathetic chain facilitates "mobilization" or "fight or flight" mode. When we experience stress and prepare ourselves to flee, several physiological changes occur, including a rise in blood pressure and a shunting of blood flow from organs to extremities.
- Some bodies react to a history of trauma by going into a perpetual state of fight or flight, while others respond with a dissociative freeze response, where they are numb. Others oscillate between the two states. These responses are how the body helped them to survive historically, but they are no longer necessary or useful once the person is removed from the situation and is safe. Over time, either one of these dysfunctional states, while never a conscious choice, can contribute to chronic, system-wide health issues.
- Questionnaires, cranial nerve testing, structural and biomechanical orthopedic testing, and heart rate variability are tools that can help us determine the status of the ventral vs. dorsal nervous system resting state.
- Individuals relying on the dorsal vagal and sympathetic chain circuits are more in-tune with lower frequency sounds (like background noise, which historically was helpful in order to hear predators) and tend to be programmed to prioritize detecting danger from their environment from modifications in muscles innervated by the trigeminal and facial nerves.
- Cranial nerves IX, X and XI pass through the jugular foramen at the base of the skull, and this close anatomical relationship has clinical implications for treatment. A combination approach that addresses the vagus nerve, the cervical spine and certain neck muscles (such as the upper trapezius and sternocleidomastoid) and the middle ear muscles is optimal for nervous system retraining for patients with chronic illness.

- The Safe & Sound Protocol is an auditory therapy designed to restore proper function of the middle ear muscles in order to facilitate increased ventral vagal state. Additional programs that incorporate breath work, meditation, dietary factors, structural/mechanical issues in the ribs and pelvic floor muscles, and supplement-based vagus nerve support can be tremendously helpful for restoring healthy nervous system balance over time.

- At a bare minimum, patients with chronic conditions should customize a comprehensive program that includes breath work, tapping, mindfulness and/or meditation, programs that focus on ventral vagal tone, and auditory therapy aimed to restore cranial nerve function and/or brainwaves that influence our nervous system. The start of new program(s) should be guided with the help of a trained professional.

- Are you in-tune with your nervous system? Do you find yourself in fight or flight or freeze states often? Out of all the nervous system retraining options discussed in this chapter, which ones have you tried? What seems to help you the most? Which options would you like to try in the future? Reflect on this topic in your Trifecta Passport worksheet.

Chapter 8:
NUTRITION

How we fuel our body can make or break how our system heals. Diet is a tricky topic in patients who have the trifecta (and in particular, MCAS, due to the tendency for foods to trigger allergic-type reactions and other systemic issues). There are a lot of opinions out there on what should be the proper approach. Low-histamine, low-salicylate, low-FODMAP, high sodium for POTS, keto, you name it... there's a lot to unpack in the world of diet.

NUTRITION FOR HEALING

Physicians often are unsure of how to advise chronically ill patients in terms of a proper dietary approach. In my experience, some doctors recommend the low-histamine diet because that is the only approach they've heard of for MCAS. Most conventional doctors have very little formal training in the area of nutrition. Only a handful of nutritionists in the United States are considered to have expert knowledge in MCAS, let alone the trifecta.

In my first book, I utilized the sentiment of "we are all different, and diet needs to be customized to the individual with the help of your medical care team." While it's true that dietary choices need to be individualized, I've come to realize how important it is to look at diet from a perspective of education combined with clinical insight as opposed to cultural trends and influences. While I still believe that it's not black and white and diet needs to take unique factors into account (particularly in the MCAS community), my opinion on diet has evolved over the years, and even more so in the past year as I completed a nutrition certification.

The bottom line is this: food can be medicine. When patients with the trifecta are severely ill, food may not be the *only* "medicine" or approach we need, but it's a crucial part of the puzzle on the journey to healing. Instead of focusing entirely on a list of "no's", let's rewrite our food story to have a different approach, one that focuses on anti-inflammatory, life-giving nutrients. Let's focus on getting excited about food and knowing that what we are fueling ourselves with will leave us feeling complete, well-nourished and healthier as a whole. Let's focus on foods that naturally restore balance and bring healing in our gut, reduce mast cell mediator release, calm the autonomic nervous system and provide our connective tissues with the proper building blocks for optimal function.

The Stable Baseline

Getting to a point of dietary diversity is not an overnight process. Some patients who have MCAS are on the extreme end of the anaphylaxis spectrum and find themselves only able to tolerate a handful of "safe" foods, while others find that food is a constant low to moderate concern among less severe (but still notable) issues. What we don't hear about as often in the social media pages and groups is how many patients with MCAS have found systemic healing of symptoms and are now back to tolerating a wide variety of dietary options. Many of these patients leave the social media groups once they improve, so while it often seems that *everyone* with X or Y condition is suffering with dietary despair, that is not a true reflection of reality. The truth is that healing is possible, food sensitivities can be reversed and dietary diversity can be achieved.

However, ignoring physical symptoms or stubbornly forging ahead is not the answer. The key to management of all three conditions that make up the trifecta is to find a stable baseline first. This may mean taking medications or supplements to reduce symptoms, taking extra precautions with exposure to triggers, wearing a mask in public to reduce exposure to allergens or toxins and eating only those foods that don't trigger reactions. Over time, the goal will be to reduce the underlying issues that up-regulate mast cells, calm the nervous system response and lower musculoskeletal inflammation so that the patient can gradually *reintroduce* more diversity into their diet. These underlying issues include topics in prior chapters (such as nervous system retraining, mold, toxins, internal health stressors) as well as topics in future chapters (such as structural and musculoskeletal issues, detoxification and emotional healing). Addressing these issues can reduce the overall inflammatory/toxic burden, which typically results in a reduction in systemic symptoms.

Why do we become intolerant to foods in the first place? Some experts suspect that factors such as hormonal changes, heavy metals, stress or an infection can be triggers for patients to develop food intolerances. Toxins and additives from our food sources and the pesticides/herbicides used on our foods also likely contribute, in addition to our total toxic burden.

Leaky gut is one of the main theorized mechanisms in the development of food sensitivities. Changes in our microbiota in the intestines (due to stress, sugar, the Western diet, medications, toxins, etc.) lead to a breakdown in the endothelial lining of the gastrointestinal tract. Specifically, as discussed in Chapter 5, the porous layers of the gastrointestinal tract remain open for too long due to tight junction/barrier dysfunction. This triggers immune activation of cytokines and other inflammatory mediators, and patients find themselves in a vicious cycle. Food and toxin molecules are then able to be absorbed into the bloodstream, and this can result in reactions and inflammatory responses. This may also lead to improper functioning of the vagus nerve, influencing the communication feedback loop and the neurological system as a whole.

Simply willing our system to tolerate more foods will be frustrating; proactive steps to reduce the true root issues are necessary to help reduce the overall load on the body that translates to most food sensitivities. Obviously, true allergies that always cause anaphylaxis are not usually reversed, but other food and gut sensitivity reactions can change with the proper approach. Many patients with MCAS find themselves reacting to some type of food today that they tolerated just fine yesterday, and this is a good example of the type of reaction that may be reversible.

Hydration

Before we dive into different dietary approaches, let's talk about one often-overlooked aspect of healing: hydration. Many patients with chronic conditions find themselves in a state of chronic, low-level dehydration. The reasons for this vary, but one common reason that patients may drink less fluids relates to the presence of abdominal discomfort and bloating. When foods are triggering abdominal symptoms or when a patient has gastroparesis, the last thing they want to do is feel fuller by drinking more water. Many patients also eliminate many fruits and vegetables from their diet, reducing food-based fluid intake. Others may focus on coffee, soda or other beverages instead of water.

Experts maintain that the general population should consume half an ounce to an ounce of water for every pound of body weight. In addition, many believe that we should consume 4–6 ounces every 15–20 minutes during vigorous exercise and roughly 16 ounces of water before and after exercising. Some sources also recommend drinking 16–24 ounces of water for every pound lost during exercise.

There's certainly some controversy around these and the "8x8" recommendations (eight 8 oz. glasses per day). One liter (about half that amount) is estimated to be obtained through our typical beverage and food consumption and amounts under 64 ounces may be adequate for some people who are following their body's signals for thirst.

Hydration has many benefits for the chronic illness patient population. Staying hydrated can help increase gastrointestinal motility and the frequency of bowel movements, which can aid in detoxification. Hydration has been theorized to cleanse the airways in asthma, dilute toxins in patients with cancer and decrease blood viscosity for patients with cardiac concerns.[1] Hydration also may improve cognitive function in both children and adults.[2,3]

Hydration also appears to positively impact the autonomic nervous system. Oral hydration triggers gastric distention, which promotes vagal tone.[1] In contrast, baroreceptor-mediated sympathetic nervous system response and neurohormonal activation to promote fluid retention are triggered by hypovolemia (low blood volume) that can occur with dehydration, so it's important to stay on top of getting enough fluids.[1]

"Liberal intake of salt and water" is a common recommendation for the management of POTS,[4] and sometimes fluids are also administered intravenously or parenterally.[5] Research consistently recommends that patients with POTS consume 2–3 liters of fluids per day,[5-9] with higher amounts when you are active and sweating. Some experts also recommend that patients with POTS drink 16 ounces of water before getting out of bed in the morning.[4]

Dysautonomia International recommends fluid intake of approximately 2 liters (~68 ounces) and salt intake of 3–5 grams per day for patients with POTS, noting that this combination can be especially helpful with blood pooling, hypovolemia, or hypotension (low blood pressure).[10] One gram of table salt contains about 0.4 grams of sodium, and this can be useful when tracking daily intake by nutrition labels specifying sodium. In addition to consuming salt in foods, some patients also carry salt sticks or use an electrolyte solution when flared. Increased electrolyte and water intake may decrease tachycardia in idiopathic POTS patients through mechanisms of increased blood volume and increased blood pressure.[11]

In spite of these recommendations, to date, scientific research has yet to determine the appropriate intake of sodium and water and their long-term effects for patients with POTS. Some sources have also expressed concern that 2–3 liters of water per day may disturb electrolyte concentrations that could, in turn, affect the heart rhythm in patients with POTS.[12] Some POTS patients report that the water and sodium strategies significantly improve their ability to be upright and functional. Patients with dysautonomia may want to think about hydration in terms of electrolyte balance instead of simply looking at fluid intake.

Patients should bear in mind that hydration and sodium approaches—while potentially useful to mitigate symptoms of POTS—are considered Band-Aid approaches that mask symptoms without addressing the root cause of the disorder. Using these strategies to temporarily raise the blood volume and blood pressure can sometimes be a slippery slope where patients become reliant on more and more salt to manage their symptoms, and this should be considered, particularly when creating a long-term healing plan.

Patients with the hypovolemic type of POTS may be more influenced by attention to hydration than the other subcategories of dysautonomia, though recommendations for hydration appear across the board in terms of POTS management. Adequate hydration also likely has a positive impact on the management of MCAS and EDS as well as the body's ability to detoxify, an important aspect of any chronic condition. External incentives and reminders to drink more fluids (such as an app like Plant Nanny, Daily Water, Waterlogged, iHydrate, My Water, Water Coach and others) can be helpful.[13] In line with an integrative approach, hydration should be one component of healing, but over time a plan that addresses root issues will hopefully reduce symptoms of POTS and restore more normal blood volume and circulation dynamics.

COMPARISON OF DIETARY TRENDS

Let's evaluate what the literature says about different dietary approaches used most often by this patient population.

The Low-Histamine Diet

By and large the most recognized dietary approach in this patient community, the low-histamine diet was popularized about a decade ago. Histamine has been in the limelight for many years now and is one of the best-known mast cell mediators due to its role in allergic reactions and the numerous pharmaceutical antihistamine medications that are available over the counter. As discussed in Chapter 1, histamine is one of the chemical mediators that contributes to the "soup" of triggers for inflammation that occur with MCAD. Histamine is released by mast cells and basophils as part of the body's immune response to invaders. It can be present in food sources and can grow in quantity on foods after they've been cooked and are not immediately ingested (i.e., leftovers).

Genetically, some people are more likely to struggle with histamine than others. There are two enzymes that help the body break down histamine: diamine oxidase (DAO) and histamine n-methyl transferase (HNMT). People who have MCAD may show genetic susceptibility to lacking the right amount of these enzymes. DAO is believed to be the main enzyme responsible for the metabolism of dietary-acquired histamine.[14] DAO scavenges the histamine outside the cells, while HNMT primarily acts on histamine inside the cells.[14] Though deficiency in either of these enzymes is not causative to developing MCAD, it can certainly exacerbate the effects that histamine has on the body.

The DAO enzyme has been shown to be effective as a supplement with the histamine intolerant population in one study.[15] DAO supplements are typically made from porcine (pig) kidneys or peas and act locally in the GI tract without systemic absorption. There are other products on the market, like quercetin and bromelain, that you can use before eating, which may also help to reduce the impact of mealtime mast cell mediators. Occasionally patients report symptom relief with supplementation of the enzyme DAO in the pill form 30 minutes before meals to help break down histamine, though from a clinical perspective, many MCAS patients report no change with DAO supplementation.

Many sources refer to a bucket theory when it comes to histamine. According to this analogy, if one is ingesting a lot of histamine-rich foods and beverages *and* experiencing stressors or injury, bodily histamine levels will continue to rise—like water being added to a bucket—until eventually over time there's spillover from the bucket and the patient experiences symptoms. The bucket baseline water level may be higher in patients who have MCAS as they may naturally have higher circulating levels of mast cell mediators. The baseline water level also may be influenced by genetic factors, the presence of a buildup of toxins, viruses, bacteria, mold or other environmental triggers that increase mast cell activation, and the predisposition to a difficulty in breaking down and eliminating histamine from the body. The offending food may not be the biggest factor, but it very well could be the *tipping point* in terms of whether symptoms occur with eating or not. If the body's detoxification pathways (like the liver, kidneys and gastrointestinal tract) are clogged, the bucket's baseline water level may hover very close to the top and make it more susceptible to frequent spillovers with minor triggers.

Symptoms of intolerance to histamine ingestion include anxiety, dizziness, fatigue, gastrointestinal issues, heart rate changes, hives, nasal congestion and swelling of various areas of the body. Many food and beverage sources increase plasma levels of histamine after consumption. Histamine levels increase in foods and drinks that are fermented, are highly processed, and contain added preservatives. A 2016 review article evaluated 14 studies of the best evidence in this area and determined that the following foods have the highest histamine levels: dried anchovies, fish sauce, fermented vegetables, cheese, fish and fish productions, and fermented sausages.[16]

Alcoholic beverages are liquid culprits associated with triggering histamine reactions. Histamine is believed to be one of the reasons why some people tend to get red or flushed when drinking alcohol. Researchers joke about whether a "red wine test" could help identify people with histamine intolerance. However, other aspects of wine (including compounds such as sulfites and tyramine or conditions such as a grape allergy) could also be playing a role in these symptoms.

An increase in histamine is more likely to occur in foods that have been overcooked or overripened, or that have spent a lot of time on the counter or in the fridge after being cooked. Reheating food more than once should be avoided, and many patients use small separate containers to freeze leftovers. In addition to food selection, meal composition and intervals between meals may also affect histamine-related symptoms.[17]

Foods that are generally considered to be naturally high in histamine, or that trigger release of histamine, include:

- Aged cheese
- All alcoholic beverages
- Canned foods
- Chocolate
- Energy drinks, soda and soymilk
- Fermented or bacterially ripened products (kefir, kombucha, yeast, sauerkraut, vinegar)
- Gluten-containing foods (breads, cereals, wheat pasta, etc.)
- Nuts, legumes
- Preserved meat (dried, marinated, or smoked) i.e., bacon, cold cuts, dry-cured ham
- Shellfish and other fish

- Specific fruits: strawberries, raspberries, citrus fruit, pineapple, banana, etc.
- Specific vegetables: spinach, tomato, eggplant, avocado, etc.

Interpreting histamine numbers in food sources can get a little confusing. There are dozens upon dozens of web resources, books and studies that cite histamine numbers for different foods. It seems that there's quite a bit of variability in these numbers. Foods like spinach, dark chocolate and avocado generally tend to have very low measured histamine content (0–62 mg/kg) compared to foods like ripened cheese (up to 2,500 mg/kg) although they still show up on website lists as being "high" in histamine, which further confounds dietary decisions.[18-21]

There are no universally agreed upon values for histamine in different foods. The numbers are not uniform, and a multitude of factors can impact measured histamine content in food. Testing parameters and conditions, phase in ripeness, handling conditions and temperatures for storage, geographical location, and many other factors could cause variability between published numbers.

Another factor to consider with these numbers is the difficulty in comparing quantities, since the numbers are not cited based on serving sizes. As an example, one kilogram of spinach certainly looks different than one kilogram of dark chocolate.

One commonality, however, is that one type of food can have a wide range of published histamine levels within the same food category. Cheese is a great example of this. According to one source, brie cheese has 2–87 mg/kg histamine, whereas cheddar cheese has 1,710 mg/kg.[21] Cottage cheese and young edam cheese have less than 5 mg/kg histamine,[21] whereas the more aged cheeses will most certainly, by nature, have higher histamine levels. One source noted that Swiss cheese has 500 mg/kg histamine, but when it's been ripened for 24 weeks, it has 750–1,290 mg/kg histamine.[20]

Research indicates that fresh fish has significantly less histamine content than frozen fish.[19] This observation appears to be supported in the literature.[22] However, histamine levels rise on fresh fish very quickly with improper handling and storage due to the increase in histamine-producing bacteria,[22] so fish that is fresh may not always be ideal, depending on a number of specific details surrounding its timeline and protocols for the time from ocean to table. Fish that is flash-frozen or fileted immediately after it's been caught while on your fishing boat in Alaska is going to be safer than fish that had delays between these steps. In some cases, fresh fish that was *immediately frozen* may be safer than the unfrozen form at the supermarket, but the numbers show that, in general, frozen fish is at higher risk. It is completely case-dependent, making it very difficult to make decisions unless you are getting the food directly from the source.

Organic vs. nonorganic food sources may also make a difference. When comparing regular dark chocolate to organic dark chocolate, there was a difference in histamine content cited by one source: 2–4 mg/kg for organic, and 10–20 mg/kg for conventional dark chocolate.[20] Notable discrepancies in histamine values are reported between a large number of studies, books and websites.[19-25]

The low-histamine diet has been challenged by the literature and clinicians alike, particularly when it is performed for a long-term time frame or when it is followed "blindly" without attention to individual-specific intolerances. ("Blindly" in this case refers to making decisions based on a concept instead of based on your own body's specific response.) In these instances, it's common to observe patients who experience the frustration of getting down to a small handful of "safe" foods because they've cut so many options out simply because they were on "the list." Many newly diagnosed patients initially follow website lists and may radically eliminate all foods on the lists they find, including nutritious fruits and vegetables, which is where I have a problem with this approach.

Most of the existing studies have only evaluated short-term effects of reducing histamine in the diet. One study found that ~75% of patients with gastrointestinal issues and the diagnosis of chronic urticaria had a reduction in symptoms following a low-histamine diet for three weeks, but they were not followed beyond that point.[26] When considering the low-histamine diet, a lack of standardization in both the research methodology and clinical tools further complicates conclusions.[16] Various researchers have questioned the connections between ingestion of histamine and adverse reactions as well as the fact that there is no reliable laboratory test for objective diagnosis of a label like histamine intolerance, making it difficult to research this topic.[15,17,27-28]

The late Yasmina Ykelenstam, also known as the "low-histamine chef" and creator of healinghistamine.com, suffered from MCAD and advocated for several tactics to reduce the overall histamine load. She recommended minimizing triggers by avoiding certain foods that are especially high in histamine, avoiding certain beauty products that may trigger reactions, adapting lifestyle factors to reduce stress and filling the diet with healthy antihistaminic nutrient sources.[29]

Ykelenstam summarized her stance on low-histamine diets in a 2013 publication. "Once you understand that histamine is just one of many inflammatory mediators leaked into our bodies by unstable mast cells, you begin to reach the root of the issue. I no longer see the point in solely focusing on low histamine or diamine oxidase: I choose to address the more general problem of mast cell instability and inflammation that creates a fertile environment for mast cell degranulation and the subsequent release of pro-inflammatory agents like histamine, prostaglandin D2, heparin, tryptase, serotonin and others."[30]

Regardless of whether research shows that symptoms can be alleviated in the short-term with the diet, many question its long-term appropriateness. Is the low-histamine diet simply a temporary solution for symptoms, while the underlying MCAS cause continues to go on undeterred? Is focusing on numbers and charts and lists helpful for your mental health, or could it set people up for disordered eating? Should we be focusing on putting a positive spin on nutrient-dense foods instead of a negative spin on others, and does this mental self-talk influence our mast cells and level of reactivity? And further, does long-term avoidance of important nutrients set patients up for more health problems down the road?

Foods that are considered high in histamine or that facilitate the release of histamine also include healthy options like the aforementioned spinach and avocado, as well as ripe bananas. For someone who has MCAS, POTS or EDS, the combined list of the foods that you are truly allergic to, the ones that seem to trigger other mast cell symptoms, and the ones that are high in histamine, salicylates, etc., can eliminate a great deal of food options, leaving the diet devoid of nutrients that are important for healing.

While foods may serve as the immediate trigger to a reaction, it's wise to consider the other factors that may have caused the bucket to fill up and overflow. When envisioning a pie chart, histamine is just one small slice of the whole picture and focusing solely on histamine may keep a patient in a vicious cycle of reactions and eliminations and a false sense of control that becomes a slippery slope into more dietary restrictions.

Patients often pick apart food or supplement recommendations without trying them simply because they are claimed to be high in histamine or block the DAO enzyme. One example of this is the research on epigallocatechin gallate (EGCG), the main active constituent in green tea, as a supplement supported for its antiviral effects against coronavirus (in addition to dozens of other beneficial effects against inflammation and diseases including cancer). Some websites state that EGCG blocks DAO, the enzyme that breaks down histamine in our bodies. However, research supports that EGCG is actually an inhibitor of the histamine-producing enzyme histidine decarboxylase.[31] In addition, with its polyphenol

273

properties, EGCG has potent anti-tumoral, anti-angiogenic, and anti-inflammatory properties.[31]

In this example, while many patients don't tolerate caffeine from green tea, the bioactive compound of EGCG is available in other forms that contain minimal to no caffeine. In addition, there's a difference between fermented tea leaves and traditional tea leaves and their impacts on histamine levels and DAO. Even if EGCG does impact the enzyme DAO, the plethora of systemic benefits may outweigh this small detail, and the impacts of EGCG on the histamine-producing enzyme likely negate this concern anyway.

It's one thing to stop drinking green tea or taking an ECGC supplement when you know that it triggers anaphylaxis or other symptoms for you every time you have it. It's another thing to avoid it simply based on principle. The take-home message is this: weigh out the pros and cons and reevaluate where you are drawing the line in the sand. If we zoom out and look at the big picture and the overall benefits (instead of having tunnel vision on one particular chemical mediator), we may find that we have more healing options available to us than we realized.

Researchers conclude that maintaining some degree of histamine-containing foods in the diet is helpful in order to establish a proper histamine baseline level and to work to improve thresholds over time.[16] A 2017 review determined that research surrounding the low-histamine diet was inconclusive, avoidance of histamine liberators (substances that have a histamine-releasing effect) is not warranted, and an approach that utilizes individualized nutritional therapy with a focus on nutrient optimization (as opposed to generalized, restrictive diets) is recommended.[17] They also recommended expert nutritional counseling in order to help patients avoid diets that "result in an unnecessary reduction in their quality of life."[17] Similarly, well known MCAS experts agree that diet should be individualized[32] and that the focus should be on a well-balanced diet that includes fruit, vegetables and protein sources and on avoidance of triggering or allergic foods.[33]

It amazes me that there have been no studies conducted to date to investigate the effects of a low-histamine diet in patients with MCAS, POTS or EDS. The few studies that exist are focused on chronic urticaria, and while this can be a symptom for some patients (especially patients with MCAS), it's astonishing that so many medical professionals are recommending this diet without scientific backing. Likely they are finding it beneficial in their own experience in certain patient cases, they are wrapped up in the cultural popularity of the diet or they simply don't have any other idea how to counsel these complex patients. Or perhaps it's a little bit of all three!

Don't get me wrong, there are many well-educated doctors out there who truly believe that this approach will help their patients. And many patients feel that following this diet helps calm things down initially. Indeed, some of the biggest high-histamine culprits (like alcohol, aged cheese and cured meats) may be beneficial to remove from the diet for other, bigger-picture toxicity/inflammation reasons. But I encourage you to reconsider the status quo when it comes to using this approach for long-term healing.

The Low-Salicylate Diet

More and more patients are presenting with the label of salicylate intolerance, and this is concerning for a number of reasons. Salicylates are found in all sorts of foods, beauty products, perfumes, preservatives and medications. It's nearly impossible (well, some would argue impossible) to avoid them completely in daily life in the U.S. Naturally occurring in plants, salicylates are derivatives of salicylic acid. Fruits, vegetables, teas, herbs and spices contain natural salicylates. Their role is to protect plants against diseases, bacteria, fungi and insects.

The beneficial effects of salicylate-containing fruits, vegetables and herbs are well established and documented in the literature. Some studies even suggest that the reason fruit- and vegetable-focused diets reduce cancer risk is *because* they contain naturally occurring salicylates.[34]

It's important to point out that most experts maintain that salicylate sensitivity is not technically an allergy. It's not mediated by IgE-type allergic reaction pathways. An intolerance or sensitivity is believed to be caused by lack of enzymes and/or abnormalities in other biochemical processes. Some medical experts voice concern that people are being placed at a high level of nutritional risk due to the belief that salicylate sensitivity is at the root of their problems.[35] I honestly am worried about this as well.

Symptoms of salicylate intolerance have been reported to include headaches, irritable bowel symptoms, joint pain, palpitations, rhinitis, urticaria, wheezing and potential neuropsychological symptoms including anxiety, depression, inattention, irritability, panic attacks and restlessness,[36] making it difficult to distinguish from "classic" MCAS symptoms at times.

The concept of salicylate intolerance is not new; researchers and clinicians have examined this idea over the past 50 years. Anne Swain popularized the discussion about salicylate intolerance in Australia back in the 1980s. The Feingold and Failsafe diets are the eating plans most traditionally prescribed for patients who are suspected to exhibit salicylate sensitivity.

Originally developed in the 1970s by Benjamin Feingold, the Feingold diet has been studied for treatment of ADHD and autism, but not in patients with MCAS and not specifically in patients demonstrating salicylate intolerance. (Part of the research difficulty lies in the fact that there's no clinical test to "diagnose" someone with salicylate intolerance, though some clinicians will do an oral provocation test using aspirin.) Feingold's development of the diet stemmed from noting behavioral problems in patients who were sensitive to aspirin, artificial flavoring and food coloring.

However, the Feingold diet focuses on elimination of other substances beyond salicylates. The few studies evaluating variations of this diet have not focused on natural salicylates in food and instead have generally included a focus on eliminating preservatives and artificial food additives, so our ability to extract insight is somewhat limited. The research about whether the Feingold diet is effective with conditions such as ADHD and autism appears to be muddy and inconclusive. Likewise, no compelling evidence exists yet to support or refute the theorized link between salicylates and depression or schizophrenia. Like histamine, there also appears to be a lot of discrepancy in terms of scientific data reporting salicylate values in different foods.[37]

A 2014 review[37] concluded that:

- Limited research exists to isolate the effects of salicylates, and naturally occurring plant-based salicylates have not been studied.
- Pharmacological doses of salicylates are unlikely to be achieved by diet alone, so a dietary approach that eliminates them based on principle, as a form of treatment, lacks logic.
- A diet low in natural (plant-based) salicylates is likely to be deficient in some of the essential nutrients of an otherwise healthy diet.
- Logically, the creation of diets that restrict food sources like salicylates should only occur after a causal link has been established connecting dietary intake of salicylates and exacerbated symptom severity.
- It's clear that more research is needed to more properly investigate this topic.

Similar to the concept of avoiding histamine in foods, for some patients, the logic in avoiding salicylates dietarily seems flawed. Obviously not all cases are the same. There's a big difference between a patient who has severe anaphylaxis to ALL salicylates vs. the one who just reacts to higher content sources like aspirin vs. the patient who has mild to no symptoms but tends to react spontaneously to random foods.

Some patients react only to synthetic salicylates and have no discernible issues with natural salicylates but still decide to eliminate all sources from their diet, which can lead to problems. There are many nutrient-dense salicylate-containing fruits and vegetables and they pale in comparison to the salicylate content of medications and beauty products. Experts maintain that a typical daily diet is not expected to exceed the salicylate levels of 325–650 mg of aspirin.[34]

Just like histamine, the growing conditions, food preparation techniques and level of ripeness can influence salicylate levels on food sources. Just like histamine, salicylates are found on many healing, antioxidant-rich food sources (like fruits and vegetables) that are (in my mind) essential to restore homeostasis and reverse disease inflammation. Salicylates themselves are anti-inflammatory and cutting them out blindly can be extra restrictive and detrimental to healing in most scenarios. And just like histamine, patients with MCAS often confide that trying a low-salicylate diet on top of an already restrictive list of options makes them more and more sensitive/reactive over time, and more and more sick, until they are down to very few "safe" foods.

The lists of salicylate-containing foods on the internet make me cringe. One website advocated that patients focus on consumption of breads, cereals and noodles/pasta while having to completely avoid sweet potato. Replacing fruits and vegetables with grains like gluten and with sugar, preservatives and processed foods does not seem to be sound medical advice. I believe that we have way too much tunnel vision here, and we need to look at nutrient factors and healing potential as a whole, instead of having patients memorize ridiculous lists of yes and no foods. Again, I realize that some patients are severely ill/sensitive and must remove certain foods on the basis of anaphylaxis and what they personally react to, and that is certainly justified. But, again, I discourage patients from blindly following internet food lists regardless of what their body is telling them.

Experts affirm that "because a salicylate exclusion diet restricts many fruits and vegetables, it is important patients do not continue the diet as a long-term measure."[38] While some patients opt for strict avoidance once they are certain that they are salicylate intolerant, research has shown that—with the help of the medical team and in a hospital setting—patients may be able to desensitize to salicylates including aspirin, though more research is needed in this area.[36] Arguably, an integrative approach that reduces systemic inflammation and mast cell reactivity may also help patients desensitize to salicylates.

The Low-FODMAP Approach

Some patients who have MCAS and gastrointestinal issues or irritable bowel syndrome (IBS) stick to a low-FODMAP diet. Examples of some of the more "notorious" foods that are higher in FODMAPs—fermentable oligosaccharides, disaccharides, monosaccharides and polyols—include garlic, cauliflower, onion and asparagus. Several other vegetables and fruits are also considered high-FODMAP foods. The low-FODMAP diet is not intended to be followed for long-term time frames but can reduce inflammation, bloating, digestive issues and gastrointestinal discomfort.

A 2016 systematic review supported use of the low-FODMAP diet for patients with functional gastrointestinal disorders, citing improvements in bloating, severity of abdominal pain and quality of life.[39] A 2015 review by Afrin and Khoruts noted, "Dietary management is important in IBS. The most successful diet (FODMAP) decreases colonic gas and SCFA (short chain fatty acids) production."[40] SCFA are the end products of fermentation of dietary fibers and the breakdown process is controlled in part by the intestinal microbiota. Specifically, a low-FODMAP diet is advocated for patients with IBS, and in theory it may be useful for patients with the trifecta who suffer from poor digestion, delayed colonic transit and bloating/distention.[40] Research from 2017 found that a three-week low-FODMAP diet reduced circulating histamine levels by eight-fold, so this approach certainly has appeal for patients in the MCAS community.[41]

Unfortunately, many of the irritable high-FODMAP foods are also the important foods that boost our detoxification pathways and promote healing. Additional research has noted that dietary FODMAPs may actually suppress the release of histamine.[42] Furthermore, potentially unfavorable impacts on the gut microbiota are a theoretical consequence of following this diet for long-term time frames. Researchers have also noted that due to its restrictive nature, the low-FODMAP diet carries risks of nutritional inadequacy and potential to foster disordered eating.[42] It's possible that this dietary option is another approach that reduces symptoms without addressing the root issues behind the gastrointestinal distress, but many patients with the trifecta report that they are in significantly less abdominal discomfort when following a low-FODMAP diet.

The Low-Nightshade Approach

Nightshades are members of the family *Solanaceae* and include white potatoes (sweet potatoes are not in this family), peppers, tomatoes, eggplant and spices made from peppers (paprika, cayenne pepper, red pepper flakes). For some people who are sensitive to nightshades, these foods may act as toxins that increase inflammation. However, the chemical compounds in nightshades bring anti-inflammatory benefits to people with healthy digestive systems.

People who suffer from issues like autoimmune disease or leaky gut are typically the ones who report sensitivity to these foods.

Nightshades have been reported to trigger joint pain, skin issues, gut problems and generalized inflammation in susceptible individuals. However, a 2019 article put out by Tufts University dispelled myths about nightshades and maintains that they are rich in nutrients like vitamin C and carotenoids and should be a worthy addition to most diets.[43]

Patients with the trifecta who note a marked change in symptoms when consuming nightshades often eliminate them, but the question should be whether this elimination still allows for plenty of additional vegetable options to choose from to maintain nutrient diversity and quantity. This dietary approach is much less restrictive than others as it only eliminates four vegetables, but its impacts on long-term health indicators is unknown. A holistic approach that eventually reintegrates nightshades into the diet is often possible once patients experience greater systemic healing.

The Low-Oxalate Diet

Oxalates are compounds found in some foods, and they are also produced as a waste product by the body that we eliminate through the urine. Foods and beverages reported to be high in oxalates include beans, beer, beets, berries, chocolate, coffee, cranberries, dark green vegetables, nuts, oranges, rhubarb, soda, soy, sweet potatoes, tea, tofu and wheat bran. Some medical sources and handouts recommend substantial restriction to complete avoidance of 75+ different types of fruits and vegetables![44]

Some research has found that dietary oxalate restriction is useful for kidney stone prevention.[45] Beyond kidney stones, pain and neurological symptoms are the most commonly reported issues for patients who are sensitive to oxalates, though it's unclear that these symptoms resolve with low-oxalate dietary intervention. Some experts suggest that urinary pain can be alleviated by following a low-oxalate diet.

Interestingly, determining food content of oxalates appears to have similar flaws and limitations as the histamine and salicylate content of foods already discussed. A 2014 review found that wide variations exist in the reported oxalate content of foods, including several substantial differences that can have a sizable impact on the determinants of a low-oxalate diet.[46] Another study found that a "DASH" style diet (Dietary Approaches to Stop Hypertension) may be an effective alternative to the low-oxalate diet in terms of reducing kidney stone risk factors. The DASH diet is high in fruit, vegetables, whole grains, and low-fat dairy products and low in fat, refined grains, sweets and meat.[47] Thus, it's questionable whether the removal of fruits and vegetables in the low-oxalate diet is truly helpful. More research is certainly needed to investigate the impacts of the low-oxalate diet within different patient populations.

Similar to the cons associated with the low-histamine and low-salicylate approaches, the low-oxalate diet recommends removing certain fruits and vegetables that could be important for healing, without addressing other root issues. Depending on the source, the low-oxalate diet can be tremendously limiting. Kidney stones are undeniably excruciating, and patients who are prone to kidney stones typically trial and error foods to determine which ones may impact them the most; for these patients, the relief of pain may be worth the sacrifice, but there are still concerns over long-term impacts and nutritional status. For other conditions, the scarcity of research on the low-oxalate diet merits caution, and patients should proceed carefully when following food lists from the internet.

An extremely small proportion of patients may have a genetic defect in the ability to process foods containing oxalates, and functional medicine testing can confirm this (via glyceric/glycolic metabolites and genetic testing) and help guide dietary decisions. Other issues such as intestinal dysbiosis, candida, vitamin B6 deficiency, mycotoxins and extremely high doses of vitamin C (when free copper is high) can increase oxalate metabolites and are more likely culprits that need to be addressed when someone experiences sensitivities to oxalates and/or the predisposition to kidney stones. Slightly elevated oxalates on organic acid testing can be dietary, but higher elevations (more than 150 mmol/mol creatinine of a metabolite called oxalic, for example) are usually due to an underlying mold or fungal issue. Oxalates can trap heavy metals in tissues and a short-term low-oxalate diet may be warranted for patients with certain functional medicine test results; following a low-oxalate diet blindly without personalized testing is generally discouraged.

The Gluten-Free and Grain-Free Diet

Mast cells have been implicated in the pathogenesis of celiac disease, and they increase in number in addition to contributing to the pro-inflammatory environment in the gut in patients with celiac disease.[48] Symptoms of gluten intolerance are not limited to the gut and often include bloating, brain fog, depression, diarrhea or constipation, fatigue, headaches, joint pain, nausea, numbness, skin issues and smelly feces.

Regardless of whether patients with MCAS, POTS or EDS have a true diagnosis of celiac disease or the inkling of the presence of gluten intolerance, removing gluten from the diet can provide symptomatic relief and reduce systemic inflammation, without the added concern that the diet will result in fewer healing nutrients. An abundance of literature exists supporting the gluten-free diet for a variety of conditions for patients with and without documented gluten issues. True adherence to a gluten-free diet is tricky as gluten is a common hidden ingredient in many processed foods, sauces and dressings; it's much more complicated than simply avoiding bread and pasta.

The more restrictive grain-free diet eliminates all gluten and non-gluten grain sources, including barley, corn, farro, oats, rice, sorghum, spelt, wheat and other cereal grains and can also be helpful for patients with chronic illness. There are many great resources available on this topic, but for the sake of this book, I will keep this section short. Many patients with MCAS, POTS and EDS find that eliminating gluten and other grains (particularly corn) can be very helpful for reducing systemic inflammation.

Further, it's a sound approach because removing gluten does not sacrifice important healing nutrients, and the reduction in fiber can be compensated for with other foods.

The Ketogenic Diet

The ketogenic ("keto") diet focuses on a low-carb, high-fat diet similar to the Atkins diet. Food choices typically consist of cheese, avocado, meat/poultry/fish, eggs, yogurt, and low-carb vegetables. This approach translates to 20–50 grams of carbohydrates daily (5%–10% of the total energy intake) as opposed to the typical 150–250 grams (up to 50% of total energy intake) consumed by individuals in developed countries.[49] Instead, individuals following a ketogenic approach consume around 70% of their daily calories from fat sources.[50] This dramatic reduction in carbs results in the production of ketones in the liver. This switches the body's fuel source from glucose to fatty acids. This diet is often used in conjunction with different types of fasting or caloric restriction.

Research behind the ketogenic diet supports its use for seizure control in patients with epilepsy.[51] Small human studies have noted that the ketogenic diet may benefit patients with dementia.[52] Research also indicates that the diet may promote weight loss and decrease BMI (body mass index) and other metrics,[53] although other research has indicated that the weight loss of approximately one kilogram may not be clinically significant.[54] Furthermore, it's apparent that the weight loss may be trumped by the increase in all-cause mortality noted in low-carbohydrate diets.[55]

Some experts believe that "the enthusiasm for its potential benefits exceeds the current evidence supporting its use for these conditions."[50] Indeed, concerning research exists that the diet poses serious risks to several systems, including the gastrointestinal tract and gut bacterial balance.[56] Specifically, the diet reduces microbial diversity and lowers concentrations of beneficial bacteria, most likely due to the reduction in carbohydrates and lowered content of vegetables and other foods that impact gut health.[49] It's unclear whether probiotic and prebiotic supplementation improve this side effect to optimal levels.[49] Additionally, gut-related side effects such as constipation, vomiting and abdominal pain occur in 30%–50% of individuals who try the ketogenic diet.[49] And because the approach limits major food groups (like certain fruits, vegetables and grains), it's much more difficult to obtain all required nutrients and fiber.[49] Experts recommend extreme caution in people who are already at risk of nutritional deficiency, as well as those who may be concerned with the risk of heart disease and bowel cancer.[49]

The ketogenic type of high-fat diet increases omega-6 fatty acids, which increase inflammation in the body. Omega-6 fatty acids are present in foods like corn, eggs, meat and certain oils. While there has been debate about this topic, recent reviews in the last few years continue to show that high-fat diets and approaches with a high ratio of omega-6 fatty acids (such as the ketogenic diet) increase the risk of heart disease and cancers.[57,58] Consumption of foods high in omega-6 fatty acids before or during pregnancy may have detrimental effects on fetal development as well as the long-term health of offspring.[59]

In contrast, a diet rich in omega-3 fatty acids—found in cold water fatty fish, nuts, seeds, plants, and some fortified foods —and low in omega-6 fatty acids provides protection against certain conditions like metabolic syndrome and also appears to reduce certain mast cell mediators like prostaglandins.[60] Alpha-linolenic acid is a plant-based omega-3 fatty acid that is found in foods such as brussels sprouts, chard, chia seed, flaxseed, hemp seed, kale, linseed, seaweed, soybeans, walnuts and some algae. The body converts a percentage of alpha-linolenic acid (omega-3 source) into DHA (docosahexaenoic acid) and EPA (eicosapentaenoic acid), which play a role in anti-inflammatory protective properties against heart disease and other conditions.[61] Linoleic acid, on the other hand, is termed the "bad" omega-6 fatty acid that's found in products like canola oil, corn oil, fried food, processed food, safflower oil and sunflower oil.

The ideal ratio for omega-6 to omega-3 fatty acids has been reported to range from 5:1 (reducing asthma symptoms) to 2–3:1 (inflammation suppression), but the typical Westernized diet often looks more like 15:1 to 16.7:1![61] Because the ketogenic diet has an even higher fat content than the Westernized diet, it's likely that it increases this ratio, depending on food sources.

Experts argue that people should focus on *reducing* omega-6s from their diet (which are commonly severely elevated in the standard American diet) instead of *increasing* omega-3s (which is more like a Band-Aid approach). A Whole Foods Plant Based approach can certainly help remedy the fatty acid imbalance noted with the typical Westernized diet and will be discussed later in this chapter.

A big part of the ketogenic diet focuses on consumption of animal products in ratios that are much higher than that of other dietary approaches. Regardless of the source, when meat is prepared, it creates toxins called advanced glycation end-products (AGEs), and they accelerate the aging process, contributing to disease all over the body. In contrast, vegetables, fruits and whole grains contain few AGEs, even after they've been cooked.

A 2019 systematic review found that weight status, energy metabolism and systemic inflammation were worse in the conventional (meat and dairy) diet group in patients with obesity or type II diabetes, as well as in healthy participants.[62] Meta-analyses of randomized controlled trials indicate that glycemic control in the keto diet appears similar to that of low-fat diets.[54] Some argue that the keto diet reduces LDL cholesterol and increases HDL cholesterol, but there's conflicting research on this point; these factors do not appear to translate to reductions in cardiovascular events.[50]

Further, the reports of harm caused by the ketogenic diet cause great concern. The "keto flu" describes the induction period of dizziness, fatigue, gastrointestinal issues, mood swings and weakness common to newcomers to the diet. Reports of deadly cardiac arrhythmias from selenium deficiency have also been noted.[50] Bone fractures, constipation, diarrhea, fatal and non-fatal pancreatitis, headaches, kidney stones, muscle cramping, restricted growth, and vitamin/mineral deficiencies have also been documented with the ketogenic diet.[50] The diet is not recommended for patients who have any internal organ issues, including gallbladder, gut, kidney, liver, pancreas or thyroid problems.

Experts also point out concern over the lack of health-promoting benefits of fruits, legumes, vegetables and whole grains with the keto approach, since the ratio of fruits and vegetables is generally substantially below daily recommendations.[50] With such a heavy focus on meat and dairy, patients are increasing the ratio of their dietary exposure to substances like growth hormones, steroids, stress hormones, and additives for color/to preserve freshness—even when they try to stick to organic, grass-fed and pasture-raised sources.

There's no research to date on how this approach impacts the trifecta conditions, and the long-term effects of the keto diet (>2 years) have yet to be studied, including its risk of bowel cancer (which is generally increased by diets that have high red meat intake and low fiber) and cardiovascular disease (which is generally increased by high-fat diets).[49] While the ketogenic diet may provide benefits that outweigh the negative consequences for patients who experience seizures, leading authorities maintain that all other individuals should proceed with caution with this eating trend.[63]

The Anti-Candida Diet

Candida albicans was discussed in Chapter 5 as a type of fungal infection that can serve as a significant health stressor in situations of overgrowth.

Candida is part of the normal gut flora, but it can leave the gut when a patient's immune system is compromised, wreaking havoc in other parts of the body. Because it originates in the gut, gastrointestinal factors and the status of the microbiome and leaky gut are extremely important in the treatment of candida.

Treatment of candida typically involves a combination of supplements or anti-fungal medications and short-term dietary modifications. It's very difficult to eradicate candida without significant dietary changes. It's important to note that this type of eating plan is NOT to be completed for long-term time frames. The goal is to reduce foods that tend to feed candida overgrowth in the gut. Once the candida load is back to healthy levels, typically within two to three weeks, patients will begin to reintegrate additional foods into the diet. Examples of foods that are believed to "feed" candida include simple sugars, carbohydrates, yeast, fermented foods, malt and vinegar.

While several books exist on this topic, there's a scarcity of research evaluating the efficacy of this diet for patients with candida fungal overgrowth issues. Many patients attest that they have reduced gastrointestinal and systemic symptoms in short- and long-term time periods following the anti-candida diet. While it's restrictive, because it's performed for such a short time frame (generally a number of weeks), the benefits of reduced candida colonization may justify the removal of certain fruits and other foods for a few weeks' time.

Alpha Gal Considerations

Galactose-alpha-1,3-galactose or "alpha gal" is found in beef, pork, lamb and venison, and may also be present in dairy, gelatin, vaccines and some medications.[64] Patients with alpha-gal allergies often have a history of a lone star tick bite; the tick is believed to have alpha-gal sugar in its gastrointestinal system, which is then passed to the host when bitten.[65] When the antibody cross-reacts during future meat ingestion, a delayed allergic reaction is triggered.[65] The IgE response to alpha gal can result in the loss of tolerance to foods that have been safely consumed for years.[66]

Patients with MCAS (particularly those who also suffer from Lyme disease, bartonella, or other types of tick-borne illness) have reported alpha-gal allergies. Alpha-gal sugar is most commonly found in red meat, and patients with an alpha-gal allergy may have delayed allergic reactions (often anaphylactic) two to six hours after consumption of the offending food.[65] Research also shows that alpha-gal is also present in intravenous cetuximab (a form of chemotherapy) and may trigger immediate anaphylaxis in exposed patients.[65]

This is a unique concern for certain patients, but it's important that you are aware of this phenomenon and the potential for it to trigger delayed anaphylaxis. Strict avoidance of alpha gal-containing foods and medications is important for this subgroup of patients and appears to be the mainstay of treatment.[67] It's unclear whether this condition can be reversed over time, as very little research is available that follows patients for long-term time frames. It's also unclear whether an integrative approach to wellness can reduce or halt these reactions.

Collagen Supplementation

Collagen peptide supplementation has become an increasing topic of interest in patients with the trifecta. First of all, collagen supplementation *does not* translate to changes in the collagen properties of your connective tissue. Collagen is an amino acid that may play a key role in healing gut damage, increasing antioxidant capacity and repairing leaky gut.[68] Collagen purportedly works to help seal the gaps in the intestinal lining, which reduces waste products leaking into the bloodstream that result in chronic inflammation,[68,69] though there's a surprising lack of studies evaluating these effects in human subjects. Collagen may also support joint health and skin appearance.[70-73]

In theory, a diet that supports the building blocks (like glycine, lysine, proline and vitamin C) would support natural collagen synthesis.[74] Some resources voice concern over collagen supplementation due to it's potential to increase the level of oxalates in the body. To date, no established research supports the supplementation of collagen peptides in patients with MCAS, POTS and EDS. However, many of these patients do suffer from gastrointestinal dysfunction, skin problems and joint issues; ultimately, the jury is still out on whether collagen peptide supplementation is appropriate for humans.

Avoidance of Lectins

Avoidance of lectins has gained popularity in recent years. Lectins are a type of carbohydrate-binding protein that stick to the cell membranes in the digestive tract. They are reportedly found in highest amounts in legumes, nightshades, grains including barley, wheat, rice and quinoa, and dairy products. One study found that they are present in up to 30% of our typical diet.[75] Lectins have been implicated as a cause of gastrointestinal distress due to the nature of these foods being undigestible and bound to cell membranes in the digestive tract. It's possible that they can cause nutrient deficiencies, intestinal damage and disrupted digestion.[75]

Most people find that proper cooking of these foods enables good tolerance, as heat inactivates lectins. Some will also soak foods like legumes and grains before cooking to reduce the lectin content, though it's unclear how effective this is. Lectins can activate and degranulate mast cells through a cross-linking mechanism,[76] but it's unclear whether this process warrants a substantial concern in terms of the big picture of health and symptoms. Information from human studies is lacking and the jury is still out on whether avoidance of lectins would be beneficial for patients with chronic illness. Critics voice concern over the lack of nutrients and the lack of fiber in this diet.

The Whole Foods Plant Based (WFPB) Approach

The Whole Foods Plant Based (WFPB) Diet is not a new concept, but it's recently been re-popularized in the chronic illness patient community and beyond. The WFPB Diet emphasizes whole, minimally processed foods and avoids animal products. Plants including vegetables, fruits, whole grains, legumes, seeds and nuts make up the majority of what is consumed. Some people consider a plant-based diet to be 80% plant and 20% meat/egg sources. Others are stricter and follow adherence to vegan standards by completely eliminating all animal products including meat, fish, eggs, butter, etc. Some people also remove oils completely when following the WFPB diet because they are heavily processed. These decisions are made on a case-by-case basis.

Many patients are afraid to cut out meat, dairy and gluten because they feel that with their _____ (insert foods here) allergies they won't be able to get enough protein. That may be the case for people who stick to processed food or have very restricted diets. However, plant-based eating, when done the right way, naturally provides the body with ample building blocks for physiological functions (except for vitamin B12, which may need to be supplemented). Some sources also recommend extra support for choline, iodine, omega-3 fatty acids, taurine, zinc and vitamins A, D and K when following a vegan diet.

Proteins are chains of amino acids that have important roles in our body. They form enzymes, hormones, antibodies and new tissue. Proteins help transport nutrients, break down toxins and regenerate cells. Out of the 22 amino acids that make up proteins, nine of them (known as "essential" amino acids) are not manufactured by the body and need to be obtained dietarily.

The Dietary Reference Intake (DRI) recommendations for daily protein consumption are 0.36 grams of protein per pound of body weight (or 0.8 grams of protein per kilogram of body weight). Someone weighing 140 pounds (~63 kilograms) would need approximately 50 grams of protein per day based on these recommendations. This equates to approximately five servings of plant protein per day or one to two servings of meat (depending on the type). Restaurants in Westernized cultures often present animal product portions that vastly exceed a single serving size and the recommended daily intake of protein. Excess protein cannot be stored in the body and eliminating it puts strain on the kidneys and liver. There's a huge misconception about how much protein we really need. It turns out we need less than we think—but of course, it's become an industry and it's ingrained into our culture, so people often refute this.

A proper plant-based diet is chock-full of non-meat protein sources like beans, lentils, nuts, seeds, hummus, tofu and whole grains. Combining grains and beans as part of daily protein intake may help provide the body with the full array of amino acids in addition to fiber sources. Fruits and vegetables also contain relatively small amounts of protein that can add up to support the total intake. For example, one ¼-cup pumpkin seeds, one cup of quinoa, one sweet potato and one cup of chickpeas is equivalent to approximately 50 grams of protein.

It's very plausible to obtain the DRI recommendations for dietary protein without consuming soy and many of my patients choose to avoid soy completely; however, there are many misconceptions about soy products. Tofu is not the soy/estrogen monster that some people make it out to be. Evidence supports that soy actually lowers the risk of reproductive cancers![77-79]

Robust evidence exists that significant beneficial effects are noted with plant-based diets when compared to conventional diets. Plant-based diets also appear to increase the diversity of the gastrointestinal microbiome (compared to those on the standard American diet), which has protective effects.[62] Epidemiological studies, including research evaluating upwards of 96,000 participants, note that people who eat plant-based diets have lower rates of cardiovascular disease and lower all-cause mortality compared to participants eating conventional (meat and dairy) diets.[80-82] A

2019 study found that the risk of heart failure decreased by 41% in individuals eating more plant-based foods.[83] Whole, plant-based foods, such as fruits, vegetables and whole grains, are high in protein and fiber, which helps slow the digestion of carbohydrates so we don't experience a sudden spike in blood sugar followed by a crash. Going plant-based can even control glucose levels/diabetes without the need for medications in many cases.

Removing fish from the diet may also have positive impacts on health. Based on literature systematic reviews, toxic levels of arsenic and lead have been noted in sources like shellfish and tuna.[84,85] Mercury is commonly studied due to its ability to be absorbed up the food chain in all types of fish-eating species, and it can create toxic bioaccumulation in humans.[86] On the global scale, persistent bio-accumulative and toxic pollutants continue to equate to ongoing consumer risk with exposure to fish. Reviews confirm that pollutant levels exceed EPA (Environmental Protection Agency) screening values.[87]

Wild caught fish (as opposed to farmed) can reduce the risk of things like antibiotics and parasites in sources, but this does not offer as much protection as we originally thought against toxins. Polycyclic aromatic hydrocarbon (PAH) toxins are present when fish are cooked in certain ways. PAHs are present in alarming levels on fish, regardless of the type of environment, the fish habitat and the exposure route, and this significantly increases oxidative stress and inflammation in the body.[88]

Westernized cultures associate the idea that the ripped and attractive macho man (or woman) eats a lot of meat. But many of the world's top elite athletes are plant-based and find that the diet improves performance, recovery and overall health. Muscle mass has to do with loading and the way the body is exercised. Further, our ancestors were mostly gatherers who very rarely had meat as a treat. While some people were hunting, others were gathering and living off the land, and the fruits of the gathering labor are what sustained the hunters to chase after animals for days on end.

Another misconception is that plant-based eating is not flavorful and filling. This is far from the truth! Interestingly, plant-based groceries can actually save money. Even when shopping organic, less junk from the aisles and from the meat/dairy section typically translates to savings. When following a WFPB Diet, it's important that you don't gravitate toward the "replacement" foods like processed dairy and meat substitutes, vegan cheese and ice cream, etc. Those products can definitely add up financially, and they are often filled with additives and unhealthy substances.

Physicians from the American College of Cardiology, the Physicians Committee for Responsible Medicine and the World Health Organization support a WFPB diet or a similar option such as the true Mediterranean diet where meat is only consumed 1–2 times per month.[63] However, it's noted that heart disease can still progress on the Mediterranean diet, and the WFPB diet is the only approach shown to reverse heart disease.[63]

The WFPB approach has yet to be studied within the trifecta conditions, but many patients find that a modified/individualized version of this can be tremendously helpful. Plant-based eating includes the most nutrient-dense food we can find. It fuels the body with rich antioxidants and healing nutrients and has indicators of better gastrointestinal absorption in the long run. The literature on the WFPB diet is a stark and refreshing contrast from other dietary trends that cite conflicting evidence and concerning stories of adverse events and escalating disease.

Other Approaches

Many patients in the migraine community follow low-tyramine diets. Tyramine is an amino acid commonly found in aged and fermented foods. Certain medications containing monoamine oxidase (MAO) inhibitors block the breakdown of tyramine, so some patients are advised to a follow a low-tyramine diet for this reason too.

A low-glutamate diet is often utilized for patients who have autism spectrum disorders, sensory processing issues and other conditions. This approach eliminates food additives such as monosodium glutamate (MSG).

A number of additional dietary approaches are popular in the chronic illness patient community, including the Paleo approach, the Autoimmune Protocol (AIP), the Mediterranean diet, the MIND (Mediterranean-DASH Intervention for Neurodegenerative Delay), and the Whole 30. In this chapter I chose to focus on the ones that I currently get the most questions about from patients, but the meat/dairy vs. plant-based logic can be applied to other dietary variations.

As you can see, there are many dietary trends and approaches out there and there are many patient-specific factors to consider when making dietary choices. There's no silver bullet dietary approach for managing the trifecta. I am not here to tell you to suddenly go vegan overnight. The Whole Food Plant-Based (WFPB) Diet has the best scientific evidence and appears to be the safest and most fruitful approach (pun intended!). Integrating components of the WFPB Diet into your healing diet plan may be a good goal to work toward over time.

Don't be too hard on yourself if you're not able to integrate colorful dietary diversity just yet. Not everyone can dive into a fruit- and vegetable-heavy nutrient focus due to sensitivities and reactions. However, no matter where you're at in your own journey, you may want to—at a bare minimum—follow a low-toxin dietary approach.

THE LOW-TOXIN DIET

Hopefully after Chapter 6 I don't need to explain why we should be avoiding toxins. It's not realistic to go about our lives living in a bubble, but reducing the overall toxic burden can have a tremendous impact on helping restore the system so that it is better able to heal and reduce the inflammatory burden over time. Over the years I've compiled some of the best practices that help to reduce dietary exposure to toxins.

Low-Toxin Diet principles include the following suggestions:

- Focus on organic fresh vegetables and fruits.
- Focus on lemon water and decaf herbal tea for beverage choices.
- Focus on foods to help with the detoxification process (as tolerated), such as cruciferous veggies, cilantro, onion, garlic and parsley.
- Focus on healing herbs, fruits and vegetables that naturally reduce inflammation and mast cell mediators. (See Tables 20 and 21 of this chapter.)
- Avoid processed foods, food additives/preservatives/dyes, GMOs, etc. If the label contains more than just the food name itself (this even goes for frozen fruit/vegetables and pre-chopped fresh greens!), then find another option.
- Use organic local honey or maple for a sugar source (no cane sugar, beet sugar, fructose, etc.).
- Avoid gum, packaged snacks, candy, etc.
- Avoid processed sauces, dressings, and condiments. Make your own simple salad dressings and sauces from scratch.
- Avoid toxic beverages including alcohol, soda, etc.
- Avoid coffee, peanuts and chocolate due to high mycotoxin contamination (and caffeine in the case of coffee and chocolate). Some coffee brands have third party testing for mycotoxins, but avoiding caffeine is also important while focusing on detoxification.
- Avoid most grains including gluten and corn. Some individuals will continue to ingest organic/gluten free rice, oats or quinoa (as long as arsenic is not an issue—with rice).
- Avoid all dairy products.
- Ensure plenty of water/hydration.

- Pay attention to your water source (filtered is recommended) and container (glass or stainless steel are advised).
- Pay attention to food containers. Avoid storing food in plastic. Avoid canned food and the use of aluminum or nonstick cookware.
- Avoid charring or deep-frying foods.
- If using oil, stick to cooking with organic olive, avocado and coconut oils.
- Avoid or limit fish and meat intake.

Note: Some patients continue to eat meat/eggs in smaller proportions, seeking out grass-fed, organic, pasture-raised options. If opting to continue eating fish, seek smaller, non-farmed sources. Some patients prefer to avoid soy products as well.

It's very possible that you are already following these principles, and if so, that's fantastic! If you still feel you have work to do in this area, sometimes it's easier on the body (and mind) to work up to gradually following these principles.

Breaking these suggestions into bite-sized goals can help. For example, on week one, you could remove dairy products and set a goal to increase your daily fruit/vegetable intake by two servings. On week two, you could phase out your processed salad dressings and replace them with olive oil and salt. The following week you could focus on reducing sugar intake, and so on. If you are feeding a large family, it can help to start with small steps, such as prioritization of purchasing the "dirty dozen" foods in the organic section.

If you're unsure where to begin, you could start with elimination of preservatives, food dyes and flavorings. In the United States, there are over 3,000 FDA-approved preservatives.[89] They are added to prevent the spoilage of food in transit. Essentially, the only "safe" foods are those grown in a home garden, or perhaps those organic sources found in a local farmers market. Reading labels can seem like a daunting task, and many words are coded in a "healthy" way to disguise that they are preservatives; "natural flavoring," "citric acid," "sodium nitrite," "sulfur dioxide," "potassium sorbate" and "benzoic acid" are some examples.[89]

The more straightforward and ideal option is to buy only organic foods and avoid shopping in the packaged grocery aisles, instead sticking to the fresh produce sections. Use fresh herbs instead of purchasing "seasoning" type spices, which often contain hidden ingredients. Make your own homemade juice, sparkling water and loose-leaf tea. If a product contains a label, make sure to read it to avoid additives.

It's best to avoid "replacing" foods that you miss from the standard American diet with other processed products that are laden with additives. A great example of this is vegan cheese, which often contains several chemicals and unhealthy ingredients.

The exception to this may be coffee, where you may experience physical withdrawals. There are some great herbal teas that taste and look very similar to coffee, and this can be helpful if you're attempting to reduce or stop your coffee intake.

As a general rule of thumb, it's best to increase your ratio of fruits and veggies instead of substituting processed comfort foods for the comfort foods you may decide to remove. Physical withdrawal symptoms and cravings can also occur when reducing processed sugar intake, and fruit-based snacks like a few dates or a bowl of blueberries with honey can help reduce these cravings.

I know there are a lot of "no's" in this list, and the overarching idea is to focus on healing and life-giving choices as opposed to a list of things that are off-limits. However, there are a lot of marketing schemes and misinformation out there, so it's definitely important to avoid the most common pitfalls that make it hard to find healing.

To promote maximal healing, the following foods and beverages should be avoided:

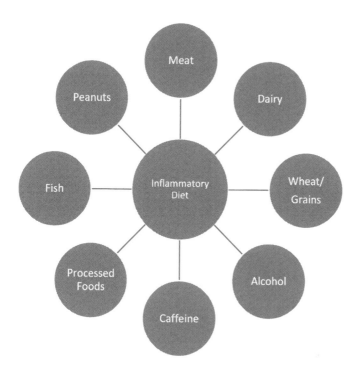

- Meat slows digestion and clogs up the bowels, breeding bacterial overgrowth in the gut. It is often contaminated with hormones, steroids and grains.
- Dairy products lead to poor cell function, the slowing of detoxification, and an increase in chemicals and inappropriate hormones in the body.
- Wheat is harmful to the intestinal lining and leads to poor nutrient absorption. Corn, rice and other grains can also be inflammatory to the GI tract and sometimes contain toxins/heavy metals. Wheat

should be 100% avoided and other grains should be kept to a minimum.

- Alcohol strains the liver and other detox organs and reduces key nutrients like magnesium and zinc.
- Caffeine can increase the level of toxins in the body. Coffee beans are often contaminated with mycotoxins. Coffee can be contaminated with mold-related toxins in the way that it is processed, stored and transported,[90] and bean harvesting location, practices, altitude, climate and other factors influence each batch.
- Peanuts are a big source of aflatoxins and defective/deteriorating peanuts are often used to make peanut butter.
- Unfortunately, many fish sources are polluted with heavy metals and need to be avoided during a detox diet. If you are going to eat fish, occasional ingestion of the more acceptable wild-caught smaller fish (like salmon, monkfish and tilapia) may provide less fish-based exposure to toxins. Some people use the acronym "SMASH" (salmon, mackerel, anchovies, sardines and herring) to refer to the smaller types of fish that are high in omega-3 fatty acids and less likely to be contaminated with mercury.
- Processed foods contain many additives, preservatives, sugar, dyes and toxins. Sugar alternatives/artificial sweeteners also should be avoided.

The bottom line is, don't find foods to "replace" your comfort foods. Change your focus and your taste buds will change with you!

Focus on healing vegetables, fruits, beans, legumes, nuts and seeds. These foods are high in fiber and help move toxins out of the body through the gut. Shop organic as much as possible. Vegetables and fruits contain enzymes that help improve digestion and detoxification, in addition to their high concentration of phytonutrients and antioxidants. Aim for at least 10 servings a day of fruits and vegetables! Keep in mind that protein needs have been misguided culturally, and plant-based healing foods can provide the body with ample protein for daily needs. (This is, of course, describing a scenario where individuals can tolerate these options. Many patients may need to follow modified versions as opposed to complete adherence to one specific approach, particularly until addressing root issues helps to expand dietary options.)

Find the right balance. Moving toward a Whole Food Plant-Based Diet is the way to go for a sustainable long-term plan, but keep in mind that you may have to progress slowly, listen to your body and make customized adaptations. Because of the complexity of food-related issues in patients with the trifecta, working with a nutritionist who is an expert in your conditions can be an extremely valuable resource. Some patients are so limited in their fruit and vegetable choices that eliminating meat, fish, and eggs or grains leads to malnutrition, improper calorie intake and disordered eating. Obviously, each individual must proceed with caution and honor what their body is telling them. Dietary changes can have a profound impact not only on inflammation and overall homeostasis but on tissue healing, vascular dynamics, detoxification and mast cell mediator release—key areas for patients who experience symptoms of the trifecta.

Detox Diet Guidelines:

An extreme diet change can be unpleasant and too straining on the body, so unless you're already eating a clean diet, you may need to start with avoidance of processed foods and then remove other unhealthy food sources in a stepwise manner. When you suddenly cut out high sugar levels and processed foods, you may find the first few weeks to be tough as your body has been accustomed to these foods. Keep faith that you will reap the improvements in higher energy, lower fatigue and reduced symptoms if you commit to eating cleaner. Supplements and ample hydration can help to improve detoxification. Two bowel movements per day are very important so that toxins don't recirculate. It's also useful to get daily exercise and to sweat to aid the detox process. (See Chapter 11, "Detoxification," for more strategies.)

The Low-Toxin Diet may not be realistic for every patient for the long haul, and this is not necessarily the goal. The problem with many eating approaches is that they are only followed for a few weeks or months before people tend to fall off. Commit to following this for three to six months and then check in to see where you're at with your health. The idea is to reduce toxic load on your system so that your organs have time to heal; ultimately, the goal is to provide your body with more energy availability for healing functions without being as inflamed, reactive and bogged down trying to process your everyday toxin exposure. Reduced sensitivity to food and other triggers is often a welcome side effect of the Low-Toxin Diet. It certainly requires discipline and a commitment to making most of your meals at home, and the benefits are not typically immediately obvious overnight. Many patients start this eating plan with the intention to try it for three to six months and end up sticking with it longer because of how good they feel.

Table 21. Examples of Foods in a Low-Toxin Diet[91,92]

	Encouraged	Advised to Avoid
FRUIT	Fresh fruits that aid detox: apples, avocados, lemons, melons, oranges, pears, peaches, pineapple, plums, tomatoes Neutral fruits: all remaining fresh fruit	

	Encouraged	Advised to Avoid
VEGETABLES	Veggies to aid detox: cruciferous veggies (broccoli, cauliflower, kale, brussels sprouts, cabbage, cauliflower), garlic, ginger, onions, radish, raw greens (red and green lettuce, romaine, spinach, endive), watercress Neutral veggies: green beans, peas, legumes, yams and sweet potatoes, all other fresh veggies not on the avoid list	Corn White potatoes Soybeans/soy products Possibly: Other nightshades (tomatoes, eggplant, bell peppers)
PROTEIN	Ideally, protein should come from plant sources such as lentils, quinoa, chickpeas, spirulina, almonds, chia, hemp, black beans, broccoli and gluten free oats. Some patients may still choose to eat: organic chicken, pork, turkey or lamb, wild caught fish	Anything processed with preservatives, nitrates or nitrites (sausage, bacon, lunch meat, etc.) Eggs Red meat

	Encouraged	Advised to Avoid
NUTS & SEEDS	Almonds, walnuts, pecans, cashews Sesame (tahini) Sunflower, pumpkin seeds Flax seeds, chia seeds, hemp seeds	Peanuts Peanut butter Sweetened nut butters
GRAINS	Gluten-free brown rice, millet, quinoa, buckwheat, gluten free oats	White rice, wheat, rye, barley, potato flour
SWEETENERS	(In moderation) Stevia, agave, honey, pure maple syrup	Refined sugars, artificial sweeteners, cane sugar, corn syrup, glucose, sucrose, dextrose
BEVERAGES	Water, non-caffeinated herbal teas, lemon or lime water, unsweetened milk substitutes (almond, coconut, oat, hemp, etc.)	Alcohol, coffee, caffeinated tea, soda, sports drinks, dairy milk, soymilk, non-dairy creamers
SPICES & CONDIMENTS	Fresh and dried herbs and spices (organic preferred), oils (olive, avocado, flaxseed, sesame, coconut, etc.), vinegar (except malt)	Canola oil, corn oil, malt vinegar, processed dressings/sauces/condiments, soy sauce, prepackaged seasonings

A HEALING APPROACH

Meal Hygiene

"Meal hygiene" is an often-overlooked aspect of healing from chronic illness. It's not just about *what* we eat but *how* we eat it. Be sure to chew your food more than you normally would, to slow down, to eat sitting in a relaxing environment away from screens/electronics (and never while on the road or when you're about to leave the home). (I know, easier said than done, right!) If you still find yourself eating too quickly, stop and do three deep, diaphragmatic breaths in between each bite of food and consider taking smaller bites.

Most patients with the trifecta have a high level of sympathetic nervous system activation and do not spend enough time in "rest and digest" mode. Building the time and space to promote better digestion is crucial. Be sure to avoid emotional eating of comfort foods in reaction to sadness, fatigue, anxiety or depression. Also avoid eating when you are in the middle of a fight or stressful moment. It's also really important to avoid eating a large meal before bed because the digestion process will cut into the hours in the middle of the night where the liver is in prime repair mode.

Factors that influence gastrointestinal digestion and absorption may need to be considered. Some patients do better with produce that is cooked compared to raw. Some individuals do better with juice made at home, smoothies or pureed foods compared to whole foods, particularly early on in the healing process. Patients with gastrointestinal issues sometimes find that nutritional formulas, such as Kate Farms or Metagenics Ultra GI Replenish, can help give the digestive system a break and restore proper nutrients in order to heal. Again, trial and error are important to find an optimal way to maintain individualized healing nutrients in the diet.

The Elimination Diet

Some patients find that an elimination diet is necessary at the beginning of their healing journey in order to discern which foods are triggering immediate and delayed reactions. Research supports that a very short-term diet that eliminates certain types of foods will make it more likely that the patient can resume dietary variety, ensure nutritional adequacy and minimize impact on the gastrointestinal microbiota when compared to longer-term restrictive diets.[93] The key here is that this process is very short, less than four to six weeks in total, if possible, in order to avoid increasing your food sensitivities. At the same time, some experts recommend waiting two to three days between the introduction of another new food in order to determine if delayed reactions may occur. The goal is to keep careful track of symptoms in order to determine what food(s) may be triggering a response during an elimination diet. Delayed reactions due to IgG antibodies can occur one to two days following exposure to a trigger and may not be recognized as the causative factor.

You should avoid using spices, oils and other additions to foods during an elimination diet—the aim is to piece-by-piece determine one specific item at a time. It's crucial that while doing an elimination diet, only organic foods without additives are utilized. The most accurate results will be reflected if you avoid processed foods and items that could be cross-contaminated. During an elimination diet, experts also recommend the bare minimum in terms of vitamins, supplements and medications (within reason) in order to figure out what is causing flares.

This is different from the Low-Toxin Diet. An elimination diet essentially strips you down to one or two staple foods and then one new food is reintroduced at a time. This process should definitely be guided with the help of your medical team. If you opt for an elimination trial, the ultimate goal is re-diversification of healthy dietary components. Creating a healthy lifestyle plan isn't necessarily all about taking things away—it's about adding healthy practices to enhance healing potential, with proper attention to avoidance of toxins (in the diet and environment) that may serve as barriers.

Both food and chemical sensitivities can trigger similar symptoms in some patients. With different triggers eliciting the same response, it can be tricky to determine what a patient is reacting to. Once you find a "baseline" diet, it may be useful to expand the concept of the elimination diet to include one-by-one introduction of nondietary sources of chemicals, such as products used regularly (like toothpaste, shampoo, skin care and makeup) in order to best isolate the findings and address as many potential triggers as possible.

Flare-Reducing Practices

It's recommended that individuals who are sensitive to certain foods provide an environment for the least amount of cross-contamination and "pollution" by using clean kitchen practices, eating organic high-quality food sources, using non-toxic cookware and food storage, having allergen-free zones of the kitchen and fridge, freezing leftovers instead of putting them in the fridge, etc. Additional tips for safe food environments were discussed in Chapter 6, "External Health Stressors."

A do-it-yourself garden helps ensure that the end product on the table is clean and chemical free. Farmers markets can also make the process of adding more fruits and vegetables fun, while supporting the local economy. For patients who live in cold climates, indoor stackable gardens can be set up with a trip to the hardware store and may be a good option for winter months.

Cooking should be fun and rewarding. Certain kitchen gadgets can make the process of healthy eating much more time efficient. Devices like immersion blenders, cold-pressed juice machines, garlic presses, and vegetable spiralizers can be helpful for meal preparation.

I encourage patients to view the topic of food with a focus on nourishment and healing from the inside out. The body is responsive to our thoughts and knows when we are coming from a place of anxiety or negativity. Too often, patients develop a fear of food after being hyper-focused on elimination diets and long-term restrictive eating. (This is not to say that you should never try an elimination diet; they can be helpful initially for identifying inflammatory culprits.)

Having a healing diet full of diverse options is not as simple as it sounds, particularly for complex patients who are reactive to much of what they try. Some individuals become so inflamed and struggle with toxins and other health stressors to the point where they are down to a handful of "safe" options. For these individuals, a root issues approach and a big focus on retraining the nervous system are often essential before dietary diversity can be achieved again. In other cases, the diet may be restricted from voluntary removal of options based on internet food lists as opposed to individual tolerance, and reintegration of healing nutrients comes easier.

Culturally, we need to reframe the way we look at food, change what we are putting into our bodies as part of a long-term lifestyle plan, and consider eating as an investment into our health and longevity bank account. Success isn't returning to a "normal" diet or finding substitutions for comfort foods. Rather, success is changing our taste buds and nourishing ourselves from the inside out as a healing way of life, and never looking back.

Healing Through Diet

Part of changing our food narrative and the message we tell ourselves (and our mast cells) relies around focusing on nutrient-dense foods that naturally support our body's clearance of toxins, mast cell mediators and other inflammatory compounds.

Below is a chart based off multiple scientific sources listing natural fruits, vegetables and grains that *may be* beneficial for someone who suffers from food allergies, food sensitivities, hives, anaphylaxis, inflammation, etc. Keep in mind that much of the available research is test-tube and animal-based and does not necessarily reflect a human patient's symptomatic response. *The chart below reflects a literature investigation for each listed food with theoretical benefits but is not considered all-inclusive.*

Several foods—including apple, beet, black rice bran, citrus fruit, cucumber, garlic, mangosteen, onion, peach, pomegranate and watercress—consistently have literature support implicating careful consideration of their *potential utility* for patients who experience symptoms consistent with MCAS. However, some of these foods may fall into certain classes (such as the birch family) that sensitive individuals may react to; *as always, an individualized approach is advised.*

Table 22. Fruits, Vegetables and Other Foods That *May Be* Helpful for the Patient with Chronic Illness[94-128]

FOOD	PROPOSED BENEFIT(S)
Amaranth	inhibits anaphylaxis, IgE production and cytokines
Apple	antihistaminic, suppresses mast cell activation, antiviral
Apricot	anti-allergy, anti-inflammatory, antiviral
Artichoke	source of rutin/luteolin (mast cell stabilizing), anti-inflammatory, antiviral
Avocado	aids skin rashes, antibacterial, antiviral
Beet (root and leaves)	reduces bradykinin-mediated swelling, anti-inflammatory, reduces cytokines
Black rice bran	suppresses mast cell mediators, reduces edema
Broccoli	anti-allergy, anti-inflammatory, antiviral
Buckwheat	inhibits histamine and cytokine release
Butternut squash	suppresses IgE antibody production
Cabbage	reduces airway inflammation
Capers	antihistaminic, inhibits mast cell mediator release
Carrot	reduces inflammation, boosts the immune system, assists with skin and wound issues
Cherry	anti-allergy, anti-inflammatory, antiviral
Chicory	anti-allergy, anti-inflammatory
Cilantro	reduces food allergies, boosts the immune system, aids detoxification
Cucumber	reduces prostaglandin/histamine/serotonin/bradykinin/proteases, antioxidant, analgesic, aids skin conditions, reduces respiratory ailments
Fig	soothes respiratory ailments, reduces inflammation
Garlic (fresh)	anti-allergic, immune boosting, reduces airway inflammation, reduces IgE-mediated swelling
Grapefruit	assists respiratory problems

Green Pepper	anti-allergy, anti-inflammatory, antiviral
Lemon	reduces airway inflammation, anti-allergy, source of flavonoids
Lime	reduces chest and throat inflammation, boosts the immune system
Mangosteen	antihistaminic, inhibits mast cell degranulation, reduces prostaglandins, leukotrienes, interleukins
Oats	antihistaminic, antioxidant, boosts the immune system
Onion	reduces food allergies, antihistaminic, stabilizes mast cells, reduces airway inflammation
Orange	reduces airway inflammation, anti-allergy, source of flavonoids
Parsley	antihistaminic, anti-inflammatory, analgesic
Pea sprouts	source of flavonoids, antioxidant
Peach	anti-allergy, antihistaminic, reduces cytokines
Pomegranate	antihistaminic, reduces prostaglandins, inhibits mast cell derived cytokines, anti-inflammatory
Sweet potato	antihistaminic, anti-inflammatory, analgesic
Tangerine	anti-allergy, anti-inflammatory, antiviral
Watercress	antihistaminic, immune-boosting, anti-inflammatory
Zucchini	anti-inflammatory, analgesic, antihistaminic

There are also many plants and herbs that are purported to have similar benefits, as depicted below in Table 23. Black cumin seed, chamomile, coriander, echinacea, elderflower, ginger, goldenrod, holy basil, lotus root, marshmallow, nettle, peppermint, red ginger (galangal), saffron, thyme and turmeric are supported by multiple literature sources as *theoretically beneficial* for patients with symptoms of MCAS. Many of these are available in organic tea form as well as in powdered spice form for use with cooking.

There has been some recent concern about the potential for turmeric to reduce diamine oxidase (DAO) levels. As previously discussed, DAO is an enzyme that breaks down histamine levels in the body. A 2016 study noted a reduction in DAO levels when rats with acute enteritis had seven days of the supplement turmeric.[129] However, the same subjects showed a reduction in TNF-alpha and certain interleukins, indicating a reduction in overall inflammation.[129]

As is often the case with foods, natural substances can induce many different properties on the physiological level. The concern over turmeric and DAO levels is an example highlighting the importance that though these are "natural" supplements, their physiological effects are still being determined, so a general level of caution is warranted. At the same time, it's best to look at the big picture, as discussed in the earlier example of green tea and mast cells.

Patients with MCAS are far from uniform in terms of tolerance to difference foods and supplements, so these charts should serve as a starting point from which to evaluate on a case-by-case basis.

Table 23 reflects a literature investigation for each listed plant/herb with theoretical benefits but is not considered all-inclusive. Herbs, plants and spices can interact with other medications and certain parts of plants can be toxic, so experimentation in this area should be closely guided by your medical team.

Table 23. Plants, Herbs, and Other Sources That *May Be* Helpful for the Patient with Chronic Illness[96,117,130-187]

PLANT/HERB	PROPOSED BENEFIT(S)
Agrimony	reduces long-term food allergies
Ajowan	reduces food allergies
Aloe vera	aids skin rashes
Alpha lipoic acid	anti-allergic, mast cell stabilizing
Annato	antihistaminic, reduces vascular permeability
Ashwagandha	reduces mediator release/vascular permeability
Astralagus	assists with multiple allergies
Baikal skullcap	reduces allergic rhinitis and hay fever
Basil	boosts the immune system, reduces sinus and chest inflammation
Berberine	reduces prostaglandin synthesis
Black cumin seed	reduces food allergies, antihistaminic, suppresses prostaglandins and leukotrienes
Boneset	reduces allergic rhinitis and hay fever
Boswellia serrata	mast cell stabilizing, inhibits degranulation, anti-asthmatic
Burdock root	aids skin rashes
Butterbur	reduces seasonal allergies
Camu camu	mast cell stabilizing effects of vitamin C
Cardamom	aids respiratory problems
Caraway seeds	antihistaminic
Catnip	reduces seasonal allergies
Chamomile	antihistaminic, reduces allergies and rashes
Cinnamon	reduces airway inflammation
Clove	reduces airway inflammation
Common plantain	relieves allergic rhinitis and hay fever
Coriander	stabilizes mast cells, inhibits mast cell mediators, assists respiratory problems, hay fever and allergies

Cumin	boosts the immune system, reduces severe allergies
Devil's claw	reduces seasonal allergies
EGCG (green tea)	inhibits mast cell degranulation, antihistaminic, inhibits vascular permeability
Echinacea	reduces allergic rhinitis and hay fever, boosts the immune system, reduces throat inflammation
Elderberry	reduces respiratory issues, reduces oxidative stress, improves detoxification and blood sugar regulation, antiviral and antibacterial properties
Elderflower	relieves allergic rhinitis and hay fever, sinusitis
Evening primrose	reduces seasonal allergies
Eyebright	relieves allergic rhinitis and hay fever
Fenugreek	reduces skin rashes, airway and sinus inflammation
Feverfew	anti-allergic, antihistaminic, anti-inflammatory
Flaxseed oil	reduces skin inflammation, antihistaminic
Galangal (red ginger)	reduces food allergies, suppresses mast cell degranulation, prevents anaphylaxis, lowers prostaglandin E2
Ginger	inhibits leukotrienes and prostaglandins, soothes throat inflammation
Ginkgo	reduces airway inflammation
Goldenrod	reduces allergic rhinitis, hay fever and respiratory inflammation
Holy basil	antihistaminic, anti-anaphylactic, stabilizes mast cells
Honey	reduces allergic rhinitis, throat inflammation and respiratory issues
Khellin	mast cell stabilizing
Lemon balm	reduces allergies, aids respiratory issues, antihistaminic
Lemongrass	boosts the immune system, antioxidant
Licorice root	anti-allergy, reduces airway inflammation, aids rashes
Lotus root	stabilizes mast cells, anti-inflammatory
Luteolin	mast cell stabilizing

Marshmallow	reduces allergic rhinitis, hay fever, throat and skin irritation
Melatonin	mast cell stabilizing, cytoprotective effects
Milk thistle (silibinin)	reduces food allergies and inflammation, stabilizes mast cells
Mint	reduces food allergies
Moringa	inhibits mast cell degranulation, antihistaminic
Neem	antihistaminic, anti-inflammatory, antioxidant
Nettle leaf	reduces food allergies, rashes, allergic rhinitis, hay fever and seasonal allergies, antihistaminic, stabilizes mast cells
Olive (fruit/leaf/oil)	stabilizes mast cells, antihistaminic
Oregano	antihistaminic, may inhibit prostaglandin release, anti-inflammatory
Peppermint	antihistaminic, reduces sinus and lung inflammation
Plantain leaf	reduces allergies and aids rashes
Pycnogenol	inhibits histamine release
Quercetin	anti-inflammatory, mast cell stabilizing
Red clover	anti-allergy, reduces skin reactions
Resveratrol	antihistaminic, mast cell stabilizing
Rosemary	aids skin issues, antibacterial and antifungal
Saffron	antihistaminic, reduces throat and airway inflammation
Sage	aids recurrent coughs and allergies
Schisandra	inhibits mast cell cytokine release, antioxidant
Slippery elm	reduces food allergies
Spirulina	antihistaminic, anti-inflammatory, reduces allergic rhinitis, inhibits anaphylaxis
St. John's wort	aids skin rashes
Tarragon	anti-inflammatory, analgesic, may inhibit mast cell mediators
Thyme	reduces food allergies, rashes, itching, allergic rhinitis and hay fever, stabilizes mast cells, inhibits anaphylaxis, boosts the immune system
Turmeric (curcumin)	reduces food allergies, antihistaminic, inhibits mast cell reactions and anaphylaxis, reduces airway inflammation

Vitamin C	antihistaminic, mast cell stabilizing
Vitamin D	mast cell stabilizing
Yarrow	aids sinusitis, hay fever and allergies

Nutritionist Resources

One of the most overwhelming aspects of daily life for patients with trifecta conditions lies in dietary decisions, particularly when the gastrointestinal system is inflamed or dysfunctional. A patient survey published in 2018 noted that only 10.7% of patients with MCAD reported being referred to a dietician, highlighting the dire need for more clinical attention in this area.[188]

As apparent in a quick glance at the above charts, navigating the nutritional world with chronic illness—particularly when patients who have any of the trifecta conditions can be seriously reactive to different foods—is extremely tricky. Nutritionists can be an important resource for the initial and ongoing management of the trifecta. Just like any discipline, it's useful to call ahead and verify that a practitioner is knowledgeable in your medical condition(s).

Nutritionists, naturopaths and functional medicine providers well versed in MCAS, POTS and EDS typically focus on reducing toxic load and allergic foods, replenishing deficient nutrients, ensuring adequate fiber intake and gut motility, healing the gut lining, enhancing digestive enzymes and optimal acid levels, re-populating the microbiome and supporting the body with substances that will naturally reduce mast cell mediators and inflammatory compounds. Often, reactivity to a particular food one day that was previously well tolerated is more of an indicator that the body's pathways are struggling; when the pathway is in disorder, a bigger buildup of inflammatory mediators can result.[189]

It's very helpful to work with a professional who is well-versed in all of the above in order to find a healing dietary approach. Visit http://www.mastcellsunited.com/telehealth to view a listing of providers (including nutritionists) who are well-versed in the trifecta and who offer telehealth appointments.

NUTRITION & THE TRIFECTA: TAKE-HOME MESSAGES

Due to cultural popularity of trends not backed by evidence, we are faced with the choice of turning down the flame on one chemical mediator like histamine (one of the hundreds released by mast cells) OR removing other systemic burdens and fueling the body with crucial nutrients to find healing and re-diversify food choices. Do we want to focus our food story on one area, or on overall systemic healing from toxins that we encounter in foods and beverages? Do we choose to eliminate all sorts of healing vegetables and fruits in order to appease one naturally occurring food category, or would we rather zoom out to see diet from an overall inflammatory burden perspective? Granted, the choices aren't the same for everyone and aren't simple when you're in the midst of a flare and are reacting to everything. But over time, with the right approach, healing of dietary issues is possible.

- Avoid comparison. Be in tune with your body. Do what feels right for your body.
- Find a stable baseline first before experimenting with new foods.
- Short-term elimination diets can be helpful, but they are not long-term solutions, and long-term restrictive diets that eliminate healing fruits and vegetables can cause harm.
- Avoid "blind" elimination of foods for the long term because they are high in _____ (histamine, salicylates, etc.) on internet lists

(unless they are foods that have toxic/inflammatory effects or the obvious allergic reaction).

- Practice mindful eating. Slow it down!
- Have patience with yourself. Know that there will be ups and downs until you find a healing eating plan that works for you.
- Keeping a food log can be helpful in the first months to determine trends but avoid over-focusing on reactions in the long run.
- Consider utilizing a Low-Toxin Diet and Whole Food Plant-Based eating for long-term healing.
- Consider enlisting the help of a nutritionist who is well-versed in MCAS, POTS and EDS.
- Reframe the way you think about food. Focus on bringing life-giving, healing nutrients into your diet instead of a list of "no's."
- The more that underlying root issues are addressed, the greater the tendency to enjoy a diverse diet with minimal food reactions. (Root issues that typically influence patients with the trifecta include internal health stressors like bacterial/fungal/viral infections and an unhealthy gut, external health stressors like mold and toxins, nervous system dysregulation, structural and musculoskeletal issues, lack of exercise, poor detoxification and emotional trauma/stress.)
- Dietary healing is influenced by so many factors beyond the gut! At the same time, gut health is so important for systemic healing, so don't neglect this area.
- What types of dietary approaches have you tried, and what has been the most helpful for your body? Are there root issues that still need to be addressed to help expand food options? Are you following a Low-Toxin Diet? Reflect on this topic in your Trifecta Passport worksheet.

Chapter 9:
STRUCTURAL &
MUSCULOSKELETAL ISSUES

As noted in Chapter 3, many structural and musculoskeletal issues can arise in patients who experience hypermobility and connective tissue abnormalities. This subject alone could be the topic of an entire book. In my own clinical practice, three recurrent structural/musculoskeletal themes consistently arise in patients with the trifecta: craniocervical instability, pelvic floor muscle issues and dysfunction of the ileocecal valve [which is often connected to iliopsoas muscle tone abnormalities, small intestinal bacterial overgrowth (SIBO) and a history of emotional trauma]. This chapter will dive into these topics, and at the end I will summarize some trifecta toolbox options for managing pain. Keep in mind that there are many other different types of structural and musculoskeletal issues that commonly occur in this patient population, and a physical therapist can be a great ally in addressing concerns as they arise.

Craniocervical Instability (CCI)

Craniocervical instability (CCI) is a condition where the ligaments of the neck are injured, damaged or become loose from congenital factors, leading to unstable movements of the head on the neck at the craniocervical junction, where the skull meets the spine. The term CCI is often interchangeable with occipitoatlantoaxial hypermobility, Barre

Lieou syndrome, posterior cervical sympathetic syndrome and upper cervical instability. Instability can also occur between levels C1 and C2 (the upper two vertebra of the spine) which is known as atlantoaxial instability (AAI). CCI and AAI together are referred to as cervicomedullary syndrome.

CCI is a well-documented finding in connective tissue disorders including lupus, down syndrome, rheumatoid arthritis and osteogenesis imperfecta. Some experts note that while CCI appears to be more common in patients with hypermobility spectrum disorders, the conventional medical community has been hesitant to accept the idea of pathological instability for individuals with hEDS,[1] and CCI is not widely appreciated by the medical community.[2]

The excess motion and translation that occurs with CCI often results in neck pain, headaches, tendon inflammation, nerve irritation, and tight muscles, which act to compensate and attempt to add stability to the spine. CCI can also result in arthritic changes in the upper neck joints and alterations in posture and body position that can affect the entire body from the head down. It can also lead to abnormalities of the upper spinal cord, brainstem and cerebellum, as well as stretching of the lower cranial nerves and vertebral arteries.[1]

Symptoms of CCI include:[3]

- Neck pain
- Visual changes (blurred vision, double vision, abnormal eye movements called nystagmus)
- Dysautonomia
- Headache
- Dizziness or vertigo
- Loss of balance and coordination, difficulty walking, clumsiness
- Difficulty swallowing (dysphagia)
- Difficulty speaking (dysarthria)

- Fatigue
- Muscle weakness
- Feeling spacey or disoriented
- Facial/tongue pain or numbness
- Ringing in the ears, hearing loss
- Nausea and vomiting
- Memory loss
- Anxiety/depression
- Raynaud's phenomenon
- Sensory loss
- Irritable bowel syndrome
- Urinary dysfunction
- Gastroesophageal reflux disease

Headaches are sometimes described as the head feeling heavy. Others note pressure-type headaches that worsen with coughing or straining (that may be associated with impaired cerebrospinal fluid flow and intracranial pressure abnormalities). Sleep apnea also appears to be strongly connected to excessive translatory movement of the cervical spine, such as what's observed in CCI.[4] Sleep apnea may also be influenced by EDS-associated laxity in soft tissue structures like a soft trachea that can impede air flow when laying down.[5] Chronic hypoxia (reduction in oxygen) can be a powerful driving force of inflammation and fatigue, and it can impact the body's ability to handle everything from toxic insults and healing from an injury/surgery to recovering from a viral infection. Sleep studies to rule out sleep apnea are important for patients who have chronic inflammatory conditions and/or concerns about CCI.

If the brainstem becomes compressed, patients may also experience autonomic nervous system symptoms that may worsen with changes in head and neck position, such as low blood pressure when standing, heat intolerance, rapid heart rate, extreme thirst, fainting or near-fainting, and delayed gastric emptying. Abnormalities of the upper cervical spine such as those seen in cervicomedullary syndrome can mimic the symptoms of dysautonomia or can trigger true autonomic dysfunction.[3]

Keep in mind that there are many different issues that can cause these types of symptoms. A thorough differential diagnosis process with an expert is essential. Chiari malformation, intracranial pressure abnormalities, cervical arterial dysfunction, and vestibular issues can also result in similar symptoms, and sometimes more than one of these processes is occurring simultaneously. Cerebrospinal fluid leaks, basilar invagination, ventral brainstem compression, and tethered cord may also need to be considered.[6]

From the patient history, symptoms such as dizziness, double vision, difficulty speaking, difficulty swallowing, sudden fainting, visual changes, nausea and vomiting, sensory changes, and abnormal movements of the eyes called nystagmus warrant further investigation.[6] Patients with CCI often report feeling as if they cannot hold the weight of their head up, and they may frequently rest their head on their hands or an external support. They may also report frequent headaches or a "bobble head" feeling. Symptoms of CCI are typically worse at extreme ranges of neck extension and rotation. Rotational misalignments of the upper cervical spine not only affect the jaw position but also can impinge on various anatomical structures, leading to symptoms such as air hunger, heart palpitations, nausea, food getting stuck when swallowing, referral pain to lower areas of the spine, and pain above and behind the eye.[7] The symptom of air hunger—a feeling of severe breathlessness—is an interesting one. In addition to CCI, it's also been associated with Chiari malformation, dysautonomia and certain infections like Bartonellosis. So any one of these symptoms in isolation is not necessarily indicative of CCI, but the whole picture can help lead clinicians in the differential diagnosis process.

Physical therapists can perform tests to gain an idea of the laxity in the alar and transverse ligaments in the upper spine, and some patients with

CCI will also report improvements in symptoms with gentle manual traction, but CCI is typically diagnosed with an upright MRI. (According to some experts, the supine MRI does not show the anatomy in a normal physiological position and often lacks the precision to detect CCI. The upright MRI [a type of dynamic imaging] also allows for flexion and extension measurements but is not always widely available.) The positioning for the MRI remains a controversial topic.

As part of the diagnostic process, many static imaging measurements are assessed, most commonly the Grabb-Oakes measurement (to evaluate the transverse ligament stability), the clivo-axial angle (to determine function of the ligaments on the back of the head) and Power's ratio (shows whether the head has moved forward on the upper neck).[8] The Harris measurement is also frequently used.[1] These measurements are not routinely used in diagnostic imaging, which can create practical challenges for patients and clinicians.

It may also be helpful to assess the cerebrospinal fluid (CSF) flow. Another dynamic imaging option, the digital motion X-ray, also helps to visualize the stability of the alar and transverse ligaments; however, dynamic imaging is not always available at all facilities. Dynamic imaging is more likely to show any potential ventral brainstem compression in cervical spine flexion, which often appears normal on routine imaging. This is important because some patients may be diagnosed with Chiari malformation without a full CCI assessment, and Chiari surgical decompression failures often reveal underlying CCI or recurrent cerebrospinal fluid obstruction.[9]

Surgical fusions for CCI are high-risk procedures, and complications including adjacent segment disease, cartilage and bone damage, misguided screws impacting the vertebral artery or spinal nerves, nonunion and paralysis can occur.[10] While some patients find relief with surgery, others find that they got worse or did not improve, and surgery is considered the last resort for CCI.[2] Newer procedures such as the Percutaneous

325

Implantation of CCI Ligaments (PICL) offer a nonsurgical, injection-based approach that inserts a person's own stem cells in the neck ligaments in efforts to help them gain stability, but research is needed on this approach.

Conservative treatment for CCI often includes physical therapy, bracing or a cervical collar, injections and pain management. Manual therapy to specific segments of the cervical spine can be helpful, provided that it's performed with caution and expertise. Exercises with a laser headlamp and a target, clock or maze are sometimes utilized in addition to strengthening the supporting muscles and reducing postural strain.

Craniosacral therapy and strategies to improve fluid dynamics may help with the symptoms of CCI. Craniosacral therapy is a gentle technique that utilizes light touch to release restrictions in the head and pelvis regions in order to improve the functioning of the central nervous system. This treatment may impact the fluid around the brain and spinal cord (cerebrospinal fluid) which often has functional impairments in patients with the trifecta.

Slight variations in the position and rotation of the upper cervical spine vertebrae can certainly impact multiple aspects of health through mechanisms that involve the cranial nerves and the autonomic nervous system. Some patients report that a treatment called Atlas Orthogonal spinal corrections is a useful adjunct to conservative muscle stabilization programs, and one case report found that this type of treatment improved vertebral artery blood flow to the head, though this has not been studied specifically with CCI.[11] Atlas Orthogonal techniques utilize X-rays or other diagnostic images before and after to determine alignment. Patients with hEDS who pursue any treatments involving cervical vertebral alignment should ensure that their practitioner is well-versed in hypermobility and CCI; caution is warranted.

Treatment programs incorporating attention to the vagus nerve, cranial nerve X (discussed in Chapter 7), may also be of value here, given that there are inherent connections between cranial nerves IX, X, and XI as they exit the skull. Thus, when there is dysfunction in one nerve, there's often dysfunction in the other two. Many patients with chronic neck tension will also experience abnormalities in heart rate, respiratory rate, digestive function, and swallowing due to these anatomical connections. While addressing the vagus nerve does not address the hypermobility occurring with CCI directly, for certain patients, it can help alleviate symptoms that arise from the complex connections between the joints, arteries, muscles and nerves in the cervical spine.

Dry needling is an incredible evidence-based modality utilized by physical therapists. Traditionally it's utilized for patients with orthopedic injuries, but it also has tremendous value for patients suffering from chronic illness. Cranial nerve XI, the spinal accessory nerve, innervates the upper trapezius and sternocleidomastoid muscles, and dry needling these muscles appears to have a positive impact on autonomic nervous system balance.[12]

Stanley Rosenberg is the author of "Accessing the Healing Power of the Vagus Nerve," which is an excellent resource for patients who may experience symptoms related to the complex interplay between the cranial nerves and the cervical spine. His book provides examples of simple and gentle exercises that can be performed at home to address upper cervical alignment and breathing abnormalities, neuro-fascial techniques, trigger point release and much more. I utilize his "basic exercise" and several other strategies with many patients and highly recommend his book as a resource for both patients and practitioners.[13]

Pelvic Floor Muscle Dysfunction

This topic is an area that is overly prevalent yet under-discussed. The simplified popular belief that "kegels fix all" is typically inadequate to help patients who are suffering from pelvic symptoms. A specialist-guided, detailed and comprehensive approach will better equip patients to find lasting healing. Many patients with the trifecta and other chronic conditions note a correlation between urinary symptoms and overall systemic symptom flare-ups, and some also experience ongoing concerns in this area.

The pelvic floor is comprised of three layers of muscles that sit like a sling. They run from the pubic bone to the tailbone. The coccygeus and levator ani muscles make up what we refer to as the pelvic floor. These muscles help to control the movement of urine and feces, support the internal organs and pelvis, are part of a complex relationship with the respiratory diaphragm and trunk muscles, and are involved in sexual function. Pelvic floor muscle dysfunction (PFMD) is generally divided into two categories, low-tone or high-tone. Abnormalities in these muscles can surface in the form of pain, muscle spasms, weakness, muscle shortening or impaired coordination. These issues can occur in all sexes.[14]

PFMD is diagnosed by a specialist (certain physical therapists have training in this area) through an internal vaginal exam or internal rectal exam. Tone, symmetry, strength of contraction and endurance are typically assessed to determine whether the patient has low-tone or high-tone issues. Other evaluations can include ultrasound, surface EMG testing and other diagnostic imaging. Most people assume that urinary issues are only caused by weak muscles, but the opposite problem of high tone and the inability to relax the pelvic floor muscles can also be problematic.

When the findings show *low tone*, or hypotonicity of the pelvic floor muscles, the muscles may have poor recruitment and decreased ability to hold the contraction for very long. This is more common among patients who experience conditions like urinary incontinence, pelvic organ prolapse, low back pain, orgasm dysfunction, and a history of childbirth trauma.[14] Low tone pelvic floor muscle dysfunction appears to be more common in patients who have genetic hypermobility syndromes including hEDS, and it's also associated with pudendal nerve issues.[15] Incontinence, urgency and frequency issues are commonly noted with low pelvic floor muscle tone.[15]

Just like any other muscle in the body, the pelvic floor muscles can develop painful trigger points. When the patient has *high tone* pelvic floor muscle dysfunction, they may also experience muscle shortening, spasms and tightness. High tone pelvic floor muscle issues appear to be more common in conditions like endometriosis, interstitial cystitis, dyspareunia (painful intercourse) and other pelvic pain issues.[14] There are various theorized mechanisms for as to why high-tone issues occur in the pelvic floor. Dysfunctional voiding of urine or feces, injury from surgery or trauma, history of sexual abuse, visceral pain syndromes and gastrointestinal issues may be connected to symptom development.[16] Postural abnormalities and prolonged sitting are other theorized contributing factors.[16] Patients with high-tone issues may note additional lower urinary tract symptoms including bothersome urgency, stress incontinence and increased voiding frequency.[15]

Treatment for pelvic floor muscle dysfunction is individualized and specific to the type of tone issue that's occurring. The cornerstone of treatment typically utilizes specialized physical therapists who rehabilitate these muscles with neuromuscular education and biofeedback, lifestyle strategies, lumbopelvic and spinal techniques, manual therapy and core stability exercises.[16] Acupuncture, trigger point injections, vaginal steaming, herbal supplements, The *Arvigo®* Techniques of *Maya Abdominal* Therapy, cognitive therapies and neuromodulation therapies are also sometimes utilized in addition to conventional medicine strategies to reduce pain and improve alignment and resting tone.[16]

It's also important to address the relationship between breathing and the diaphragm when pelvic floor muscle dysfunction is occurring. The diaphragm is closely related to the function of the vagus nerve and the muscles of the back, abdominals and pelvic floor. On inhalation, the diaphragm muscle moves down, pushing the organs down. The pelvic floor stretches as we breathe in and contracts slightly as we exhale.

If you imagine the cylindrical shape of a soda can, you can visualize the 3D anatomy of these muscles. There's a layer of muscles that create the front of the cylinder called the transversus abdominis. This corset-like muscle is the deepest layer of your abdominals. On the back side of the cylinder, the multifidus muscles are deep spinal muscles. The diaphragm is the top of the can (with the vagus nerve entering through the small opening) and the pelvic floor muscles are the bottom of the can. Together, these four muscle groups act like a closed cylinder in the trunk.

When pressure increases in the abdomen, such as with a cough or a shout, the abdominals contract, increasing pressure on the pelvic floor, which can trigger incontinence when there's abnormal tone in the muscles that control the flow of urine, leading to leakage. On a chronic basis, alterations in posture can change the pressure and degree of tilting of the pelvis and can also impact the ability of the diaphragm to expand, which can result in the pelvic floor muscles not getting the gentle exercise that they need, causing them to grow weaker over time. Surgical procedures, spine pain and disengagement of the deep back and core stabilizer muscles can also alter the pressure dynamics of this cylinder, leading to further dysfunction. From the opposite perspective, both weakness or hypertonicity in the pelvic floor muscles can alter the pressure balance in the cylinder, leading to dysfunctional movement patterns in the spine, diaphragm and ribs. It's clear that these areas go hand in hand, and a comprehensive program should include attention to all of these anatomical factors.

There are many other sexual/reproductive health issues that occur outside of pelvic floor muscle dysfunction, and conventional medicine often offers an incomplete approach to addressing the root cause of these issues. To find a directory of therapists who have advanced training in sexual/reproductive health and pelvic floor muscle function, visit https://pelvicguru.com/, https://ptl.womenshealthapta.org/ or www.pelvicrehab.com.

The Ileocecal-Psoas Connection

The iliopsoas musculotendinous unit (often described as the "psoas") is comprised of the iliacus muscle and major/minor psoas muscles. This large muscle group has attachments on the thoracolumbar spine vertebral bodies and transverse processes (T12–L5) as well as the iliac fascia and the femur. These muscles can act separately or together and are responsible for movements like hip flexion, spinal side bending and hip hiking, stabilization of the lumbar spine and stabilization of the femoral head in the hip joint.[17] The psoas creates a shelf-like support for the organs in the abdominal cavity in addition to having musculoskeletal functions. The psoas can sometimes cause referral pain into the stomach and groin areas, and some patients also feel back tightness when it is hypertonic due to its spinal attachments. It's also associated with posterior pelvic pain, sacroiliac joint dysfunction, and the sensation of a (typically painless) popping or snapping in the hip joint. Two other muscles, the piriformis and the quadratus lumborum, have a complex functional relationship with the iliopsoas and may also be relevant myofascial players in patients experiencing chronic pain in this area.[18]

The ileocecal valve is located at the lower right quadrant of the abdomen and serves as the juncture between the small and large intestine. A dysfunctional ileocecal valve is theorized to be one of the mechanisms responsible for small intestinal bacterial overgrowth (SIBO) by allowing the large intestinal bacteria to have a backflow migration into the small intestine, which not only displaces microbes where they shouldn't be, but also alters the normal cleansing wave of the small intestine. This may also lead to chronic dehydration as the body tries to flush the area with water to remove the bacterial overgrowth from the small intestine.

Some theorize that a tight psoas muscle may also influence sacrum (and in particular, sacroiliac joint) alignment which, when occurring on the right side (our typically dominant side), can influence the ileocecal valve due to its anatomical location. Adhesions from abdominal scar tissue or inflammation resulting from factors like repetitive sitting, repetitive motion, trauma to the abdomen, or dehydration may also influence the function of the ileocecal valve, the psoas and its connection to internal organs. Thus, it's easy to imagine a vicious cycle between a tight psoas, subsequent spine and sacrum factors, and chronic gut inflammation.

Most people do not realize that the fascia that the psoas connects to extends to the internal crus of the diaphragm muscle. Fascia is a sheath of fibrous connective tissue with tremendous tensile strength. This is important because dysfunction of the psoas muscle can influence the diaphragm, and vice versa.[17] This often presents as someone who does a lot of desk work or driving and has a chronically shortened psoas muscle, which impacts rib expansion and the ability of the diaphragm to activate, creating shallow breathing, which in turn usually influences the position of the entire spine and the ability to regulate ventral vagal tone (discussed in Chapter 7).

The psoas is also one of the main muscles involved in the fight or flight (sympathetic nervous system) reaction. The psoas is sometimes considered a "bridge" between our different nervous systems (particularly the central, autonomic and enteric nervous systems). Clinically, patients with PTSD or high levels of stress or emotional trauma almost always present with tightness in their psoas muscle(s) and neck muscles (particularly the upper trapezius and sternocleidomastoid). An improperly functioning vagus nerve, injuries impacting rib expansion and an impaired diaphragm may also elicit compensatory shortening of the psoas muscle. Due to the proximity of the ureter to the psoas, kidney stones may also trigger psoas inflammation.[17] Individuals with leg length discrepancies and runners/cyclists who frequently use the psoas muscle may also find hypertonicity and chronic inflammation in the iliopsoas musculotendinous unit.[17]

Psoas Reset

Strategies to help restore proper tone to the psoas muscle include manual therapy techniques (performed with a physical therapist or osteopath) that include counter strain, muscle energy techniques, dry needling and myofascial release. Strategies to modify ergonomic or biomechanical factors and engage the gluteal and hamstring muscles may also be helpful, in addition to attention to the diaphragm function, vagal tone and visceral manipulation of the ileocecal valve.

Long-duration static stretching of the hip flexors is not particularly useful in this patient population for chronically hypertonic psoas muscles. Many people like stretching out their hip flexors for several minutes because it can feel good, and this was the traditional "old school" approach for muscle tightness. However, static stretching has since been deemed ineffective and it also has the potential to stretch other types of tissues including ligaments, which could be a concern (particularly in patients with hEDS).[18] Static stretching may also reduce improvements in strength/force and proprioception that are needed to effect change in chronic inflammatory conditions.[18,19]

Most of the scientific literature discusses non-conservative management of psoas issues with surgical and injection-based approaches. However, conservative management of psoas-related issues is clinically efficacious and should be encouraged as first-line treatment. Certain strategies may be especially useful, such as the exercises outlined below.

Exercises to help restore proper psoas muscle tone:
Exercise 1: Self Massage in Prone

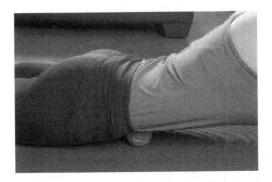

1. Self-massage in prone position: Use a softball or lacrosse ball to perform a self-release by lying prone (face down) over the ball with the ball halfway between the bellybutton and the front of the pelvis for 20 seconds. You can modify this by adding a little forward to back weight-shifting movement so that you are self-massaging the length of the psoas. If you're not feeling any tenderness, you can also bend your knee and shift more of your body weight toward the ball for a deeper release.

Exercise 2: Self-Massage in Supine

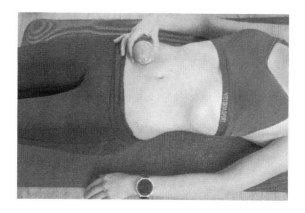

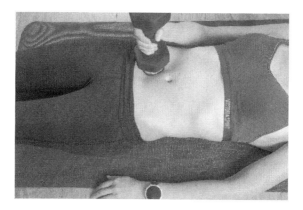

2. Self-massage in supine position: Lie on your back and place a softball or lacrosse ball in the same spot as exercise #1. Take a light dumbbell (3-10 pounds) and gently rest it on top of the ball, holding the weight with your hands. Take deep breaths for 20 seconds. You can add gentle movement of the weight over the ball to help find restrictions and self-massage the muscle. You can also have your right knee bent and your right foot resting on the ground before you start in order to work with the psoas in a shortened position.

Exercise 3: Self-Massage in Side-lying

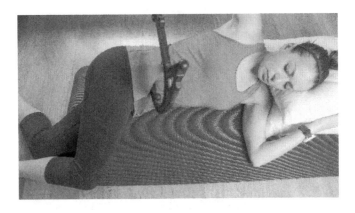

Note: easier to perform with both hands on cane, but modified so you can see what I'm doing

3. Self-massage in side-lying position: If the above positions are not tolerated, you can also try using your hand or a trigger-point massage stick (like a Thera Cane) to release the psoas while lying on your side with your top knee bent and your top hip flexed (between 45 and 80 degrees) while the top leg is resting on the bed, ground or treatment table. Laying on the side shifts the abdominal contents out of the way, so this position may be a better option for those who experience chronic abdominal discomfort. Self-massage the psoas for 20 seconds (you can also work up and down the length of the muscle) while performing deep breathing.

Exercise 4: Self-Massage in Side-lying with Movement

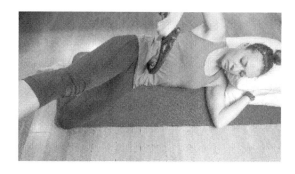

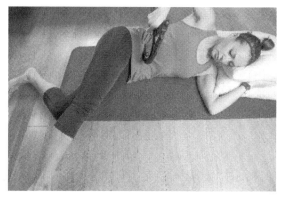

Note: easier to perform with both hands on cane, but modified so you can see what I'm doing

4. Self-massage in side-lying position (exercise #3) with movement: Once pressure is on the muscle, lift your top leg straight up toward the ceiling to 45 degrees, pause and rotate the toes out slightly, and then lower the leg in a controlled motion back to the surface. Repeat slowly for 40–60 seconds.

Exercise 5: Active Stretching with Reach or Rotation

5. Active stretching: Kneel on the ground in a lunge or "runner's stretch" position with the left foot planted in front of you with the left knee bent to 90 degrees and the right knee and foot on the floor behind you. The right knee should be behind the right hip so that a gentle stretch is felt on the front of the right side. Make sure that your trunk is upright and that you are not arching your spine. From this position, you can add one of two movement options:

Reach Away Motion

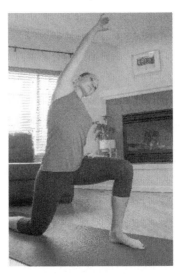

    a. Reach away: Reach the right arm overhead and to the left side, leaning your trunk to the left slightly. Pause for 2–3 seconds and return to the starting position. Repeat this motion for 30–60 seconds.

Rotate Away Motion

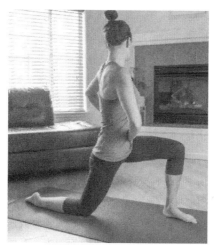

b. Rotate away: Clasp your hands together with your hands near your belly button and rotate your entire trunk and head to the left side. Pause for 2–3 seconds and return to the starting position. Repeat this motion for 30–60 seconds.

The above instructions can help restore normal tone to the right psoas. To reset the left side, perform the same steps to the opposite side. While one side is generally more hypertonic than the other, it's important to evaluate and treat the psoas muscles bilaterally (on both sides).[19] Many yoga flow sequences also help to actively release the psoas muscle and can be very beneficial. For best results, these strategies should be accompanied by addressing postural/biomechanical/alignment factors and emotional factors that may be influencing psoas muscle tension. Further, muscles that hold extra resting tone are also often weak and may need certain strengthening exercises to prevent recurrence of issues.

Keep in mind that other issues can cause discomfort in these areas, and the psoas is not tight in everyone. The best results come when a physical therapist can analyze exactly what is going on with your own body to determine the best approach.

Ileocecal Valve Reset

There are some clinical tests and indicators to determine if the ileocecal valve may be functioning improperly. If that is the case, it's fairly simple to help reset the ileocecal valve sphincter tone and function. While lying down, find the point that is halfway between the belly button and the bony prominence on the front of the hip (the anterior superior iliac spine) on the right side of your body. Use your fingers (the pads, not the nails) to push directly downward (toward your back) at this point. It is usually tender. Hold that spot for 20 seconds, taking several deep breaths, and then perform small clockwise circular motions over that point for another 20 seconds.

Ileocecal Valve Reset

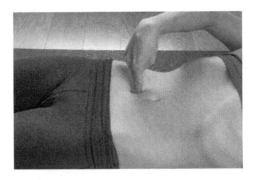

Some practitioners will perform muscle testing to ensure that this quick self-massage was effective. While some sources advocate for a decent amount of pressure on this point, others believe that less is more, and a firm yet gentle approach may be better, especially for patients who are very tender at this spot. This technique can be performed before meals.

Because the ileocecal valve connects the small and large intestine, regular preventive attention to this area may be especially helpful for patients who have had small intestinal bacterial overgrowth (SIBO) issues in the past. Keep in mind that it is possible to overdo it and elicit nausea and other symptoms, so if you feel that you'd like to consider this self-help technique, start gently and slowly.

There are other forms of self-massage that can help promote gastrointestinal motility. "ILU massage" incorporates firm but gentle pressure over the abdomen in three different patterns that stimulate different parts of the ascending, transverse, and descending colon. "ILU massage" is sometimes used in conjunction with the ileocecal valve release; helpful tutorials are available online.

Some practitioners also support the avoidance of spicy foods, popcorn, nuts, seeds, alcohol and caffeine in order to reduce inflammation around this valve. Specific acupuncture, acupressure and lymphatic points may also improve the function of the ileocecal valve.

Revisiting the connections between the diaphragm, the pelvic floor muscles and spinal muscle stabilizers serves as another reminder of how inner-connected we are, and attention to the psoas can also impact patients with urinary issues and spine pain (and vice-versa). It's clear that these entities have a close physiological relationship and optimal restoration of the function/tone of each component can have a powerful impact on pain, orthopedic alignment, digestive function and neural regulation for patients with chronic illness.

The above strategies are not intended to be medical advice. Many different conditions can cause tenderness and dysfunction in this area, and these techniques are difficult to do properly and can make some patients feel worse. It's always best to work with a physical therapist and/or professional with advanced training in visceral manipulation and body work to determine if the psoas muscle and ileocecal valve are functioning properly.

Pain

Pain activates mast cells, can lead to abnormal movements patterns (especially in the presence of the hypermobility noted with hEDS), can influence our regulation of heart rate and blood pressure, and alters our nervous system state and regulation. Pain is a big deal for patients with the trifecta and other chronic conditions. Many will experience intermittent visceral pain that can refer pain to other areas of the body. Abdominal pain or some type of gastrointestinal discomfort is usually present on a chronic basis. Orthopedic injuries and pain are often exacerbated by ergonomic and biomechanical factors in our daily routine. Patients with chronic illness often report night pain alongside neuropathy and insomnia. Migraines are common in this population and can be especially painful. Patients who have a high bacterial or viral burden often experience regular achiness and flu-like symptoms. It's also common for patients to experience joint pain and inflammation on a regular basis. These are just a handful of examples; hopefully it's clear that pain is very relevant for this patient population as something that needs to be addressed to find systemic healing.

Pain is our body's alarm system, and it's an important signal to our conscious mind so that we know when to let go of a sharp object, or when to allow our system to rest and recover. However, when pain becomes chronic, it can play into a vicious cycle scenario with cortisol, one of the body's major stress hormones, which can lead to a predominance of sympathetic nervous system (fight or flight) activation and adrenal problems, which can perpetuate the cycle.

Stress and pain most certainly feed off each other, but it's much more complex than it may seem. There are several physiological changes that occur when the system experiences pain. These influence the resting muscle length, the presence of trigger points (tight fibrous bands in muscle tissue), the circulatory system and the way we breathe, and in turn often affect the quality of sleep, which can influence the body's ability to detoxify and clean up waste, which can create a sluggish liver/gut/lymphatic system... When you add extra cortisol being pumped around due to stress, this can easily turn into a big obstacle for healing.

When the brain receives chronic pain inputs over time, several peripheral and central nervous system changes can occur. Patients can develop hyperalgesia (an exaggerated response to noxious stimulus) or allodynia (the perception of pain from normally innocuous stimuli). A systematic review on musculoskeletal pain noted that there are changes in the somatosensory, affective and cognitive processing areas of brain in response to chronic pain.[20] Morphological and functional structural alterations in the brain have been noted, in addition to less gray matter volume in frontal and temporal lobes, the cingulate cortex and insula.[20]

Pain can be viewed in light of the total load concept. Patients with chronic conditions like the trifecta are likely exposed to a tremendous amount of health stressors that may be orthopedic or visceral, internal or external. This list is not all-inclusive, but there are several factors to consider.

Factors that commonly influence chronic pain:

- Bacterial infections
- Dental issues
- Emotional stress
- Food triggers
- Gastrointestinal problems
- Health and beauty products
- Heavy metals
- Mechanical stress
- Medications and supplements
- Mold exposure

- Other environmental toxins
- Oxidative stress
- Postural impairments
- Viruses

When the body is overburdened by the above issues, it's going to try to perform triage, and if the pain signals are blaring, pain could take priority and essentially hog all attention and resources, diverting the body from addressing the other important issues. Simply put, a physiologic focus of attention to pain/inflammation in one specific area can shift the body's resources that it needs in order to support detox organs and engage in deep healing. And it is also likely putting fuel on the inflammatory fire.

There are a multitude of strategies for management of chronic pain. There's no one-size-fits-all approach, but most patients find that some combination of the modalities listed below helps reduce inflammation and calm the system. Pain management doesn't have to be expensive or complicated. It can certainly include some at home self-care strategies such as regular breathing exercises, meditation and yoga. Often, immobility or a lack of movement can increase pain, so healthy movement should be a part of the strategies to reduce (and prevent) pain.

Just as it's important to figure out the underlying issues and triggers responsible for mast cell overactivity, the same principle applies for the pain. (For example, if it's neck pain, are there postural and ergonomic factors that are perpetuating the repetitive strain?) It's also especially important to address sleep. Sleep and pain go hand in hand and "sleep hygiene" is essential. (This topic will be discussed in the detoxification section, Chapter 11.) It's also important to get regular exercise (in the right manner) and to fuel the body with clean nutrients in order to promote tissue healing and reduction in pain. The bottom line is this: Make sure that you address WHY the pain is occurring in the first place, and at the same time, be sure to make efforts to reduce the pain in order to support the entire system in healing. Below are some pain-reducing approaches to consider for your toolbox.

Modalities that may be useful in addressing chronic pain:

- Acupressure (often a good option if acupuncture is not tolerated)
- Acupuncture
- Addressing psychological stress through counseling, journaling, etc.
- Aromatherapy
- Biofeedback
- Bracing, taping and external postural feedback devices
- Breathing exercises
- Cannabinoids and other supplements to reduce pain and inflammation
- Chiropractic care
- Craniosacral therapy
- Cupping
- Customized exercise programs
- Dance therapy
- Dry needling
- Electrical stimulation (transcutaneous electrical nerve stimulation "TENS"; frequency specific microcurrent "FEM", pulsed electromagnetic frequency "PEMF")
- Epsom salt baths and mineral water/hot spring soaking
- Ergonomic assessments to reduce postural stress in the workplace
- Feldenkrais method to increase body awareness through movement
- Heating pads
- Hypnosis

- Laser/light therapy
- Lymphatic drainage
- Massage, fascial release therapies
- Meditation and visualization
- Music therapy
- Nature therapy
- Nervous system retraining programs
- Osteopathic manipulative treatment
- Physical and occupational therapies
- Prevention of repetitive stress/strain through movement analysis
- Reflexology
- Reiki
- Sauna therapy
- Sound healing
- Tai chi
- Visceral manipulation
- Yoga

Medical cannabis can play a key role in pain management for certain patients with hEDS. Experts maintain that it's important to give attention to *when* and *how* medical cannabis is incorporated into practice as well as its potential contraindications, side effects and medication interactions.[21] Cannabis may be especially useful for the treatment of insomnia, gastrointestinal disorders, and anxiety/depression.[21] Like any substance, certain dosage and timing considerations become relevant and vary depending on the type of usage (inhaled vs. consumed orally, for example). In theory, cannabis can cause certain physiological changes in heart rate and blood pressure that may also need to be considered, particularly in patients with POTS.

Conventional medicine focuses on medications for pain, but many patients with the trifecta are unable to tolerate oral pain medications (or choose not to take them because they mask symptoms, can be addictive and have potentially damaging side effects), so it's important to have alternative tools for managing pain. Patients respond differently to different types of modalities for pain, and you probably know by now which methods work better for you than others.

During acute attacks of a painful and unpredictable condition, you may find it helpful to have a routine and use a positive mantra. Whether it's a warm bath and essential oils or that favorite tea and a movie marathon, find out what works for you. Avoid "pushing through" pain until it becomes unbearable, as this can influence and flare your entire system. And remember to give yourself some grace in this aspect of your journey.

STRUCTURAL & MUSCULOSKELETAL ISSUES: TAKE-HOME MESSAGES

- Craniocervical instability is a common finding in patients with the trifecta and, in particular, hEDS.
- Conservative management of upper spine instability is encouraged for most patients and should be carefully guided with a professional.
- Pelvic floor muscle dysfunction can present as either a problem with high tone or low tone, both of which can trigger symptoms including incontinence. Both issues can be addressed with the help of a physical therapist specialist in reproductive health (often advertised as "women's health" although all people can benefit).
- There appear to be powerful connections between the psoas muscle and the ileocecal valve, small intestinal bacterial overgrowth/gut health, the diaphragm, the autonomic nervous system, emotional trauma, the spine and the pelvic floor. Addressing these areas may offer powerful improvements for patients experiencing chronic illness.
- Pain should not be ignored! The prevention and management of pain is a key part of a holistic healing plan and there are many useful options to consider.
- Do you have certain structural and musculoskeletal issues that are not being investigated or addressed? What types of providers can

help you work with these concerns? Reflect on this topic in your Trifecta Passport worksheet.

Chapter 10:
MOVEMENT

Regular, consistent physical activity is a key part of any holistic healing plan. Many patients with hEDS express fear around movement due to past painful experiences. And yet, exercise is one of the top strategies to help reduce and prevent hypermobility-related flare-ups.

Similarly, patients with POTS experience overwhelming symptoms when upright and may write off exercise altogether, but there are many exercises that can be done in more tolerable positions in order to build up to standing movement. Exercise is consistently recommended for the management of POTS, and in some cases, specific exercise programs may bring POTS symptoms into remission over time.

Patients with MCAS also often have a fear of exercise or feel that it can trigger them. By following the other strategies outlined in this book to reduce overall health stressors and toxin load, address structural and musculoskeletal issues, enhance nutrition and retrain the nervous system, most patients with MCAS find that exercise no longer provokes symptoms. However, it's important to be aware of other factors (such as the food or medication consumed prior to exercise, or environmental triggers in the exercise space) and to mitigate these issues in order to enjoy movement without flare-ups. Exercise is an important method to help us detoxify and it can also have a powerful impact on stress, anxiety, depression and mental health. Movement, when performed in the right manner, is actually a natural mast cell stabilizer!

It's time to change our movement story; it's time to move away from fear and into empowerment. For some of us, it's time to stop making excuses. For others, it may be time to stop pushing through symptoms with exercise—listen to what your body is telling you! There are certainly two ends of the spectrum. Let's empower ourselves to *think smarter* to get stronger and restore overall vitality. The benefits of exercise are well-documented and can have a profound impact on mental well-being as well as physical disease risk factors. Creating a life-long habit of movement may be the difference between survival mode and thriving; many patients find that a well-planned exercise routine is the final factor that helps them return to work and/or community activities.

There are a few key strategies that help patients to start an exercise routine—and stick with it:

1) Focus on movement or activities that bring you joy (or, at least, that you don't hate). Don't force yourself to go to the gym if you hate being there. Some patients do better being outdoors for walking or biking, while others find that they experience more triggers outside and need to stick to indoor activities. Listen to what your body (and mind) are telling you.

2) Start small and avoid the all-or-nothing mindset. Five to 10 minutes a day is better than nothing. Exercise does not need to live up to a certain standard time limit.

3) Consider your movement plan as part of a continuum. On flare days, be gentle with yourself and consider focusing on things like breathing exercises or a gentle yoga flow. Have different options available and cater them to how you are feeling each day.

4) If you don't have a lot of experience with exercise, or if you have heart or lung concerns, be sure to start a new exercise routine with

medical supervision. Physical therapists can guide you and help you get started.

5) Pace yourself. Try to avoid extremes. Many patients push themselves too hard and then find they need a week to recover. Instead, try to keep a more even-keeled approach to the exercise intensity.

6) If you have concerns about orthopedic issues related to hEDS, work with a physical therapist who can help you modify activities to your individual needs.

7) Pick movements that counteract the typical postures you find yourself in during the day. For example, if you have a desk job or spend a lot of time slouching while using electronic devices, you'll want to make sure you engage the opposite muscles. The classic "desk posture" involves forward shoulders, a forward head, a rounded spine and shortened hip flexors. Instead of focusing on exercises like push-ups (which strengthen the anterior chest muscles, perpetuating the forward shoulder posture) consider exercises to engage the muscles around the shoulder blades, the glutes and hamstrings to help bring you out of that (poor) static habitual posture.

8) Write out your goals for exercise and be sure to break them down into small and realistic short-term goals too. Whatever the type(s) of exercise, *long-term goals* should aim for the American Heart Association recommendation, which is 150 minutes of *moderate-intensity* aerobic exercise per week (the equivalent of 30 minutes x five days a week), or 75 minutes of *high-intensity* or "vigorous" exercise per week (the equivalent of 25 minutes x three days a week), or a combination of both, plus moderate-to-high intensity muscle strengthening at least two days per week.[1] Patients who tolerate shorter-duration bouts should be encouraged to split up their sessions (such as more than one bout of exercise per day).

353

Particularly in the hEDS population, many people get hung up on types of exercise: Is yoga a bad idea for me? Should I be stretching or not? Do I have to avoid all contact sports? Can I run again? The answer to any of these questions is never a simple yes or no. In general, the issue is not necessarily the type of movement, but rather, the way you may go about it. Yoga headstands are a bad idea for someone with craniocervical instability, but there are so many types of yoga and different yoga postures, most of which do not require circus act positioning. Plus, a physical therapist or good class instructor will show many modifications to different poses.

Stretching the shoulder joint to the point of putting it into further hypermobility (beyond what is functional for you) may not be a good idea, but active stretching for a tight psoas muscle from prolonged sitting in the car may be helpful. Starting a new running program or contact sport with poor endurance, stability and proprioception leading to faulty movement mechanics and compensatory patterns could be the recipe for disaster, but with the right preparations, many individuals with hEDS enjoy contact sports and can return to running safely.

Instead of thinking in black and white terms, remember that there's a lot of gray area, and these types of considerations depend on the scenario and the individual. While some research indicates that generalized joint hypermobility may increase the risk of knee injury in contact sports,[2,3] other literature suggests that the overall rate of lower extremity injury in sporting activities is similar between individuals with and without joint hypermobility.[4,5]

That being said, if you're starting exercise or continuing exercise with ongoing injuries, there are certainly some strategies to reduce the risk of joint strain. Activities that entail heavy joint loading or plyometrics (loaded jumping exercises aiming to use maximal force in order to increase power) may not be the best idea for these scenarios. Many patients find that great exercise options are tai chi and yoga nidra, which incorporate gentle movements with visualization and meditation. Some patients prefer unloaded light, rhythmic activities like a stationary bicycle or swimming. Pilates is another great option to build stability in a slow and controlled manner.

Some patients with one (or all three) of the trifecta conditions utilize mobility aids such as canes, walking sticks, crutches and wheelchairs. Experts maintain that patients with hEDS should avoid overusing these mobility aids and should have a careful discussion with their care team about considerations for their use, as the ultimate goal is to become as independent as possible through fitness and lifestyle modifications.[6] That being said, mobility devices can also empower individuals to access more community activities, and this needs to be factored in too.

Patients with POTS often find they need wheelchair transport due to increased symptoms with upright positions, but the long-term goal should be to transition to less reliance on mobility aids over time as improved movement tolerance occurs. A gradual tapering is advised as opposed to a drastic overnight change. There's a lot of difference between "use it or lose it" and unrelenting pain/dysfunction, so these decisions should be carefully weighed with a multidisciplinary care team. It's also important to note that a reliance on mobility aids or braces does not mean that you cannot exercise. Exercise can be adapted and modified to so many different scenarios and physical/occupational therapists can help you navigate these considerations.

The following sections will discuss some considerations for movement and exercise specific to each condition of the trifecta.

EXERCISE FOR POTS

Exercise has been shown to be a widely accepted key component to POTS treatment plans. Exercise expands blood volume and plasma volume, increases cardiac size and mass, and improves orthostatic tolerance. An eight- to 12-week exercise protocol is ideal, though most patients continue exercising beyond that point because of the many system-wide benefits. Successful POTS exercise programs typically have three components: cardiovascular exercise, strength training and postural training.

Below are the guidelines that I recommend specifically for patients with POTS. These guidelines are based off the Levine protocol, the CHOP Modified Dallas Protocol and recommendations from Dysautonomia International.[7,8] For a more in-depth description, these protocols can be viewed and downloaded online.

Cardiovascular Exercise for POTS

Some guidelines suggest a maximal heart rate of 75%–80% of the patient's calculated max during exercise for POTS. However, measuring the heart rate range as a guide for exercise is not very useful in patients on beta blockers and other medications, so I recommend that patients use the Borg Rating of Perceived Exertion (RPE) to determine their warm-up, recovery and base paces. The Borg is a scale from 6 through 20.

Warm up/recovery should be 10–12 on the Borg, and the base pace should be in the 13–14 range.

Figure 4. The Borg Rating of Perceived Exertion

Perceived Exertion Rating	Description of Exertion
6	No exertion (sitting or resting)
7	Extremely light
8	
9	Very light
10	
11	Light
12	
13	Somewhat hard
14	
15	Hard
16	
17	Very hard
18	
19	Extremely hard
20	Maximal exertion

If you have POTS and become symptomatic during exercise, you want to:

- Decrease the exercise intensity (or stop if you are having emergency-type reactions)
- Ensure that you are hydrating during exercise
- Lie on your back on the floor to recover, with your legs propped up on some pillows, if needed

When starting out in your cardiovascular program, you want to pick an exercise form that is in a recumbent position. Stationary recumbent bicycles are a great option. If you don't have access to a bike, you may also consider swimming or using a kickboard in the pool (once your vitals are stable), an arm bike, a rowing machine, or other supine or seated exercises.

The pressure of the water in the pool can actually decrease POTS symptoms and may enhance venous return in the legs, but cooler water temperatures may exacerbate POTS, so warmer water is advised.[9] Please talk to your PT if you have any equipment concerns or questions as to what type of exercise you should consider.

Cardiovascular exercise starting instructions:

- Begin your cardio three days a week for 20 minutes.
- Perform a 5-minute warm-up (Borg 11–12 or less), 10 minutes of base exercise (Borg no higher than 13–14), and a 5-minute cool down (Borg 11–12 or less).
- Keep in mind that patients who have been bed-ridden for a long time may need to start with 1–5 minutes per day instead of 20 minutes. This is general advice for the average patient but be sure to customize it to where you are.
- The goal for cardiovascular exercise is to build up to 30+ minutes of continuous base pace (Borg scale 13–15) exercise. Over time, you'll find yourself able to progress to more upright exercise options like the elliptical, stair stepper, walking and eventually jogging/running for some patients.
- It's common to get fatigued after exercise and it's also common to notice more symptoms of POTS initially as your body adapts to starting a new exercise routine. Remember to pace your daily activities. Avoid things like house cleaning and shopping following your exercise sessions, especially early in the program. Also avoid oversleeping and try to resist the urge to nap right after exercise.

For an advanced patient, the progression for cardio exercise can look like the following:

- Month 1 – recumbent bike, rowing, pool exercise (swimming or kicking)
- Month 2 – upright bike instead of recumbent, some patients can add walking on a flat treadmill or elliptical
- Month 3 – elliptical, walking on treadmill
- Months 4–6 – if you are doing fine at this point with upright activities, your PT may guide you in integrating jogging, running or sport activities

For other patients, the progression for cardio exercise should be slower:

- Months 1–3 – recumbent bike, rowing, pool exercise (swimming or kicking)
- Month 4 – upright bike instead of recumbent bike
- Month 5 – elliptical with arms stabilized, walking on treadmill
- Months 6–8 – more difficult upright training (adding arms with elliptical, or adding incline with walking)

Strength Training for POTS

The strength training program begins with lying down exercise and eventually progresses to seated and then standing exercise. Alternately, some patients may already be performing yoga or Pilates and may use this exercise as their strengthening each week. Upper and lower body exercises are typically included, with a greater focus on the lower extremities and larger muscle groups.

Strength training starting instructions:

- Perform strengthening two days a week, but not on the days that you are doing cardio exercise.
- Strength programs begin with about 20 minutes of exercise and build up from there. (Similar to the cardio section, adapt the total time to where you are at personally with your fitness status as you begin.)
- Begin exercises training for endurance with body weight or very light resistance and 12–15 repetitions, 2–3 sets of each exercise.

Examples of strengthening exercises:

- Supine (on your back): bridging, marching, diagonal pattern arm and leg lifts
- Prone (on your belly): superman, planking, gluteal exercises, exercise ball progression
- Side lying: side planks, hip abduction, clams, rotational exercise
- Seated: leg press, calf exercise, hamstring and quadriceps strength, hip strength, seated row, pull-downs
- Standing: squats, lunges, hip strengthening with resistance bands, step ups

Talk to your PT for a customized/personalized plan and for additional exercise ideas.

Postural Training for POTS

To work on upright standing tolerance, the third component of the exercise program involves static standing against a wall. Make sure you have a chair nearby and a watch on when you practice this progression. If nobody can supervise you while you do this, find a wall in front of a bed. You'll start out with a goal of one minute of standing against the wall at one time (or as long as is tolerated). Don't allow yourself to fidget with your legs—this is cheating! The ultimate goal is 10 minutes of static standing without symptom exacerbation; when you achieve this, you'll be graduating from this aspect of your exercise program.

Postural training starting instructions:

- Perform the postural wall standing exercise three times a day.
- If you experience any symptoms (dizziness, lightheadedness, nausea, chest pain, headache, blood pooling), you can stop before your goal time.
- Expect that some days will be better than others.
- Stick with a goal time and make sure you are stable with it for at least a week before adding on time. When the previous level of time is no longer causing symptoms, progress by adding 30 seconds to your time for the following week (or longer than one week).

Additional Suggestions for POTS

- Make sure you have enough fluid intake around your exercise. Most experts recommend that you drink at least 16 ounces of fluid 30 minutes prior to, during, and after exercise (in addition to your normal fluid intake for the day).
- Spread out or modify your house chores throughout the week.
- Make effort to remain upright as much as possible during the day. Try to get up and move a little bit every hour during the day. Avoid complete bed rest.
- No household or exercise activity should exceed 15 on the Borg scale.

- Some patients do well with elevating the entire head of the bed by four to six inches. (Move the whole bed; propping on pillows does not have the same effect.)
- It's wise to have a shower chair and grab bars available in the bathroom tub/shower area.
- Compression garments can help with poor venous return and can be used during exercise.
- Avoid alcohol, as this tends to make POTS and dehydration worse. Carefully consider caffeine intake, as some patients find that it makes symptoms worse.
- Make sure that your body temperature is well-regulated. Some patients experience a worsening of symptoms with heat. Ensure adequate ventilation in the exercise space.
- Most patients experience fatigue in the first month of this program.
- Most patients notice improvements in POTS symptoms after two to three months. This is not a "quick fix!" Exercise for POTS is a marathon and not a sprint!
- Exercise should be treated like it's a preventive supplement and maintained for life. Adherence to the exercise schedule is crucial to seeing improvements.

EXERCISE FOR EHLERS-DANLOS SYNDROME

For the hypermobile type of EDS, there are a few general considerations regarding movement. Work with a specialized physical therapist to know which joint positions to avoid. Because of the propensity of dislocation and subluxation in patients with EDS, certain activities and positions should be modified depending on the individual. For example, with the shoulder joint, you may want to avoid the baseball cocking motion (anterior instability), a scenario of distraction overpressure (such as carrying heavy groceries, an issue with inferior instability), and the push-up position (posterior instability). Work with a specialist to understand ways to modify activities and postural ergonomic alignment, decide which activities need to be avoided completely and determine strategies to protect the joints during movement.

Know which muscles to focus on for strengthening. Patients with hEDS need to strengthen muscles in order to use them as a substitute for the (typically lax and unsupportive) ligaments. It's important to create stability before advancing the movement patterns. For example, performing advanced plyometric movements or heavy loading of the knee joint without first ensuring adequate stability of the hip and core muscles can lead to issues.

Know which ways you can support the joint externally. Straps, supports, braces and taping are often helpful tools for this patient population. Their use should be guided initially with a professional who is knowledgeable in movement patterns and EDS. Note that 24-7 bracing is generally not advised outside of severe cases, but higher-level activities and exercises/positions that are known to cause joint instability are more appropriate times for bracing.

Expect that progress won't always be linear. Like trialing medications with MCAS patients, exercise can be a trial and error process for patients with hEDS. Have patience and keep in mind that the "average" patient presents with one single joint or muscular issue, compared to the tendency to see numerous widespread concerns in patients with joint hypermobility.

Don't assume every single joint is hypermobile. As we age, we (as individuals with hEDS) are not immune to the impacts of joint osteoarthritis and the tendency to have increased stiffness in certain areas over time. This typically happens selectively in certain joints. We may also develop isolated hypomobility in certain joints from improper movement patterns as a result of our generalized hypermobility. For this reason, certain physical therapy treatments like manual therapy may be useful when performed in a manner that is very customized to specific impairments. Dysfunctional movement patterns should be corrected.

Some sources recommend against massage/soft tissue work, stretching, manual therapy or dry needling in certain anatomical areas unless they are simultaneously being strengthened for patients with hEDS. This is not an outright rule for most physical therapists, but it is for some who voice concern over elongating tissue that may be shortening as a compensation to provide greater stability. Experts indicate that carefully applied and selective manual therapy and soft tissue mobilization are useful techniques for pain in this patient population.[10]

Clinically, it's been noted that certain shortened and painful muscles (often affected by improper ergonomic factors) prevent normal or neutral alignment and can ultimately prevent the patient from restoring proper autonomic nervous system tone or proper biomechanics with activities. Patients who have myofascial pain may alter their movement patterns into more faulty/harmful positions to compensate, which can trigger additional issues. Some individuals may have tight muscles pulling on hypermobile joints, which can lead to further laxity and dysfunction, and focused interventions targeting a specific muscle are often helpful for restoring proper joint alignment and functional mobility. Experts conclude that focused stretching to address muscle imbalances can be performed safely when the joint is maintained in a stable position.[9] Again, a case-by-case analysis of the big picture is important when making decisions and it comes down to more factors than a "tight vs. loose" perspective.

Postural Considerations for hEDS

When ligaments have excess laxity, the body must work harder to withstand the force of gravity in daily life. Forward head position is a very common postural impairment in this patient population, and over time it can increase strain on the joints of the upper cervical spine and the muscles that support the head and neck, increasing risk of brainstem, spinal cord and peripheral nerve issues in patients with hEDS. Forward head posture also affects our rib expansion and breathing pattern, our balance and equilibrium, and even the vagus nerve impact on our autonomic nervous system function, including digestion.[11] The classic way to visualize this is to imagine that for every inch that the head is forward, 10 pounds of weight are added to the head (which already weighs about 12 pounds).[12] It's key that posture is addressed in a way where kinesthetic awareness is increased and certain muscles are strengthened to help prevent forward head positioning.

Another common postural impairment in hEDS is weakness in the lateral hip muscles, which often presents as a pelvis tilt, knees going inward, and/or excess pronation and flat feet. Knee hyperextension can result in similar postural changes. It's important to incorporate specific muscular strengthening that addresses these types of postural concerns/imbalances as part of your exercise routine. By factoring in these impairments with the help of a physical therapist, you can maintain a more proactive role in reducing strain to the musculoskeletal system. We only get one body, so let's take good care of it and work to prevent future flare-ups as well as more serious complications!

More on Bracing

There are generally opposing opinions on the use of braces and splints to add joint stability. Some practitioners voice concern that over-bracing can lead to increased weakness, increased stiffness, increased dependency and increased risk of injury down the road. This may be a valid consideration for the general population as well as certain patients with hEDS. However, for patients with innate and *severe* global joint hypermobility issues, there can be a ceiling effect to which our compensatory muscle strengthening will only provide so much assistance to the ligaments. There's a big difference between an individual without global hypermobility who sustains a low-grade sprain to their ankle playing soccer for the first time and is still wearing a brace eight months later and a patient with hEDS who dislocates their patella weekly with everyday activities around the house. That being said, hEDS issues exist along a spectrum, and some patients are able to support the joint during the acute phase of an injury, gradually tapering away from brace use in the weeks to months that follow.

The decision for bracing should be determined by many factors including the patient's history, the presence of a genetic soft tissue abnormality, degree of joint instability, the symptoms occurring, the patient's typical activities, and the potential consequences of injury and persistent pain. The patient with a joint that is chronically and severely loose because of mechanical inadequacy of ligaments may find that bracing provides enough stability to increase overall functional mobility and restore proper movement patterns, and this should not be overlooked. In this type of a scenario, the individual may be able to significantly increase their activity level as a result of the brace, which could increase muscle strength and endurance when compared to the alternative of complete disuse. Thus, in hEDS, a brace can sometimes be considered a way to permit movement instead of restricting it.[13]

Bracing in the form of orthoses also appears to enhance proprioception in children with hEDS.[14] That being said, several sources still maintain that splints, while helpful for joint instability and pain, can makes muscle weaker through decreased load and muscle firing, particularly when they are used consistently, and this can also be a legitimate long-term concern in patients with hEDS.[15] After evaluating all the angles, the recent consensus is that while research is inconclusive, external joint supports including braces and splints may help protect large and small joints during everyday and recreational activities.[9]

If it's determined that joint bracing is appropriate for you, it's best to pursue necessary bracing with a physical therapist who can collaborate with an orthotist to create the proper set-up. Patients with hEDS in particular may need to consider lightweight braces (since braces are used for the long-term) with soft padding (due to the tendency for skin fragility) that are also strong.[13] Adjustable braces are helpful, and special care should be given when fitting patients with braces to ensure three bony points of contact, since many braces are designed for thin bodies.[13]

For neck issues and cervical instability, many experts recommend a Vista Aspen brace in order to avoid pressure and subluxation of the clavicles and upper ribs.[13] The Miami J Collar is another cervical spine support option; these neck orthoses should be fitted by a medical professional. The prescription of neck braces is a controversial topic and is typically reserved for patients with hEDS who develop severe laxity in their cervical spine. The use of a cervical soft collar is another controversial option, and while it may assist with postural training and proprioception, it does not protect an unstable spine.[16] Experts maintain that, when utilized, cervical collars should be temporary aids with the ultimate goal to improve posture and strength for better alignment of the cervical spine positioning at all times.[16]

It may be important to look into small finger splints to stabilize loose interphalangeal and metacarpophalangeal joints in the hands; SilverRing™ is a company that offers EDS-specific splint options for the hand that look like jewelry. Special purpose finger splints may be especially relevant for "swan neck" finger hyperextension deformities.[15] Mallet finger, trigger finger and Boutonniere injuries can also be stabilized with splints, and Oval Eights are plastic splints that are more affordable than the SilverRing™ splints (but less sturdy).[16]

Some specialists recommend Bauerfeind splints for other joints, as they appear to be more in-tune with the needs of individuals with permanently hypermobile joints.[13] Orthotics such as patellofemoral (kneecap) splints/braces may be useful for short-term assistance for a patient who experiences frequent patellar subluxations or dislocations.[16]

Other devices and aids like pen grips and adaptive utensils can reduce the force required in the fingers and hand and can substantially reduce pain and inflammation.[9,13] For patients with hypermobility who demonstrate pronated flat feet on weight bearing or increased valgus stress at the knee, attention to shoe design and orthotic shoe inserts may be beneficial. In 2020, research found that three-months' use of foot orthoses improved markers of pain, disability, fatigue and mental health-related quality of life in patients with EDS,[17] so this may be another option to consider.

There are many brands and options available for bracing/splinting/inserts, but some are more geared toward the athlete as opposed to the individual with chronic ligamentous laxity. It's important to work with your medical team to determine if and when an external support may be needed, and subsequently which type would be most appropriate.

Exercise Protocols for hEDS

Many experts agree that exercise is the only treatment option for hEDS that can give lasting results.[18] Of course, patients with hEDS are not immune to orthopedic concerns such as fractures, muscle and tendon tears and inflammation, ligamentous strains, meniscal tears, spinal facet and disc issues, labral tears and neurological inflammation, and these potential issues should be considered before starting an exercise program. As noted in Chapter 3, patients with hEDS also have an increased risk of conditions like Chiari malformation, craniocervical instability (CCI), intracranial pressure issues, tethered cord syndrome, cauda equina and cerebrospinal fluid leaks, and symptomatic individuals should work with a specialist to rule out these concerns.

Various physical therapists have proposed treatment protocols for hEDS over the years. Outside of one case report about the Muldowney Protocol (written by the protocol authors),[19] there's a surprising scarcity of research in regard to specific protocol-based exercise programs for hEDS. A systematic review noted that while some research shows benefits with exercise, there's no single specific type that appears more efficacious in patients with joint hypermobility syndrome.[20] Programs that incorporate progressive strength/stability, proprioception and patient education are supported in the literature for patients with joint hypermobility syndrome.[21-23] The Alexander Technique is a strategy to change movement habits and it incorporates concepts of energy conservation and re-education into movement[24] that may be useful for patients with EDS and other conditions.

Kevin Muldowney authored the book "Living Life to the Fullest with Ehlers-Danlos Syndrome," published in 2015. He presents a very detailed program of structured exercises for hEDS that can take six months to a year to complete, alongside a recommended high frequency of physical therapy visits (two to three per week, in some cases). The exercises incorporate strengthening and stabilizing the pelvis, back, upper body and lower body in a specific sequence, with eventual higher-level dynamic movements (like twisting and throwing) and a maintenance program.[25]

Experts agree that the progression of joint stability exercises should begin with exercises lying down in supine, side-lying and prone positions (beginning with static or no motion and advancing to dynamic movement patterns), eventually progressing to seated exercises (that also begin with static and advance to dynamic movement patterns) and lastly to standing exercises. The standing exercises should begin with static control before progressing to dynamic movement patterns and eventually to movement through different planes.[16] Complex patients most certainly benefit from a personalized approach, particularly at the start of any exercise program.

Most authors agree that there are several key aspects of a comprehensive exercise program for patients with hEDS:

- Include a focus on regular, consistent endurance activities. Many patients with hEDS are deconditioned. The type of activity for endurance is important; early on, exercises like swimming or water aerobics, cycling, Pilates and tai chi may be better tolerated, and adequate attention to form and biomechanics is important. Some patients with neck or shoulder issues may find swimming to be aggravating and may do better with water aerobics or water walking.

- Improve the strength and postural support of joint-stabilizing muscles through general and targeted (slowly progressive) strengthening. Low-impact isometric, concentric and eccentric exercise with an emphasis on proper alignment and posture can be helpful. Working on slow eccentric end-range control may be an effective strategy to reduce the likelihood of injury.[16] Spinal exercises and breathing exercises should also be included. Global range of motion and repetitive/forceful exercises are generally inappropriate and may make joint symptoms worse for patients with hEDS.[15]

- Include exercises for balance, motor control and proprioception (i.e., body spatial awareness). Patients with hEDS often have impaired firing patterns in muscles as well as difficulty with coordination, and exercise programs should address this with the help of a physical or occupational therapist.

- Correct for body mechanic/postural and gait impairments (and assess the underlying issues responsible for them).

- Include education about behavior and activity modification, pacing and bracing options when appropriate.

370

- Exercise programs should be goal-oriented and should eventually relate to functional everyday movement patterns as opposed to a single muscle action at a joint.
- Pain should not be ignored. Pain management and education are important components of the program. Emphasize conservative pain management as opposed to a focus on medications and injections. While there's limited evidence for modality management of pain in hEDS (utilizing devices like electrical stimulation, heat or ice), such modalities may be helpful for some patients.[26,27]
- Patient education regarding other factors such as nutrition, sleep, pacing and stress are key. Many patients with hEDS report a generalized difficulty in relaxing (both physically and mentally) because they are accustomed to maintaining some constancy of muscle tension to support the excess movement of their skeleton.

In terms of proprioception, there are several theories as to why body spatial awareness seems to be especially impaired in patients with hEDS. Some suspect that pain in the joints alters proprioception. Another theory is that excess joint mobility may damage proprioceptors. Others believe that the clumsiness and lack of spatial awareness stem from brainstem or craniocervical issues that are common in this patient population.

External feedback on body position may be important, especially at the start of an exercise program. Tactile input on the skin can help enhance proprioception, and some patients receive hands-on movement input, tape applied to the skin and tight-fitting clothing in early phases of exercise programs. Research indicates that the Feldenkrais method, a type of somatic education, may improve proprioception in patients with hEDS.[28] One study of knee proprioceptive acuity in kids (ages 8–16) with joint hypermobility syndrome concluded that *proprioceptive training* in the entire range of motion (including the hypermobile range) is encouraged, although further research is needed.[29]

Recently, some patients have questioned whether *strengthening* muscles in the hypermobile end-range of motion is important for hEDS too. One expert recommends exercising in the middle 50%–75% of the joint range of motion, with a progression to the full and hypermobile range of motion over time.[16] Another recommends starting with static exercises in the hypermobile range before progressing to dynamic and resisted work in hEDS patients who are experiencing significant pain.[30]

While it appears that there's not a consensus on this, keep in mind that unloaded static exercises in the end-range are very different from loaded dynamic exercises in the end-range of motion. The end-range and the position where the joint may be more likely to dislocate are not necessarily one and the same. Further, some patients experience pain and subluxation/dislocation in the hypermobile range, while others do not. An appropriate approach is one that also factors in the purpose of the strengthening: Is this patient preparing to return to aggressive athletics that require dynamic end-range stability, or is their goal to be able to carry the groceries in from the car? Again, a customized and individualized approach is key here.

While POTS has several reputable clear-cut programs designed to help improve upright exercise tolerance over time, hypermobile EDS is more complicated. In my opinion, with hEDS there's no single cookie-cutter exercise approach that works for everyone. Given the complexity of hEDS and the wide array of orthopedic concerns (not to mention additional concerns related to POTS and MCAS in some patients) and unique individual factors, a customized approach is essential.

EXERCISE FOR MCAS

A 2016 review on MCAS concluded, "In spite of the substantial fatigue and malaise that many MCAD patients experience, they should be strongly encouraged to exercise regularly."[31]

The biggest concern I see in patients who have MCAS is the possibility of exercise-induced flare symptoms (such as flushing, hives, respiratory issues, headache and other signs of mast cell degranulation, which very rarely include anaphylaxis).

Patients who are currently sensitive/highly reactive may find a few tips helpful when considering an exercise routine:

- Some patients need to pre-medicate with trusted antihistamines or other mast cell medications.
- Some patients do better indoors, while others are less reactive outdoors. Don't forget to factor in considerations like indoor air ventilation, molds and pollens, car exhaust and overhead power lines when considering spaces for exercise.
- All patients who have been prescribed auto-injectors of epinephrine should carry them with them while exercising.
- It's also advised to exercise with companions and wear medical alert bracelets.
- Foods and medications can trigger anaphylaxis when they are ingested in close proximity to exercise and should be avoided for two hours prior. It's best to space out the timing of these factors to reduce likelihood of reactions. On the other hand, certain patients may find that taking mast cell-specific medications prior to exercise is necessary in order to tolerate exercise.
- Many patients with MCAS find that gentle yoga and deep breathing work can be very helpful.

- On flare days at home, keep in mind that you can still exercise, even if it looks different than on good days. Some patients opt to do supine exercise, gentle spinal twists and breathing techniques or aim to walk to the mailbox and back. Be compassionate with yourself when your symptoms necessitate a change in your routine.

- If you regularly experience symptoms with exercise, be sure to delineate, in advance, what symptoms constitute halting exercise (and administering emergency medications) and what types of flare-ups may be acceptable during and immediately after exercise.

Mast Cell Mediators & Exercise

Histamine is the mast cell mediator most commonly studied with the human response to exercise. It appears that histamine increases locally in muscle tissue, as opposed to systemically (in healthy subjects) during exercise, and it may be connected to delayed onset muscle soreness.[32] A certain level of histamine during exercise facilitates important processes that affect everything from energy, endurance, insulin, blood flow and performance to post-exercise recovery.[32,33]

It's important to weigh the benefits of exercise in terms of long-term protective effects on physiological mechanisms, and not simply on an analysis of in-the-moment reactivity. While exercise is associated with short-term mast cell activation in some patients, there's also preliminary evidence in animal research that regular aerobic exercise may be a long-term protective factor for cardiac mast cell degranulation.[34]

Certain factors like blood flow, muscle recovery and energy may be generally negatively impacted by the use of oral antihistamines with exercise but delayed-onset muscle pain and excess hypotension following exercise may be improved with their use. Of course, the literature has yet to evaluate these factors specifically in patients with mast cell activation disease.

Exercise Type & MCAS

Yoga is generally a great option for patients with chronic illness, because it is low-impact and incorporates breathing techniques and stress reduction. Person-to-person modifications are encouraged to customize to individual needs as well as day-to-day fluctuations in symptoms. In the MCAS patient population, hot yoga is generally less tolerated than traditional yoga due to the potential for extreme heat to induce mast cell degranulation. There are many different types of yoga out there, and while some focus more on stability, others may increase flexibility, may focus largely on breath, or may be geared specifically toward mindset and mental health. The idea of sitting cross-legged and chanting "om" is an unfortunate stereotype that often prevents individuals from ever unlocking the healing potential of yoga. At-home videos and customized flows make it easier than ever to try yoga on your own without the environmental and financial concerns of a studio class.

Yoga may be especially beneficial for those suffering from allergies, headaches, and asthma.[35,36] Substantial evidence supports the many additional health benefits of yoga, including but not limited to: aiding walking tolerance, improving balance and sleep, increasing strength, lowering blood pressure, and improving cardiovascular health, health-related quality of life and control of chronic conditions.[37] Yoga has been shown to reduce anxiety and contribute to a more balanced autonomic nervous system.[38] Yoga practice is associated with increased intestinal blood flow and may be a great option for those who have both irritable bowel syndrome (IBS) and MCAS and those who experience intestinal discomfort with exercise.[39]

Pilates also has tremendous benefits and research indicates that it's an effective type of exercise for pain reduction and lowering the mast cell mediator prostaglandins measured in the blood.[40] Research shows that

Pilates exercise programs also appear to improve endurance, sleep quality and quality of life.[41,42]

Tai chi exercise programs have documented evidence of numerous factors including improvements in pulmonary function, airway inflammation, and inflammatory mediators like interleukin-6 and C-reactive protein.[43,44]

Aquatic centers offer options to swim laps, aqua jog, kick with a kickboard, or perform specific exercises, and there are numerous health benefits associated with swimming for the asthmatic population and beyond.[45] However, swimming is not always well-tolerated in the MCAS patient population due to chemicals used in swimming pools and the tendency for swimming pool indoor environments to be musty and moldy. Some patients find that they do better in saltwater pools, open water (lakes or ocean) or outdoor pools, while others tolerate indoor chlorinated pools without issues.

Endurance training, resistance training and high-intensity interval training (HIIT) have all been shown to improve function on the cellular level.[46-48] HIIT involves strenuous activity with brief periods of active rest. HIIT can take the form of different types of exercise. For runners, this could mean a track or hill workout that involves aggressive sprinting. HIIT approaches can also be created with gym exercises and many machines. Ultimately, the goal is to elevate the heart rate to near-maximal levels for certain intervals of time. This type of exercise is typically performed no more than three times per week. Ample research supports HIIT programs for patients with cardiovascular disease and asthma, with promising improvement in factors like inflammation, oxidative stress and insulin sensitivity, which are often prominent issues in patients with MCAS.

MOVEMENT: TAKE-HOME MESSAGES

- The best approach is one of carefully guided *modification* as opposed to total avoidance of exercise for patients with MCAS, POTS and EDS. Exercise has tremendous benefits for this patient population, and it should be a foundational component of every holistic healing plan for all three conditions.
- The Levine Protocol and CHOP modified Dallas Protocol provide guidelines for patients who have trouble with upright exercise due to POTS, and these programs are generally widely accepted as beneficial for this patient population.
- There is no universally accepted protocol for exercise in patients with hEDS. Exercise programs should be customized and guided with the help of a physical therapist knowledgeable in EDS. Joint bracing may be appropriate for some patients with chronic hypermobility.
- Patients with MCAS may have special considerations regarding exercise due to their sensitivities to different environments, but they should be encouraged to exercise while taking certain precautions. Avoidance of meals and certain medications immediately prior to exercise may be helpful, in addition to selecting optimal environments that are free of irritants or toxins.
- Programs inclusive of endurance, stability/strengthening, balance, proprioception, breathing exercises, postural and ergonomic factors, and patient education for activity modification and joint protection are key for patients with the trifecta.

- Exercise should be based on functional movement patterns mirroring your goals, and it should be enjoyable!
- What does movement look like for you right now? What are your short- and long-term goals for exercise? What types of programs and/or providers can help you work toward these goals? Reflect on this topic in your Trifecta Passport worksheet.

Chapter 11:
DETOXIFICATION

Environmental toxins and biotoxins including mold were already discussed in Chapter 6. Clinically, the majority of patients I work with who have chronic conditions, including those of the trifecta, present with detoxification organs that are not functioning optimally. This often leads to a vicious cycle scenario, as the body cannot keep up with the toxic load it is exposed to (or was exposed to historically). In addition to physical toxins, this chapter also discusses the presence of mental toxins in the form of harmful thoughts and relationships, as well as strategies to help support the detoxification pathways.

Detoxification Overview

"Detox" has been something of a buzzword lately in the chronic illness community and beyond. Detoxification refers to the process of physiological/medicinal removal of toxins from the body via certain organs. The liver is most commonly associated with detoxification, but there are several other organs that play a key role in this process.

The ability to remove toxins is especially influenced by mitochondrial function, exercise, glutathione, nutrients and thyroid function.[1] The liver and gallbladder, lymphatic system, kidneys and gastrointestinal system are the main organs associated with detoxification. Supporting these systems to do their job more efficiently and addressing root issues are key aspects of healing from a high toxic burden. Toxic by-products may build up disproportionately in patients who are genetically susceptible to physiological differences in the body's ability to process and remove toxins (such as those who have SNP mutations) and/or those who already present with higher loads of other burdens like viruses, mycotoxins, bacterial infections, parasites and other inflammatory conditions. Of particular concern is patients who have a poorly functioning gastrointestinal system. Theoretically, improving detoxification can have a profound impact on the baseline level of our mast cell reactivity, as well as flares in symptoms associated with MCAS, POTS and EDS.

Most disease stems from oxidative stress. Oxidative stress is where the production of reactive oxygen species (ROS) is greater than the body's ability to remove them. The decreased ability to neutralize ROS creates cellular damage and this damage is tied to inflammation and aging. Oxidative stress is caused by both external toxic insults and endogenous toxic insults. Endotoxins are present in the membrane of gram-negative bacterial cells and are released inside the cell as it disintegrates, as in the example of lipopolysaccharides (LPS) discussed in Chapter 5. Exotoxins, in contrast, are proteins released/secreted by certain bacteria outside of the cell.

Toxins were discussed at length in Chapter 6, but as a review, the more common toxins that influence patients with chronic illness include:

- Environmental home/workplace toxins
- Food and the standard American diet
- Health and beauty products
- Heavy metals (like mercury and lead)
- Hormonal and metabolic toxins that are not eliminated properly
- Internal toxins: bacteria, fungus, yeast, viruses
- Medications (supplements can also be contaminated!)
- Mental, emotional and spiritual toxins
- Molds/mycotoxins

- One-time major events or repeated exposure to lower levels (like carbon monoxide poisoning)
- Pesticides, fertilizers, petrochemicals
- Toxins passed during pregnancy/delivery

From this perspective, we are no longer just thinking about the histamine or mast cell mediator bucket! When the toxin bucket overflows, certain conditions such as cancer, autoimmune disease and neurodegenerative disease are more likely to develop. The ultimate goal is to lower the total toxic body burden so that body may remove stressors and restore homeostasis properly. The first step is to remove environmental toxin sources as best as possible. (This includes sources of mold and products like dryer sheets, air fresheners, perfumed candles, health and beauty aids, cleaning supplies, plastic water bottles/food storage, etc. This also requires taking a good look at your dietary food/beverage choices.) Cleaning up the diet and lifestyle will only take you so far when you have a high burden of health stressors, so the integrative treatment of components like viral and bacterial load and gut health also need to be prioritized.

Phases of Detoxification

When it comes to detoxification, most people are familiar with the importance of glutathione, an essential coenzyme in oxidation reactions responsible for helping the body complete these pathways. Not only does glutathione protect the body from harmful oxidative stress, but research supports that it also provides protection from persistent organic pollutants, alcohol, mercury and other toxic metals.[2] However, the process of aiding detoxification is much more complex than simply boosting glutathione.

There are three main phases of detoxification that occur in the liver-gut and liver-kidney systems. Phase one or "functionalization" utilizes a group of enzymes (cytochrome p450 family) that protect your cells from damage. Specifically, these enzymes make toxins water soluble for further processing and take large volatile toxins and break them down into smaller (less harmful) substances. The by-products of substances that go through phase one detoxification are free radicals, which create oxidative stress, and it's important to keep them moving so that they can be eliminated from the body. Phase one detoxification is activated by substances such as caffeine, certain fruits and vegetables, vitamins, minerals, herbs and compounds that break down fat. Cruciferous vegetables such as broccoli, brussels sprouts, cabbage, collard greens, kale and turnips especially support phase one detoxification. Some doctors advocate for supplementing antioxidants and cofactors including copper, CoQ10, manganese, resveratrol, selenium, vitamins (A, C, E) and zinc to support phase one detox.[3]

The second phase of detoxification, "conjugation," focuses on taking the water-soluble metabolites from phase one and conjugating them to help prepare them for removal via your stool, urine and bile. This is where many patients get stuck—they start the process appropriately in phase one but get hung up in phase two, which means that these harmful free radicals continue to circulate. In a healthy functioning system, harmful free radicals are either neutralized or transformed to harmless water by antioxidants. In an unhealthy liver, these intermediate substances are not able to be completely transformed by the phase two enzymes, resulting in recirculation of toxins. Substances that support phase two detoxification include amino acids, glutathione, molybdenum and vitamin B12. It's important to supplement with vitamin B12 if you're on a vegetarian or vegan diet, as most B12 comes from meat. Sulfuric food sources are also helpful here, and key dietary options to support phase two detoxification include a plethora of fruits, vegetables, legumes, nuts, meat, eggs, grains, seeds and other types of foods noted in Table 25. Flavonoids (found in a variety of fruits, vegetables and herbs) are also supportive of phase two detoxification.[3]

In the final step, phase three or "elimination," the phase two conjugates are transported to the organs of elimination (kidneys or gastrointestinal tract). In this phase, adequate hydration is key in order to support the kidneys in the final elimination through the urine. This phase also requires proper gastrointestinal system functioning and motility so that toxins are eliminated in the stool.[3]

Table 24. Detox Toolbox: Strategies to Aid Detoxification

DETOX STRATEGY	NOTES
Reduce continued toxin exposures in home and work environments, foods, beverages, personal health and beauty products.	Minimize continued exposure to endotoxins and exotoxins. (Chapter 6 has a home and workspace environment checklist that can aid in this process.)
Address "root issues."	The lower the overall total body burden of health stressors, the less strain on detoxification organs. Address underlying root issues such as the internal health stressors discussed in Chapter 5.
Ensure adequate hydration to support the kidneys.	Flush out toxins with lemon or lime water (citrus aids with phase one detoxification). Avoid sugary electrolyte beverages and make your own with water/fruit juice/salt or consider coconut water.
Focus on the breath. Work on mindfulness and meditation.	Get into nature. Get fresh air. Minimize stress. Incorporate breathing exercises. Mindfulness and meditation can lower inflammation by restoring proper nervous system function.

DETOX STRATEGY	NOTES
Sweat. Get outside.	Sweat every day. Whether through a sauna, gentle exercise or time outdoors, sweating is a process that naturally helps the body eliminate toxins. Getting midday sunlight every day is helpful for vitamin D levels and circadian rhythm, both of which aid detoxification.
Fuel your body with foods that help support detoxification pathways.	Focus on a healing anti-inflammatory, antioxidant-rich diet free of processed junk, additives, pesticides and herbicides. (See Table 25 for ideas.)
Consider juicing as a supplemental boost.	Studies support the juice of various fruits and vegetables for enhancing detoxification and improving antioxidant and vitamin levels as well as reducing cardiovascular risk factors including oxidative stress.[4,5] While juice doesn't contain the fiber content you'd get from eating produce and it shouldn't be a substitute for fruit and vegetable consumption, it can be a helpful supplemental boost for the immune system and the detoxification organs. Be sure to use a machine to make juice at home as opposed to store-bought options.

DETOX STRATEGY	NOTES
Try a castor oil pack over the liver at night.	Castor oil contains ricinoleic acid, oleic acid and linoleic acid, which work to support the liver, reduce inflammation, improve digestion and the microbiome, and help balance hormones and neurotransmitters.
Consider supplements to help support detoxification pathways with the help of your care team.	See Table 26 for specific supplement ideas.
Consider additional holistic treatment modalities that may improve detoxification.	Acupuncture and acupressure, infrared sauna, ionic footbaths, ozone therapy, intravenous infusions, hyperbaric oxygen therapy, massage and colonic (enema) therapy are sometimes considered useful adjuncts in detoxification programs.[6-8]
Consider a fasting routine.	Some sources support intermittent fasting or time-restricted eating (12+ hour intervals of fasting) to aid in detoxification, but this may not always be ideal for every patient who has chronic conditions; if curious, discuss it with your medical team.
Consider toxin binders when appropriate.	Some patients may also need to take toxin binders for mold or heavy metals if their system is physically unable to remove certain toxins on its own. Binders are substances that can trap toxins to facilitate swifter or easier elimination. Binders generally need to be taken spaced away from food, medications and other supplements. Binder efficacy may be enhanced by taking certain substances under the tongue 30 minutes prior in efforts to enhance bile and liver shunting of toxins to the gut, referred to as a "push-catch" system.

DETOX STRATEGY	NOTES
Consider strategies to boost the lymphatic system.	Skin brushing, manual lymphatic drainage with a trained professional, reflexology, light repetitive physical activity, abdominal lymph-specific hula hoops, and rebounder exercises may assist in lymphatic system optimization.
Strategies to improve mitochondrial function may assist in detoxification efficiency.	Antioxidant- and polyphenol-rich foods appear to boost mitochondrial function. Some patients experiment with intermittent fasting, cold showers and high-intensity interval training to support mitochondria, though the jury is still out on the efficacy of some of these strategies.
Consider taking Epsom salt baths to help with detoxification.	Magnesium sulfate has been claimed to lower inflammation, soothe skin and muscles, improve bowel and cardiovascular health, boost detoxification and raise serotonin levels, though there are some skeptics. It's a safe and soothing form of self-care.
Ensure adequate attention to quality sleep.	A bulk of our detoxification via the liver occurs between the hours of 1 and 3 a.m. Practice sleep hygiene strategies such as blue light-blocking glasses in the evening and avoidance of screen time 1–2 hours before bed. Make sure you are getting an extra 1–2 hours of sleep per night when you are focusing on detoxification! (Further information to come in this chapter for more sleep hygiene ideas.)

DETOX STRATEGY	NOTES
Elimination of toxins via the gut is one of the most important pathways. For patients with chronic constipation, strategies should be employed to maintain bowel regularity.	A foot stepstool may assist in reducing strain while on the toilet. Visceral manipulation and abdominal massage can help with motility. Hydration and specific supplements to maintain bowel movement regularity should be discussed with your medical team. Certain issues including dysbiosis, parasites, candida overgrowth, lack of fiber, magnesium deficiency, and food intolerances can influence gastrointestinal motility and should be addressed.
Consider avoidance of sources of electromagnetic energy, particularly if your body is already struggling against a heavy total burden.	Put your wifi router on a timer so that it's turned off at night. Consider putting devices on airplane mode when not in use. Avoid sleeping with cell phones near the bed.
Consider air and water purification devices for the home and office.	HEPA air purifiers and filters for tap water and shower heads can help reduce the presence of toxins incurred via inhalation, ingestion and skin absorption.
Include strategies to improve nervous system tone and stimulate the vagus nerve and other cranial nerves which may foster more time spent in "rest and digest" mode, equating to more optimal function of detoxification organs.	Programs such as The Safe & Sound Protocol, The Gupta Program, Heart Rate Variability Training, and Dynamic Neural Retraining System can assist in this area. (See Chapter 7 for more ideas.)

DETOX STRATEGY	NOTES
Address energetic and emotional healing.	Mental toxins (unhealthy thoughts) and relationships that deplete you have a huge impact on your physiology too! Check in with an internal self-assessment and be sure to prioritize adequate time for self-care.

Specific strategies for detoxification should always be *guided with the help of a medical professional.* Detoxification strategies should be performed *carefully and slowly,* and short-term flare-ups in symptoms may be expected for patients with MCAS and POTS as well as the general population. Massive detoxification reactions should be avoided. The topic of detoxification is shared multiple times in this book to highlight its importance in this patient population. Reducing toxic burden can have a profound impact on the resolution of things like mast cell reactivity, dysautonomia/POTS, migraines, chemical sensitivity, orthopedic pain and inflammation, chronic fatigue/pain and even other conditions like thyroid disease. Thus, it should be a big part of the foundational treatment plan for every patient with the trifecta. Work with an integrative provider to determine which phase of detoxification may be more of an issue for your body so that you know how to better support it.

Table 25. Foods That Support Detoxification Pathways[9]

Benefits	Food Source
Phase One Detoxification	Caffeinated beverages (coffee, black tea, green tea) Chicory root Cruciferous vegetables (arugula, bok choy, broccoli, brussels sprouts, cabbage, cauliflower, kale, radish, turnips) Garlic Herbal tea: rooibos Rosemary Soy
Phase Two Detoxification	Barley Citrus fruits (except grapefruit) Caffeine sources (black tea, cocoa, coffee, green tea) Cruciferous vegetables (arugula, bok choy, broccoli, brussels sprouts, cabbage, cauliflower, kale, radish, turnips) Fruit (apples, apricot, avocado, cherries, lemons, peaches, plums, prunes) Egg Ellagic acid (berries, black currant, grapes, pomegranate, walnut) Ferulic acid (asparagus, berries, citrus fruits, coffee, olives, peas, tomatoes, whole grains) Herbal tea (dandelion, honeybush, rooibos) Legumes (adzuki bean sprouts, alfalfa sprouts, butter beans, lentils, mung bean seeds) Meat Non-cruciferous vegetables (artichoke, asparagus, carrots, celery, chives, cucumber, garlic, ginger, green pepper, horseradish, leeks, lettuce, mustard greens, onions, potatoes, spinach, watercress) Nuts (almonds, brazil nuts, peanuts, pistachios, walnuts) Oats Quinoa

	Rosemary
	Seeds (sesame seeds, sunflower seeds)
	Soy

A recent scientific review concluded that the above foods are key for various detoxification pathways and that a dietary pattern favoring whole, unprocessed plant-based foods (plus removal of exposure to toxic substances) has the best scientific support.[9] Cruciferous vegetables, rooibos tea, caffeinated beverages, garlic, rosemary and soy all have scientific evidence supporting their utility for both of the first two phases of detoxification, so these foods may be the best bang for your buck from that perspective. However, it's important to have diverse options for nutrient-based detoxification support as well as a custom-tailored plan to ensure support of the phase(s) that may be more of a struggle for your body specifically. Genetic testing can shed further light onto which phase of detoxification may need more attention for you personally. Genetic testing can also help you determine whether certain pathways such as glucaronidation, methylation, acetylation, sulfation, and amino acid conjugation need extra support.

You can imagine how problematic it can be for detoxification if you decide to completely remove salicylates, high histamine foods, etc. from your diet, which leaves the body with fewer natural options for detoxification support. If you are unable to tolerate garlic, other high FODMAP foods, or other options in the above table, you may want to consider supplementation (with the help of your healthcare team) to ensure that you are providing these pathways with adequate support. Even if you tolerate a diverse array of foods, your practitioner may also guide you to specific supplements to assist in the process, particularly if you have a high toxic burden, malnourishment or persistent chronic illness.

Supplements That Support Detoxification Pathways

Table 26. Supplements That Support Detoxification[3,9]

Benefits	Supplement
Phase One Detoxification	Curcumin Fish Oil Iron Magnesium Milk thistle Most of the B vitamins Quercetin Resveratrol
Phase Two Detoxification	Curcumin Glutathione (liposomal or intravenous) or its precursors glutamine, glycine and n-acetyl cysteine (NAC) Methionine Milk thistle Molybdenum Resveratrol Spirulina Taurine Vitamin B12

The above supplements assist with detoxification in different ways. For example, some of them are precursors to glutathione, a powerful antioxidant that is easily depleted by the presence of toxins (particularly toxins from mold). You provider may also draw attention to cofactors needed for the production of glutathione, such as vitamins B2, B6, B12, folate and magnesium. Key additions to support these pathways may also include alpha lipoic acid, choline, copper, CoQ10, gingko biloba, inositol, manganese, pantothenic acid, plant-based antioxidants, selenium, superoxide dismutase, vitamin A, vitamin C, vitamin E, zinc and 5-MTHF.[3,9] Digestive support such as enzymes and betaine hydrochloride (HCl) may also be helpful, in addition to magnesium to help with bowel elimination.[3] All of these factors depend on your specific scenario and what is occurring in your body. For example, certain supplements and foods may target the up-regulation of specific genetic expressions that support heavy metal metabolism, such as cruciferous vegetables, hops, pomegranate rind extract, prune skin extract and watercress extract.[10]

It's important to keep in mind that if a patient does not control or manage their detoxification carefully and time it following repair to the necessary organs (particularly the gut, lymphatic system, liver and kidneys) in a particular sequence, more toxins can be unleashed than the body can safely process.[1] A guided stepwise approach is important, and the use of supplements can recirculate toxins and make the patient sick if the vital organs are not prepared for the process.

Any given patient may have specific genetic variants that equate to difficulties with certain pathways, and in these cases certain supplements can make them feel worse. In a perfect world, alterations in the biopterin, dopamine, epinephrine, folate, histamine, melatonin, methionine, norepinephrine, and serotonin pathways should be addressed to help guide supplement decisions and areas to support with a better understanding of your unique predispositions. Supporting detoxification is certainly not a "one supplement fits all" approach. And for patients who don't tolerate supplements well, it's important to remember that there are many other options available to support detoxification in a gentle and natural manner.

Detoxification Resources

Useful links – websites to evaluate safety of household products and foods:

Assessment Tools, Recipes and other Resources:
www.thetoxinsolution.com
Cosmetics: www.safecosmetics.org
Environmental Toxic Assessment: www.pureairpurewater.com
Safe Air: www.airnow.gov
Safe Cleaning Products: www.ewg.org/guides/cleaners
Safe Foods: www.ewg.org/key-issues/food

The Lymphatic System

When we think of the cardiovascular system, there's a giant muscle called the heart that's pumping blood, and if we increase our activity, the heart beats faster and increases the circulation. Lymph, however, is not influenced as easily and therefore needs specific strategies to help it flow through the body more effectively, particularly in patients who have stagnation or accumulated toxins. Lymph is a colorless fluid containing white blood cells, and it bathes the tissues and drains around the lymphatic system into the bloodstream. Lymphatic vessels lead into lymph nodes, and there are hundreds of these cleansing "hubs" all over the body. Lymph relies on relaxation and contraction of muscles and joints to help move it around the body.

Lymphatic tissue carries waste from the tissues and cells back to the heart. It's hypothesized that an increasing toxic/bacterial/viral load can reduce the efficiency of the lymphatic system to the point where it becomes sluggish and impaired. There are several strategies that appear to assist in fostering helpful lymphatic flow.

Lymphatic Drainage

Lymphatic drainage specialists offer manual therapies, positional considerations, compression instruction and/or light therapy machines aimed to reduce lymphedema, blockage of the lymphatic vessels leading to fluid accumulation. Reflexology lymphatic drainage aims to stimulate lymphatic reflexes in the feet and may be another resource.

We have over 500 lymph nodes in our body,[11] and lymphatic massage has shown to push stagnant lymph from these areas back into circulation. This mobilizes the toxins for clearance, lessening the burden on the lymphatic system.

It's important to find a practitioner who has adequate training and experience in this arena. The following website is a great resource for more information and lists many reputable therapist directories.

https://lymphaticnetwork.org/living-with-lymphedema/find-a-lymphedema-therapist

Additional Lymphatic System Strategies

- Hydration: As previously discussed, some experts maintain that patients should drink at least half their body weight (in ounces) of purified water per day, throughout the day. Hydration is a key practice for optimizing detoxification pathways and lymphatic flow. Adding freshly squeezed lemon juice to water a few times a day can also assist.
- Massage: Lighter types of massage can assist the lymphatic system, but deep tissue work is less useful when this is the goal.
- Skin brushing: Before showering, when your skin is dry, take a natural-bristle brush (the type used for body scrubbing in the shower) and use it to gently brush your skin with low to medium pressure. Move the brush from the extremities toward the heart to stimulate sweat glands and skin circulation.

- Rebounding: Jumping on a trampoline/rebounder may assist with lymphatic drainage. The jumping should be gentle and relaxed. I typically have patients start with one to two minutes at a time, building up to two 10-minute sessions per day, as tolerated.
- Other light rhythmic activities like swimming, hula hooping and jumping rope are also reported to be helpful for enhancing lymphatic flow. Special weighted hula hoops can assist in abdominal area lymph stimulation. Wearing looser-fitting clothing while performing lymph-targeting rhythmic activities may promote additional lymphatic flow.
- The natural rhythm of yoga facilitates contraction and relaxation of muscles, which is the primary way that lymph moves through the body. Twisting also helps stimulate lymphatic flow. Through the practice of twisting the abdomen, the organs and muscles are squeezed, forcing the lymph out of the tissues.
- Inverted positions utilize gravity to help drain the lymph toward the heart, escalating the rate in which it is cleaned and filtered. Inversion table use and inverted yoga positions are tolerated by some patients; placing the legs up on a wall while lying on your back is another alternative to gently help facilitate lymphatic flow.
- Deep breathing exercises: Diaphragmatic breathing causes the lungs to press into the thoracic duct, and this pressure aids in moving the fluid from the thoracic duct into the bloodstream. Research supports breathing exercises that spend more time on the exhale than the inhale as supportive for lymphatic flow.
- Soaks and compresses: A foot soak in warm ginger tea or five-minute use of a tea-soaked compress on the neck (where lymph nodes drain from the head) feels great and boosts the system. Saunas and Epsom salt baths are also good options, if tolerated.

- Acupuncture is a modality that can benefit the lymphatic system and it has ample evidence supporting that it's a safe option for reducing edema in various patient populations.[12]
- Consider increasing your intake of foods that may boost the lymphatic system: almonds, apples, avocado, brazil nuts, celery, chia seed, cranberries, flaxseed, garlic, green leafy vegetables, okra, walnuts, and watercress.[13]
- Consider herbalist-approved lymphatic system-supporting teas: astragalus, calendula, cilantro, cleavers, dandelion, devil's claw, echinacea, goldenseal, knotted figwort, parsley, red clover and wild indigo root.[13-15]
- Remember to avoid the following foods that may cause blockages to the lymphatic system: artificial sweeteners, conventionally raised meat and eggs, dairy, processed foods and sugar.[13]

As always, consult your medical team before starting any new supplements (including herbal teas) as they can interact with medications and cause adverse reactions. Some of the herbs recommended on the internet specifically for lymphatic support are poisonous in large doses, so it may also be important to work with an herbalist.

Sleep Hygiene

Many patients suffer from insomnia due to neurological inflammation and/or dysautonomia related to extra sympathetic nervous system activity at night. Some attest that additional factors like detoxification problems, high infectious burden, improper nutrition, lack of exercise, orthopedic conditions, the presence of sleep apnea and emotional stress also contribute to insomnia. Many patients report that no matter how many hours they spend in bed, their sleep does not feel restorative in the morning. Regardless of the unique contributing factors, it's important that sleep is addressed early on in the treatment plan.

According to 2018 research, approximately 25% of Americans suffer from insomnia every year,[16] and I imagine that statistic is actually much higher in the population of individuals with chronic illness. Sleep hygiene is becoming a catchphrase in the medical world, and it describes the concept of creating good sleep habits on a daily basis. Some of these are a no-brainer, such as avoiding caffeine at night. Others, however, are less intuitive and have more to do with our electronic devices, lighting, functional medicine concepts and use of certain spaces in the home.

Below are some suggestions based off clinical experience and expert recommendations that seem to assist in reducing insomnia:

- Address viral and bacterial issues that are affecting the entire system with the help of a professional. Many patients with MCAS also have chronic Epstein-Barr virus, Lyme disease, and other burdens that stress and deplete the system and create a perfect storm of issues, both during the day and at night.
- Address gut health issues (such as candida, SIBO, etc.) with the help of a professional. Follow a diet that focuses on whole foods like organic fruits and vegetables and avoid processed foods, alcohol, caffeine, additives, etc. Try taking your probiotic at night.
- Address mold with the help of a professional if it is an issue for you. Many patients with CIRS (Chronic Inflammatory Response Syndrome) from mold toxins experience a high number of neurological symptoms, and insomnia tends to be especially common in this patient population.
- Consider a sleep study and rule out sleep apnea.
- Address anxiety. Most people won't sleep better while their mind is racing or when they are anxious about things that happened in the past or about future events. If you lie awake thinking of things

you need to do the following day, keep a pen and notepad near the bed to jot down reminders.

- Reduce exposure to EMFs (electric and magnetic fields), especially at night. In some living scenarios this is difficult, but it can help to turn off the wireless internet router at night, turn wifi/data off the cell phones and physically remove cell phones from the sleeping area. Consider other sources of EMFs as well.

- There are several products that aim to enhance the quality of sleep and to wake you gently and at a specific time in your sleep cycle. Some products for the bed itself block EMFs, while others include vibrational frequencies and sounds that may soothe the nervous system for sleeping. Some alarm clocks utilize essential oils and a gradual light to wake you up when you are in light sleep as opposed to deep sleep so that you feel more refreshed.

- Consider stopping all screen time two hours prior to bed. Dim electronic screens in the evening. Invest in a pair of blue light-blocking glasses to use in the evenings. Also consider dimming the lights in the home for a few hours prior to bedtime. Special light bulbs that reduce blue light exposure are available for the home environment. Some cell phones have a "night shift" function where you can adjust things like screen brightness. Blue light-blocking screen protectors can also help.

- Maintain the bed as a sanctuary and avoid doing anything work-related or using the computer, TV or phone while in it. Teach the body to recognize the bed space as solely for sleeping and intimacy. Keep the room dark and use earplugs and/or white noise if needed. Consider an eye mask and a weighted blanket. Make sure you have a comfortable mattress and pillows and rotate the mattress regularly.

- Be intentional about avoiding things that trigger emotional stress before bed. For example, avoid checking emails or watching the news late at night.
- Get active. Consistent physical exercise can help, presuming it's not done within a few hours of going to bed. Interestingly, midday light exposure helps the body get into a better rhythm and produce more melatonin at night.[17] So, consider a midday walk or bike ride when able.
- Make sure pain is well-controlled. Come up a with a relaxing pre-bedtime ritual. Many people find that taking a warm bath, drinking hot tea, or reading a book helps with relaxation before bed.
- Make sure you avoid dehydration and hypoglycemia, both of which can cause you to wake up at night. Alcohol and caffeine can also influence sleep and should be avoided.
- Breathing exercises and strategies to work on ventral vagal tone can be helpful too in the time before sleep, particularly for patients with POTS and patients who experience adrenaline rushes that jolt them awake as they start to fall asleep. Certain strategies like Emotional Freedom Technique (EFT) can also help redirect the nervous system back to a calm state if you wake up with anxiety in the middle of the night.
- Many resources recommend getting into a good routine and going to sleep at the same time every night. The jury still has mixed results on napping as well as whether a light snack before bed is ideal. Some people find that intermittent fasting also has an impact on sleep issues and the frequency of waking up at night.
- Persistent insomnia can be tied to many conditions. Repeat waking in the middle of the night (particularly between 1 and 3 a.m.) can signal that certain issues with liver health or hormones, gastrointestinal infections or parasites, neurological inflammation or glucose regulation may be present. Experts recommend

evaluating toxic burden, gut health and hormones including melatonin and the cortisol awakening response in those who struggle regularly with insomnia.

- Some patients with chronic illness tolerate melatonin supplements well, while others do not. Other nighttime supplements typically include a blend of melatonin with vitamin B6, GABA, L-theanine, valerian root, passionflower, ashwagandha, lemon balm, hops, kava and chamomile. Obviously, multi-ingredient supplements can be tricky with patients who are extra sensitive, so many patients prefer to test the different ingredients one at a time first. And some of these substances can cause unwanted effects; for example, in some individuals valerian root can make insomnia worse because it acts as a stimulant. (Always consult your medical team when considering adding a new supplement, as these ingredients can interact with other supplements and medications.)

- Some patients find that taking toxin binders before bed (away from other medications) and/or the use of a castor oil pack at night can reduce insomnia. These components of a detoxification program should be supported with other steps and a customized plan for best results.

- When sleeplessness occurs, try not to get frustrated. Make an effort to avoid fixating on what symptoms may be keeping you awake (presuming they are non-emergent). If sleeplessness occurs for more than 10–20 minutes, consider moving to a different space and doing something relaxing in low light until you get sleepy again. Keeping a slightly boring book handy usually does the trick. Some patients find that listening to binaural beats (the tones specific to sleep) or recorded meditations can be helpful too. Otherwise, avoid using electronics and your phone when you can't sleep at night.

ENERGETIC & EMOTIONAL HEALING

Healing is not solely a physical entity, and unfortunately many patients (myself included) find that they've ignored this realm of healing or failed to fully tap into it early in the chronic illness journey. Some believe that mental/psychological toxins are just as powerful as physical toxins.

Many patients who have MCAS (and other conditions) note a "chemical-like" feeling to their anxiety or depression that increases when their physical symptoms are flared up. First and foremost, it's essential to figure out what underlying factors or health stressors are responsible for the systemic inflammation affecting the brain. By identifying and eliminating physiological factors such as adrenal dysfunction, environmental toxins, gut dysbiosis, hormonal imbalances, improper nutrition, mold, parasites, viral and bacterial infections and other issues, some patients find that their anxiety and/or depression improves or resolves on its own. Addressing physiological factors contributing to your mental health status is certainly an important step, but it shouldn't be the only step. Addressing the neurological system (discussed in Chapter 7) can also really help in this area. Needless to say, it's also very important to address mental health concerns with the help of a licensed healthcare provider.

Professional Resources

Professional mental health resources are a huge priority for the patient newly diagnosed with a chronic condition and can also be helpful for ongoing assistance when living with chronic illness. Many people think of psychological trauma in the past as a potential trigger for the disease, but it can also work the other way around where patients (particularly those who have experienced severe anaphylaxis or intubation) may experience trauma from emergency room visits. Many patients downplay their past experiences as insignificant when they don't involve outright and blatant physical or sexual abuse, but mental abuse and "minor" incidences can also be incredibly powerful triggers that can impact the brain and nervous system for a lifetime.

The establishment of regular psychotherapy or counseling sessions can be immensely helpful. Having a safe, non-biased place to help you navigate the physical and emotional challenges of living with medical conditions can be empowering and healing. Most patients with the trifecta put tremendous pressure on themselves in terms of their interpersonal relationships and career considerations.

Based on clinical observation, patients with the trifecta almost always experience some degree of anxiety, depression, attention deficit hyperactivity disorder (ADHD), autism spectrum disorders (ASD) and/or post-traumatic stress disorder (PTSD). Talk therapy not only provides an outlet but can also help you to learn key tools for prevention and management of symptoms. While the trifecta conditions are not caused by stress, working to reduce psychological triggers that lead to mental stress can certainly help reduce overall inflammation and flare-ups.

Some options like talk therapy and eye movement desensitization and reprocessing (EMDR) may involve conscious reprocessing of past experiences, while other treatment approaches like tension and trauma releasing exercises (TRE) address the neurological impacts of past trauma without reliving it. EMDR is a therapeutic technique used to alleviate the distress associated with traumatic injuries by utilizing bilateral sensory input (such as alternating buzzing devices in the hands) with the goal to change the way traumatic memories are stored in the brain. TRE is a type of therapy that activates a natural shaking reflex that releases muscular trauma and subsequently calms the sympathetic nervous system of the impacts of repressed emotions and PTSD.

Somatic therapy is a body-centered therapy that works from the "bottom up" to help discharge trauma and alter the autonomic nervous system through a combination of psychotherapy and physical therapies. This approach is especially useful for body-based trauma and PTSD, and it aims to heal the relationship with the body and help patients learn how to cope. There are many different types of somatic and cognitive therapies, and it's important to work with a professional to determine what type of approach is best for your current situation.

Quantitative Electroencephalography (qEEG) is a form of assessment evaluating the electrical activity of the brain and the types of brain waves in order to create brain maps. This tool can be used to evaluate brain activity and it can also serve as a neural biofeedback treatment option. Having real-time 3D imaging of brain activity can enable an individual to perform certain activities and to work with a practitioner to retrain the brain based on the biofeedback. Individuals with conditions such as ADHD, anxiety disorders, autism spectrum disorders, bipolar disorder, depression, learning disabilities and PTSD may find this type of treatment helpful.

Brainspotting is a treatment based on the concept that where you look affects how you feel. Specifically, this technique uses points in the patient's visual field in order to help access subconscious unprocessed trauma in the subcortical brain. This helps the brain to process trauma from the bottom up.[18]

Practitioners may also help patients to incorporate tools like Callahan techniques thought field therapy (TFT) and emotional freedom technique (EFT), two examples of treatments that involve tapping in order to create a balance in your energy system. EFT focuses on acupressure meridians, and TFT focuses on sequential tapping as a code to balance the body's energy system. Tapping as a part of EFT is believed to work by helping adjust the amygdala fear response that occurs with our thoughts so that we are better balanced in a place of safety and acceptance.

Chronic illness can be very hard on your loved ones, who often feel helpless and can also grow frustrated with daily limitations, inconveniences and stressors. Early on, family members may experience something called "research fatigue," which can also morph into sadness, grief and "compassion fatigue." Counseling is also strongly encouraged for partners and caregivers, as they can feel helpless when adapting to the daily challenges that their loved one faces.

A Healing Mindset

There are several additional factors that can help promote emotional healing. When it comes to chronic illness, it's important to remember that "you can't ride a bike going backward" (author unknown). Too great of a focus on past wounds—on diagnoses and labels and symptom clusters, for example—can certainly be detrimental, but most patients are already so deeply embedded in the chronicity of their issues and their typically long-standing quest for answers (especially by the time they receive a diagnosis that best describes everything) that it seems impossible to *not* dwell on it.

That being said, progress is best facilitated when you are ready to let go of the past and move forward with a positive mindset for healing. Letting go of people who have wronged you in the past (including those in the medical system) and releasing regrets pertaining to your own actions are key to getting back on that bicycle with forward momentum. Letting go of past wrongs can be tough, particularly if you were told that your illness is all in your head by a loved one or doctor. But consider those experiences to be a big pile of unwanted baggage; let them go.

Many public figures and speakers have described *unforgiveness* as a toxic poison that we drink in the hopes of hurting others. Often, the things that you hold on to are most damaging to yourself and not the other person. Regardless of your religious perspective, many cultures and communities (and resources like Alcoholics Anonymous) incorporate forgiveness into the approach for physical and/or mental healing.

In order to foster deep emotional healing, forgiveness of self and others can be a key foundation. Release of past hurts and wounds may have a benefit in assisting the body to release physical manifestations of toxins and disease. In some cases, a lifespan assessment of emotional baggage can be followed by conversations with people who either 1) wronged you or 2) you wronged. However, some scenarios render a face-to-face conversation unsafe or impossible; journaling and prayer can also assist in this process of an inward shift and release. Exercises that involve the physical releasing of unforgiveness (such as letting balloons go or burying paper with words) offer another symbolic and unique way to express emotional release more literally.

Another helpful approach is to reframe the situation. For example, we can get wrapped up in a lot of negativity about our mast cells or our collagen properties. Many websites depict mast cells in a negative manner when considering MCAS. Instead of thinking of the mast cell as an evil entity that is aggressively going into attack mode—this is going to sound strange, but try it—remember to thank your mast cells! Be grateful that they are signaling that something is off in the body. Individuals who have silent, stealthy forms of cancer are often not so lucky to be afforded the time to recognize and remove triggers. Have gratitude for the incredibly complex set of properties and functions of your mast cells. MCAS reflects an intelligent immune system that is crying out for help, signaling an alarm system and trying to get the body back to homeostasis. When mast cells flag the system to a buildup of underlying factors and toxicities that are detrimental to your health, you can identify root issues and foster changes that, thanks to the sensitivity of the mast cell, should provide somewhat clear responses as to whether the change is effective over time.

Similarly, our unique collagen deficits with EDS can be viewed as a painful hindrance, or we can choose to focus on the fact that our skin stays soft and our faces seem to age more slowly than our peers. (OK, this one may be a stretch... awful pun intended!)

Mast cells are like a home security system, but if the focus is solely on symptoms (or is too negatively embedded into the role of mast cells), you may remain stuck in a vicious cycle of surviving and reacting to crises, rather than thriving. Therefore, optimal management of MCAS goes far

405

beyond medication management and far beyond the mast cell itself. (And the same goes for POTS and EDS.) Lifestyle changes needed to reduce inflammation/underlying root issues and promote healing should be continued for the long term; it's important that you are aware of this and mentally prepared for the challenges, changes and endurance that are necessary to reap healing rewards. This is a marathon and definitely not a sprint; consider each healing lifestyle change an investment for your future.

Another helpful approach lies in setting appropriate boundaries—with yourself and with others. Healthy boundaries are important in any relationship, but especially in ones where you may be sensitive to certain environmental factors, fatigue quickly or require adaptations for daily activities. Evaluate relationships in your life and determine which ones bring you joy and which ones may be toxic. Surround yourself with individuals who bring you joy.

As hard as it can be, try not to worry about pleasing others. Stand firm in what you know you need and be an advocate for yourself. Follow your intuition and trust your body. You know your body best, so remember to honor that in your conversations with peers and medical providers. And be compassionate toward yourself. We are often our harshest critics.

When I work with parents and particularly mothers, I find that many feel insecurities surrounding their ability to parent in the way that they want to. Many will also carry a lot of self-blame for scenarios where their child(ren) may also have chronic health issues. They feel responsible for passing on certain traits or obsess over what they did or didn't do prenatally and during pregnancy and nursing. This is usually accompanied by a great deal of negative self-talk. Reversing these constructs is absolutely essential for healing from chronic illness, yet this is one area that is often neglected. In these scenarios it's important to have regular reminders that 1) this is not your fault and 2) you are doing the best that you can. Taking care of yourself first so that you can then take care of your family is non-negotiable and the very opposite of selfish.

Social media can be a double-edged sword, so be cautious about how much time you spend online. Patient group pages often have wonderful and well-meaning leaders, but it can be emotionally draining to navigate through your own challenges, let alone those of others. And sometimes advice on those pages may be misguided. Many patients in this community have empath tendencies with immune and nervous systems that are easily activated by the slightest emotional stress or excitement.

Remember to pace yourself with activities of daily living. Approach setbacks in the trial and error process with gratitude, since they help you gather valuable information that can guide your decisions in the future. Work on fostering acceptance of your situation and cultivating joy no matter what circumstances come your way, while also allowing yourself to acknowledge and feel tough emotions when you have a bad day. Try to avoid perseverating on the things that are out of your control. Let go of the uncontrollable and try to recognize when your actions persist simply to gain some form of control over the situation.

Consider using mantras or reversal statements, as described in Chapter 7. Come up with positive mantras to use throughout your day. Keep in mind that while mantras can be a helpful tool, there's a fine line between infusing positive thoughts into our mindset and utilizing what some refer to as "toxic positivity," which can deny an individual's experience or reality. It's important to acknowledge the challenges and low moments and to validate what you are going through while remembering that change and healing are possible. Focus mantras on the antithesis of harmful mindset variables that, deep down, you know are untrue, such as "I am a failure" or "I am not enough."

Practice self-love, forgiveness and gratitude daily. Prioritize self-care in your daily life. Figure out what the best-case scenario of self-care would look like for you. Write it down and post it somewhere visible.

Self-care looks different for everyone, but here are some ideas of activities that my patients commonly report as helpful and rejuvenating:

- taking a warm bath
- listening to music
- journaling
- reading
- meditating
- gardening or tending plants
- cooking
- getting a massage
- diffusing essential oils
- watching TV or movies
- painting
- knitting or sewing
- drawing
- growing an herb garden
- counseling services
- going on walks
- getting into nature
- singing
- dancing
- emotional freedom technique (EFT) tapping
- coloring
- playing a game
- listening to podcasts
- praying
- grounding

- playing a musical instrument
- writing
- specific types of exercise
- deep breathing exercises
- photography
- book club
- church group
- coffee date or phone call with a friend

For some patients, spending time with family and friends is really recharging, while for others, it can be draining. The same goes for activities like travel. Figure out what works best to help recharge your own battery. Carving out self-care time in your schedule is essential.

Finding a balance in daily life is so important, alongside patience. Chronic illness does not equate to giving up on your passions or goals entirely, but it can mean modifying them or changing your timeline expectations. Set short- and long-term goals. Strive to maintain an identity beyond the chronic illness, label or diagnosis.

We are innately relational beings, and chronic illness often forces us into isolation. Find ways to connect with others and contribute to an outside project or purpose, but—this is important—once you have the "spoons" to do so. In the chronic illness community, the concept of "spoons" refers to how much energy a person has per day for their activities. If you have few "spoons," you'll be exhausted from simple tasks like personal hygiene and getting dressed and won't have energy left for other activities.

The point here is to avoid engaging in new projects or activities if they mean that you will have to recover for several days (or weeks!) afterward because you depleted your energy reserves. There is an art to finding this balance. Pacing of everyday activities is of the utmost importance. We cannot take care of others unless we first take care of ourselves. Stay aligned with a higher calling beyond the realm of chronic illness and over time (when you are ready) you will find that you can enjoy a combination of self-care and outreach to others without feeling depleted.

Emotional Healing

The energy we give out to the universe matters and can influence what we receive in return. Reframing our perceptions about things like mast cells, collagen and our immune system certainly helps, alongside ensuring that we have a solid identity outside of our illness, labels and diagnoses, as discussed above. But if we approach situations with a mindset of "bad things always happen to me," then chances are, it will be harder to see what is going well in our lives and where the possibilities might be. In order to change our future, we must change our thoughts and our approach. Be confident in yourself and honor your experiences and intuition, aim to find inner balance and recognize that not everyone needs to know the full story—and that's okay.

In my practice, I encourage patients to complete themed mini "retreats" that focus on specific areas of emotional healing and mindset change. For example, for a patient who struggles with finances and debt, I have them pick out a book that interests them on the topic and then they complete a 4-6-week process of reading and reflection/meditation, followed by initiation of at least one measurable goal that relates to it. [In this example, it could be opening up a high-yield bank account as a self-care or travel fund where you can deposit a small amount (even just $5) each month.] Proactively working on something like that can be extremely empowering on multiple levels. Healing is a complex process that is interwoven with our subconscious thoughts and working on areas that trouble us (even if they seem completely unrelated to our health) can have a profoundly positive impact on the journey.

Cultivating inner peace and acceptance is a lifelong journey for most people, and the energy that we live in matters. Having a home environment that sparks comfort, joy and creativity is very helpful, especially since patients with the trifecta may spend more time at home than the average person. Likewise, the set-up of our workspace and other living spaces also matters. Many believe that a clean and clutter-free living environment has a tremendous impact on our physical and mental health, with some going as far as to look at the color schemes and shapes in rooms.

The energy that we take in also matters. Many patients with MCAS, POTS and EDS consider themselves empaths and/or exhibit unusual characteristics such as emotional sensitivity, high intelligence and psychic-type tendencies. An empath is a person who is innately in tune with the emotions of those around them, often to the point of feeling those same emotions themselves. Empaths are highly aware of others and tend to see the world from a different perspective. This can be a wonderful gift in some scenarios, but it can also leave that person feeling drained emotionally on a personal level. Whether it's fasting from news, only connecting with others on a certain schedule each week, limiting time on social media, etc., make sure that you set up the right boundaries and adhere to them, with a special focus on limiting exposure to toxic individuals or previously acknowledged mental triggers.

There are several types of treatment approaches that utilize the concept of energy for physical and emotional healing, and many were already discussed earlier in this book. It can be helpful to embrace both Eastern and Western philosophies in terms of trying different forms of healing.

Reiki is a popular form of energetic healing (considered alternative medicine) that is conducted through placement of the palms of the hands near the body, where a universal energy is transferred from the practitioner to the patient to encourage healing. Reiki may be useful for relieving pain, improving quality of life, and decreasing anxiety and depression in older adults, though more research is needed.[19] Reiki appears to promote statistically significant reductions in post-operative pain as well general pain.[20,21] A recent review found that reiki appears more effective than the placebo treatment and may facilitate enhanced parasympathetic nervous system tone.[22]

Crystals and gemstones are also believed to promote the flow of good energy and help rid the body, mind and soul of negative energy, and some people also use them to attempt to block the harmful effects of electromagnetic pollution. While anecdotal reports have suggested value, scientifically speaking, this approach to energetic healing has no evidence in the treatment of disease.

Sound healing has also been used since the times of ancient medicine and may be of great benefit. In theory, certain sound frequencies are believed to help rewire the brain and connect the right and left hemispheres for healing of anxiety and depression that may stem from a history of trauma. The use of tuning forks, chanting, bowls and humming are examples of techniques offered by practitioners for sound healing. Sometimes these techniques are combined with other strategies like meditation. One study found that Tibetan singing bowl meditation improved anger, fatigue, depressed mood and tension among participants.[23] Recent approaches (such as a strategy called HUSO) combine vocal sounds from experienced sound healers with modern technology that adds beneficial waveforms and harmonics along with vibrating pads at acupuncture points for a healing sensory experience.[24] Biofield tuning is a practice that utilizes the power of sound and electromagnetic energy to provide a therapy targeting the nervous system through specific frequencies of a tuning fork.

Binaural beats are a simple at-home option for sound wave therapy. Binaural beats are a type of sound therapy that can be accessed using headphones and an internet connection. Two pitches of sounds are utilized that are different in each ear; these are close in pitch but are not quite identical. This fosters a brain-level interference that is akin to the brain waves that occur during certain states like meditation. Different frequencies are available that target different goals like relief of anxiety, reduction in depression, improved memory/concentration, or enhanced relaxation and sleeping.

Research has noted attention improvements in as little as three minutes of binaural beats exposure at certain frequencies, as well as reduced depression and improvements in heart rate variability and blood pressure in older adults who listened to 30 minutes of alpha binaural beats for five consecutive days.[25,26] The sounds have also been shown to significantly reduce preoperative dental anxiety.[27] It's plausible that regular use of binaural beats may assist patients with chronic illness. Binaural beats are theorized to work on the premise of differences between the right and left ear sound frequencies, and this mechanism is different from the auditory therapy discussed in Chapter 7.

"Grounding" or "earthing" refers to direct physical contact through bare hands or feet with the earth's surface. Barefoot walking has been touted as a key to health for centuries. One potential mechanism for the beneficial impacts of this phenomenon has to do with the ground's electrically conductive free electrons that enter the human body through direct contact with the skin. In theory, if the electrical energy of the organs, tissues, cells and molecules is stabilized, the immune system may function more optimally.[28] This ties back to the studied effects of electromagnetic fields (EMFs) that were previously discussed. Direct earth contact has been suggested as a therapeutic antidote for people who are exposed to high levels of EMFs (such as following airplane travel or long periods of occupational exposure). Grounding may be a way for the body to recalibrate after exposure to the harmful effects of EMFs.

Barefoot yoga on the earth's surface may be a way to enjoy the benefits of grounding and combine it with breathing techniques and exercise. Research has associated increases in barefoot grounding with improvements in aging, blood glucose regulation, cardiovascular function, cortisol levels, diabetes, inflammation, osteoporosis, pain and sleep quality.[28] The quality of the earth and the proximity to metropolitan areas

413

and sources of electromagnetic radiation may influence the efficacy of this phenomenon.

Aromatherapy and the use of essential oils may also positively impact our mental and physical well-being. Essential oils are a natural liquid substance that's been extracted from plants that can be ingested, used on the skin or inhaled from a diffuser machine. Research supports the use of aromatherapy from essential oils in the treatment of depression, pain, post-operative nausea/vomiting, sleep quality and other conditions; it may also be effective against symptoms of dysmenorrhea (painful periods).[29-34] Diffusion of essential oils into the air is generally the best-tolerated route for patients with environmental, food, supplement/medication and chemical sensitivities (as opposed to topical or oral use), and certain essential oils should never be used internally.

Not all essential oils on the market are appropriate for patients with the trifecta. For example, clove, cinnamon and nutmeg are histamine-liberating, and juniper, pine, spruce and chamomile can cause irritation if you're allergic to certain trees and weeds.[35] Many companies mix chemicals or odors/fragrances in with essentials oils, so brand selection is extremely important. And for some complex patients, essential oils are simply not tolerated in any formulation.

Table 27. Potential Benefits of Specific Essential Oils

Essential Oil	Benefits
Eucalyptus (Eucalyptus radiata)	Analgesic, anti-inflammatory, reduces edema and histamine-induced vascular permeability[36]
Frankincense (Boswellia – various varieties)	Anti-inflammatory, antifungal, anticancer, antibacterial, reduces edema;[37] anti-asthmatic, anti-arthritic[38]
Geranium (Pelargonium graveolens)	Antioxidant and anti-inflammatory effects, inhibits mast cell degranulation and cytokine release[39]
Ginger Root (Zingiber officinale)	Bronchodilatory effects;[40] antioxidant, anti-inflammatory, antinociceptive;[41] antimicrobial, anticancer, neuroprotective[42]
Holy Basil (Ocimum sanctum)	Antihistaminic and mast cell stabilizing;[43] antioxidant, antidiabetic, antiulcer, anticancer, antibacterial, antifungal[44]
Lavender (Lavandula angustifolia)	Calms nervous system inflammation and reduces insomnia;[45] suppresses airway inflammation;[46] reduces cytokines, histamine and edema[47,48]
Myrrh (Commiphora myrrha)	Analgesic, anti-inflammatory;[49] antihistaminic[50]
Peppermint (Mentha piperita)	Reduces histamine-mediated airway inflammation;[51] inhibits histamine release and may alleviate allergic rhinitis;[52] antimicrobial[53]
Turmeric (Curcuma longa)	Bronchodilatory effects, more powerful than cromolyn sodium for mast cell degranulation when combined with ginger and galangal;[40] anti-inflammatory and antinociceptive[54]

Mindfulness and meditation both have strong support for positively impacting our physical and mental health. Mindfulness is the active awareness of your thoughts, feelings, behaviors, movements and environment. Through this awareness, you are present in the moment and fully engaged in the here and now. Mindfulness training has been shown to be effective in several different medical conditions. For example, in patients with irritable bowel syndrome, mindfulness appears to attenuate the harmful impacts of stress on the gut barrier.[55]

Mindfulness activates the frontal lobe of the brain. In contrast, the back of the brain is more active in times of fight or flight. On both sides of the thalamus, the limbic system is the part of the brain responsible for behavior, emotions, memory, motivation, and our sense of smell, and it regulates autonomic function in response to emotional stimuli. Within this system, the amygdala is the structure responsible for perception of emotions and it also stores memories of events and emotions in order to quickly recognize (and potentially seek or avoid) similar events in the future. This is one of the reasons that certain smells can elicit emotions like nostalgia or anxiety.

This limbic system characteristic has a complex interplay with our mast cells and chemical sensitivities. Mast cells release chemical mediators near nerve endings in the limbic areas of the brain. While a heightened reaction to a trigger (such as someone's perfume or walking into a moldy building) initially serves to protect us, when the amygdala stores this data and references it often, it can present as a vicious cycle of sensitivity. For this reason, it's so important to combine nervous system retraining and exercises to restore ventral vagal tone with practices like meditation, mindfulness and tapping (Emotional Freedom Technique).

Practicing mindfulness decreases the activity of the amygdala,[56] the brain's "smoke detector."[57] When the frontal lobe of the brain is activated more often, the amygdala shrinks because you are using it less, and your nervous system spends more time in a relaxed ventral vagal state instead of a state of hypervigilance or shutdown. Restoration of executive functioning (controlled by the frontal lobe of the brain, which lights up during mindfulness and meditation) and the capacity for self-confidence, playfulness and creativity are important aspects of recovery from trauma.[57] Restoring a proper balance between the rational and emotional parts of the brain is one of the many benefits of these practices.

Mindfulness can be practiced anywhere. Some people find it helpful to practice mindfulness periodically throughout the day. For example, if you find yourself mentally spiraling or fixating on something, find an object in the environment and mentally describe its appearance (color, texture, size, etc.) to help bring yourself back into the present moment. This basic practice can help shift the entire system into a better resting state.

Mindfulness is one form of meditation. Meditation refers to a formal, typically seated practice that focuses on a specific area (such as calming the mind, experiencing inner peace, opening your heart, etc.). Examples of meditation include guided single-focus meditation, visualization, mantra-based meditation and breath-awareness meditation. Some types of meditation incorporate mindfulness, such as those that draw attention to areas of tension in your body or the breath. Other types of meditation aim to help quiet the brain in order to focus on "nothing."

Meditation has been shown to alter our brain waves, which can impact our cognitive function as well as our resting nervous system state.[58] It appears that as few as five minutes of meditation per day may improve stress levels.[59] A meta-analysis of 47 studies determined that mindfulness-based meditation programs have moderate evidence of improvements in depression, pain and anxiety.[60]

Some patients are not open to trying tools like mindfulness and meditation due to stigmas and preconceived notions. However, most practices look very different from the stereotypes. A great number of smart

417

phone apps and websites offer guided meditation and mindfulness options, and they can be very calming both during a flare and in prevention of a flare. Many of the formal nervous system retraining programs incorporate these tools as part of their comprehensive approach. For gear junkies, EEG devices worn on the head (such as Muse) aim to provide feedback on what's going on in the brain, offering a novel approach to meditation. On a cellular level, these approaches have the potential to reduce inflammatory cytokines and mast cell mediators, foster ventral vagal-dominant nervous system tone, facilitate more optimal physiological function at the organ and tissue level, reduce oxidative stress and enhance detoxification, reduce the nervous system sensitivity to pain, improve sensitivity to triggers and much more.

It's important to note that meditation can be very overwhelming or intense for people with trauma histories and PTSD. In this scenario, it's wise to seek support from a mental health professional in order to incorporate mindfulness-based practices in a trauma-informed manner.

Scientific research has attempted to uncover more information about spiritual healing—for example, the healing power of prayer.[61] While it's a difficult area to "research," for many, spirituality cannot be adequately explained by science or quantified. Some patients are open to visiting healers who may pray over them or include structured spiritual healing sessions. Holistic retreats that involve a period of isolation in nature or in other spiritual environments may provide resources for patients wanting to jumpstart the healing process with a more structured mind–body focus.

Worship in the form of music or organized gatherings, group and individual prayer, and community activities may be very beneficial for the patient suffering with chronic illness. In this digital age, there are many options for patients who are homebound. Podcasts, websites, books and apps can help bring faith and spirituality resources into the home. Incorporating quiet time into your daily routine for prayer, reflection and/or meditation can be challenging at first, but many patients find that these practices serve as pillars for their individualized healing plan.

Therapy incorporating art, nature, music and dance can provide tremendous healing. Some individuals find it very helpful to address a history of trauma or PTSD by expressing their feelings in artistic manners instead of words, and this can assist in helping the body to finally grasp and realize that the trauma happened in the past. Instead of reliving the trauma regularly, creative or expressive arts therapies can help show the system that the person is now in a safe place and can relax and express who they are without fear.

Trauma is stored in the right side of the brainstem (back part of the brain), which means that the more artistic and creative right brain modalities can be effective for providing pathways to healing. Music, for example, integrates the whole brain and uses neuroplasticity to rewire pathways. Singing can also have a powerful positive impact on the nervous system. Improvisational theater ("improv") and acting are great avenues to incorporate vocalization with movement, which can help rewire the brain, presuming the individual is able to feel at ease on stage. Dance as a form of movement also incorporates retraining parts of the brain impacted by trauma. Spending time in nature incorporates all our senses and it's no secret that shinrin-yoku ("forest bathing") has been practiced for centuries in Japan. This gentle and contemplative method incorporates simply being present in nature and experiencing the sights, sounds, smells, textures and even tastes that occur away from our modern world.

Regardless of what approach you take, addressing the mental aspects of chronic disease should be at the top of the priority list in this journey. The combination of psychotherapy and other therapies that target autonomic nervous system regulation and mind-body energy may offer an added benefit for patients who have MCAS, POTS and EDS or other comorbidities.

Various online search engines can help patients find a therapist who is the right fit. Consider looking at psychologytoday.com, inclusivetherapists.com, and openpath.com for more resources. Patients can search for therapists based on their identities, what they are struggling with, and factors like insurance source and sliding scale payments. Most communities will have a therapist who specializes in working with chronic illness. Be sure to have a consultation with several therapists before choosing someone that you feel a level of comfort and safety with.

DETOXIFICATION: TAKE-HOME MESSAGES

- The liver and gallbladder, lymphatic system, kidneys and gastrointestinal system are the main organs associated with detoxification. Supporting these systems to do their job more efficiently and addressing root issues are key aspects of healing from a high toxic burden.
- There are three main phases of detoxification that occur in the liver-gut and liver-kidney systems.
- Phase one of detoxification or "functionalization" utilizes a group of enzymes that protect your cells from damage. Specifically, these enzymes make toxins water-soluble for further processing and take large volatile toxins and break them down into smaller (less harmful) substances.
- The second phase of detoxification, "conjugation," focuses on taking the water-soluble metabolites from phase one and conjugating them to help prepare them for removal via your stool, urine and bile.
- In the final step, phase three or "elimination," the phase two conjugates are transported to the organs of elimination (kidneys or gastrointestinal tract). In this phase, adequate hydration and proper gastrointestinal motility are key for elimination of toxins.
- There are several foods and supplements that can help boost the different phases of detoxification (see Tables 23 & 24), and it's important to work with your care team to determine the best ways to support overall systemic detoxification.

- Additional strategies to boost detoxification include addressing underlying root issues and health stressors, Epsom salt baths, hydration, intermittent fasting or time-restricted eating, juicing, machine-based modalities, minimizing continued exposure to toxins, sweating, strategies to improve sleep and resting nervous system tone, and toxin binders.

- Lymph is a colorless fluid containing white blood cells, and it bathes the tissues and drains around the lymphatic system into the bloodstream. Lymphatic vessels lead into lymph nodes, and there are hundreds of these cleansing "hubs" all over the body. Lymph relies on relaxation and contraction of muscles and joints to help move it around the body.

- Strategies to help improve lymphatic system function include acupuncture, breathing exercises, herbal teas and dietary changes, hydration, inverted positions, lymphatic drainage, certain types of massage and manual therapy, rebounding on a trampoline, reflexology lymphatic drainage, rhythmic activities like swimming/jumping rope/weighted hula hooping, skin brushing, soaks and compresses, and yoga.

- Sleep hygiene is especially important for patients with chronic illness and the quality and quantity of sleep can have a big impact on the detoxification that occurs in the middle of the night.

- Emotional healing is an often-overlooked aspect of a comprehensive healing program and it should be prioritized in patients who have the chronic conditions like the trifecta. There's no cookie-cutter approach and there are many options out there that can help restore proper nervous system function following minor or major trauma in both conscious and subconscious manners.

- Self-care, aromatherapy, art and dance therapy, barefoot grounding/earthing, binaural beats, Brainspotting, Callahan thought field therapy (TFT), cognitive behavioral therapy, counseling and talk therapy, emotional freedom technique (EFT), eye movement desensitization and reprocessing (EMDR), tension and trauma releasing exercises (TRE), meditation, mindfulness, music therapy, nature experiences, neural biofeedback programs, reiki and sound healing are some of the many options that can help facilitate healing from the effects of mental toxins and underlying trauma.

- Are you supporting all the phases of physical detoxification? Brainstorm additional treatment modalities and lifestyle factors that can help your system with this area. Are you giving adequate attention to mental and emotional healing? What are some resources that you can tap into in this area? Reflect on these topics in your Trifecta Passport worksheet.

CHAPTER 12: SUMMARY & CASE EXAMPLES

This chapter describes three examples of patient cases that show the integration of a multidimensional Trifecta Passport plan into practice. This information is NOT intended to be medical advice, nor should it be considered a blueprint to follow. Working one-on-one with an integrative provider to put all the puzzle pieces together is essential.

Note: The following case stories are being shared with permission, but names and identifying information have been changed.

CASE #1: AN MCAS-HEAVY HISTORY

Jen was in despair because she felt like she was getting worse and worse. She was down to a handful of "safe" foods mostly consisting of chicken, rice and coconut milk. She'd had a few dozen systemic symptoms since her early teenage years, but now, in her thirties, she was in the process of applying for disability because she could no longer work. Jen was extremely sensitive to her environment and she was pretty much homebound. She would experience anaphylactoid reactions to car rides (vibrations), foods, secondhand smoke and medications, and she would break out in hives with other triggers like exercise, beauty products, exposure to sunlight, emotional stress and radiocontrast media used in diagnostic imaging. She was hospitalized one time following a severe reaction to an insect sting. Her symptoms would consistently worsen when she was ovulating as well as when she was on her period.

Her biggest concerns were gut issues (cramping, bloating, gas, constipation), shortness of breath, anxiety and depression, migraine headaches, interstitial cystitis, brain fog, fatigue, itching and hives, and poor tolerance to warm climates. She was chronically constipated and only had a few bowel movements per week. She also experienced a consistently low blood pressure and had occasional near-fainting episodes. She reported sensitivities to foods containing histamine, gluten, soy, oxalates and salicylates.

Jen had previously been living in a home with a mold issue, but they had relocated about six months ago which was somewhat helpful. She was going on walks for 10–15 minutes one to two days per week at baseline while using her face mask to avoid contact with triggers. She fell asleep fine but tended to wake up in the middle of the night, typically between the hours of 2 to 3 a.m. Jen enjoyed painting and found art therapeutic but she would react to the paint fumes so she had stopped this hobby about a year prior. Patient goals included improving her tolerance to more food options, reducing gut pain, investigating more natural options to stabilize her mast cells and starting a yoga exercise program.

Jen had mast cell mediator testing on two occasions, which confirmed high urinary prostaglandin and histamine levels with normal tryptase and leukotrienes. She had trialed several prescription and over-the-counter medications with her physician, including H1/H2 blockers, montelukast, cromolyn, ketotifen, Xolair injections, steroids, cannabinoids and lorazepam and found that the generic version of Zyrtec, dye-free liquid Benadryl and CBD oil were the only things she could tolerate. Her medical records showed mildly elevated liver markers over the last three years. Thyroid testing from her primary care doctor was within normal limits. She had abdominal tenderness, brittle nails and a white coating on her tongue.

Jen decided to pursue some functional medicine testing, which revealed:

- SIBO: positive (methane dominant)
- Comprehensive diagnostic stool analysis: dysbiotic *Klebsiella pneumonia* (susceptible to berberine and oregano, resistant to ampicillin), *Blastocystis hominis* parasitic infection, low secretory IgA, low butyrate and short chain fatty acids, and a candida yeast infection (most susceptible to undecylenic acid and nystatin)
- Visual Contrast Sensitivity: positive, 26% for right eye and 22% for left eye, suggestive of biotoxin illness and nutritional deficiency (though not diagnostic in itself)
- Mycotoxin urine test: elevated gliotoxin, ochratoxin A and mycophenolic acid metabolites

It was clear that Jen was suffering from an immune response to mycotoxins, an abundance of gastrointestinal issues (including leaky gut, SIBO, poor motility, candida and parasites), a high toxic burden and other systemic health stressors.

Jen worked with her integrative provider for the next seven months to come up with a holistic healing plan and to trial and error solutions. Jen's initial wellness plan focused on removal of offending toxins and microbes to restore a more stable baseline. She completed an environmental toxin screening tool, which helped her to remove certain products from her home environment and beauty routine. She decided to get rid of her permeable belongings and air purifier that were previously exposed to mold, noting about a 20% improvement in symptoms from that decision alone. She found that her shortness of breath and fatigue were especially impacted by discontinuing the use of belongings from the prior building.

She began supplementing with magnesium, increased her fiber intake and started having daily bowel movements. She switched to organic hormone-free chicken and organic rice and after a few weeks was able to begin incorporating some zucchini squash and leafy greens into her diet. She increased her hydration and began going on walks four to five days a week at the coolest times of the day. She also started turning off the wifi router at night and noticed that she was waking up less during the night. With the help of her care team, Jen worked on the concept of meal hygiene and mindful eating, mindset and breathing exercises to enhance parasympathetic nervous system tone.

Because she was so sensitive to oral supplements, she started by opening the capsules of activated charcoal and sprinkling a fraction of the typical dose into water as a mold toxin binder. Over time, she was slowly able to increase up to half of the capsule taken on an empty stomach, and she was advised to avoid taking a higher dose than that because she found it would trigger symptoms consistent with toxin recirculation. After about three weeks of activated charcoal, she had an allergic reaction to it and switched to bentonite clay, which was not well tolerated. Following the trial of bentonite clay, she opted for the probiotic *Saccharomyces boulardii* and eventually added in use of a powder form of N-acetyl cysteine, both of which were well-tolerated for mold toxin binding. After a few months of this approach, she found that she was significantly less reactive to her environment and was able to tolerate more foods and supplements.

Over the next several months, Jen found that she was able to add a 20- to 30-minute vinyasa flow yoga routine three days a week. On days she was flared she stuck to basic breathing exercises, and on the other days she continued to increase her endurance with walking. From there, once mold had been addressed and she was more stable overall, her provider focused on the removal of remaining unwanted pathogens (candida overgrowth, dysbiotic gut bacteria, parasites, SIBO) through a combination of short-term dietary modifications and oral supplements. This process involved some trial and error until she found certain natural substances that were effective without triggering a reaction. She noted that in the past another provider had tried to treat her for candida, but that she had been extremely reactive to the medication. However, this time around, after addressing mold and helping her body reduce her toxic burden, Jen had a different and more positive experience with her candida cleanse.

Jen was then able to add digestive enzymes and quercetin into her routine and noted that she was not needing to use Benadryl as often. She also expanded her diet to include more fruits and vegetables without any indication of salicylate, oxalate or histamine issues. She focused on a gluten-free whole foods approach with minimal use of processed foods, sugar, additives or artificial sweeteners. She began to incorporate more aspects of self-care into her daily routine and decided to create art again on her deck in a well-ventilated area while wearing a mask. At this point she also began a nervous system retraining program called Dynamic Neural Retraining System (DNRS).

Jen continued to work on her gut health and was able, after a period of trial and error, to add a probiotic to reinoculate the gut with friendly bacteria and certain supplements to assist with repairing the intestinal mucosa, boosting immune system health and aiding detoxification. She began to integrate more self-care into her routine including acupuncture and massage. She planned to continue with the DNRS program because she felt it was helpful.

CASE #2: DYSAUTONOMIA, WITH A SIDE OF LYME & HORMONAL ISSUES

At age 23, Natasha had already been previously diagnosed with POTS, Lyme disease and Bartonellosis infection. She also reported a history of small fiber neuropathy and was recently diagnosed with polycystic ovarian syndrome (PCOS). Natasha suffered from regular heartburn, severe depression, fatigue, nerve pain, insomnia, digestive issues and difficulty concentrating. While she was not formally diagnosed with autism, Natasha described symptoms such as intolerance to loud noises, difficulty concentrating with background noise, adrenaline rushes with noises, misophonia (intolerance to sounds like dripping water, chewing, gum chewing), anxiety with flashing lights, sensitivity to certain textures, intolerance to physical touch, and avoidance of social interactions. These symptoms would worsen when her other issues were flared up. She noted a history of sexual abuse as a child that she was currently in counseling for.

Natasha's medical providers would observe that she often had a low affect with blunted facial expressions and a monotonous voice. Natasha's main goal included improving her tolerance to standing so that she could continue to work at a dog boarding facility where she assisted with exercising and bathing the dogs, a job that was physically demanding. She was currently on a short-term leave from work due to standing intolerance and POTS symptoms. She also wanted to improve her insomnia, sensory sensitivities and hormone-related issues. Natasha had previously tried Lyme-specific antibiotics (both prescription and herbal), which she felt made things worse. She had also tried several prescription medications for POTS but had not found one that was effective.

Natasha saw a new functional medicine doctor who ordered a dried urine hormone panel, cortisol testing and organic acid testing, which showed several abnormalities:

- Dried urine hormone panel:
  - Estrogen dominance, a higher 4-OH ratio in phase one estrogen metabolism (which can damage DNA), low methylation in phase 2 estrogen metabolism (which can increase the buildup of estrogen metabolites)
  - Androgens showing a preference for 5-alpha reductase (associated with insulin resistance and PCOS)
- Cortisol testing: Impaired cortisol awakening response with diminished morning values at 1) awakening and 2) awakening plus 30 minutes; high level of cortisone metabolites
- Organic acid testing: high oxalates, signs of yeast/fungal infection, clostridia bacterial markers, low B vitamins and glutathione, low metabolites of the neurotransmitter serotonin

Natasha's provider suspected that the combination of clostridia and low B vitamins may be influencing her depression, and clostridia could also be connected to symptoms of autism. They utilized natural substances to address the clostridia bacterial issues. She began supplementing with liposomal glutathione, vitamins and minerals. She addressed candida with an antibiotic and candida cleanse diet for a few weeks. Her provider had her start on licorice root and adaptogen supplements for the adrenal system. She also educated Natasha to reduce her exposure to sources of estrogen and had her begin supplementing with diindolylmethane (DIM). She began taking melatonin and other natural herbs at night for insomnia and worked on stress reduction. She also started taking digestive enzymes and hydrochloric acid. Natasha's provider also helped her address the potential influence of insulin resistance in her PCOS symptoms and suggested that she make some dietary changes.

Natasha was referred to a nutritionist. She was coached to remove sugar, dairy, gluten and antibiotic-containing meat products. She also began a trial of a low-oxalate diet, which was mildly helpful, but once she finished the candida treatment, she was able to re-integrate oxalate-containing food sources without issues. In addition, she had previously been consuming large amounts of artificial sweetener in her coffee and she began to replace it with small amounts of honey instead. Natasha was encouraged to increase her hydration and electrolytes. She was also advised to avoid processed foods and food additives.

Natasha was working with a physical therapist for shoulder pain/hypermobility concerns, and they began to address her POTS and exercise goals. They began with a program that incorporated swimming and a recumbent bicycle for endurance exercise, a daily standing program against a wall at home, and supine exercises targeting her core, hip and lower extremity strength. She started with about 45 seconds of standing tolerance and gradually worked up from there. She also worked with her physical therapist on breathing exercises and the concept of sleep hygiene. Natasha decided to decrease her screen time in the two hours before bed and reduce her caffeine intake, and she began a more relaxing pre-bedtime ritual.

One of Natasha's providers suggested that she try an auditory program like the Safe & Sound Protocol for her sensory stimulation concerns. She completed the program in 10 days and noticed significant improvements, particularly in her sensitivities to noises and her ability to concentrate. Her provider taught her exercises to help her reset her nervous system back to the ventral vagal state, and she learned how to be more in tune with her body's signals. Whenever she felt herself freezing up or going into an adrenaline rush, she would perform her breathing and nervous system exercises and self-soothing techniques, which helped immediately.

After ten months since Natasha's integrative program began, she reported that she was no longer avoiding social situations and that she had started dating. Her periods were less heavy and her heartburn had resolved. She was sleeping better and had more energy and less nerve pain. When she did become fatigued, she used pacing and self-care techniques that she had learned from her care team. She reported her depression to be about 50% less severe than her first visit. She returned to work and was able to tolerate standing for up to 30 minutes at a time, and she planned to continue exercising every day. She continued to work with her functional medicine doctor to support detoxification, gut health, and hormonal and neurotransmitter balance.

CASE #3: EHLERS-DANLOS SYNDROME & CCI

Aliyah, a 42-year-old mother of three children, had previously been a competitive collegiate gymnast and an avid CrossFit aficionado. Since her youth she had experienced an abnormally high rate of orthopedic pain and injuries, and she was eventually diagnosed with hEDS in her mid-20s. Aliyah was experiencing regular neck pain and intermittent dizziness that flared up with computer use and exercise at her gym. She also complained of headaches, fatigue, susceptibility to getting sick with a cold or the flu, weight gain, hair loss, constipation, sensitivity to the cold, fevers and chills that would come and go, blurred vision, skin rashes, chronically swollen lymph nodes, sensitivities to chemicals and muscle weakness. Aliyah had previously been diagnosed with MCAS and felt that ketotifen and vitamin C were helpful in reducing her symptoms. Her husband encouraged her to have a sleep study done and she was subsequently diagnosed with sleep apnea. Aliyah confided that she had a very high stress level and that she did not have a lot of time for herself. Her husband traveled a lot for work and in addition to her parenting duties she was also working full time. Her goals included returning to weightlifting, reducing neck pain/dizziness/headaches and improving overall immune health.

Aliyah saw an orthopedic doctor who ordered imaging of her cervical spine and referred her to a physical therapist with the diagnosis of craniocervical instability (CCI). They began to work together to improve her postural awareness, strength and endurance, proprioception, balance and body mechanics. Aliyah began neck exercises that utilized a laser headset aimed at posters on the wall and eventually her dizziness improved. She also shared that she was experiencing symptoms of urinary incontinence, and they began a program that addressed the function of the pelvic floor muscles, diaphragm and core muscles. As her headaches and neck pain resolved, she was educated on a modified weightlifting program. She also worked with her physical therapist on strategies to reduce stress, restore her nervous system balance and improve mindfulness. She began the Gupta Program and due to her schedule, she started out with 10 minutes a day, building up over time. She eventually began using a CPAP machine for sleep apnea and found that it was helpful for sleep quality and feeling more refreshed in the morning.

Aliyah found that she often used caffeine and sugar to help her through the workday, and she was counseled in ways to clean up her diet. She also switched to more natural toothpaste, shampoo, deodorant and make-up products. She was already using natural cleaning agents in the home, but they had recently put new carpets in the house that were off-gassing, so she purchased a HEPA air purifier to reduce exposure to volatile organic compounds.

Aliyah was also encouraged to a see a naturopathic doctor to address underlying health stressors. The naturopathic testing revealed hypothyroidism, gastrointestinal dysbiosis, vitamin and mineral deficiencies and chronic Epstein-Barr virus. She worked with this provider for nearly a year to find the right combination of iodine and other natural thyroid support, immune support, natural antivirals, probiotics and natural supplements for the gastrointestinal system. The provider also focused on detoxification and over time this program was able to reduce Aliyah's chemical sensitivities.

Aliyah's healing path was not linear. She tended to overdo it with work/exercise/household activities and had several flare-ups along the way. She was very hard on herself and was referred to a therapist to help her find more strategies to cope with the high stress in her life. She had to endure some trial and error in order to find the right naturopathic supplements that didn't flare up her MCAS. She had several periods where she simply did not have the time to complete the Gupta Program or self-care strategies at all. However, over time, this combined multidisciplinary approach helped her to reach her goals and she felt that she was then able to be more present with her family and was able to return to her group exercise classes.

Limitations to the Trifecta Passport

One of the biggest limitations to the Trifecta Passport approach is that it can offer some fairly unrealistic solutions for individuals who find themselves lacking the time or money to pursue healing like it's a full-time job. I often reflect on the socioeconomic barriers to care (and in particular, naturopathic and functional medicine care, which are not typically covered by insurance) with great frustration. How can I tell people to do more self-care when they are hanging on by a thread? This is a huge problem and some leaders are advocating that instead of shouting "self-care," we should be focusing more on community approaches.[1]

Of course, there are several tools and solutions that won't necessarily break the bank. Sometimes we need to start with one simple thing that we can focus on. Whether it's 2 minutes of breathing exercises, tapping once a day, focusing on healthy boundaries, removing dairy from your diet, joining a support group, journaling, or listening to a guided meditation on your commute, there's always something free and simple that can be integrated into daily life... if you prioritize it.

For many of my patients, the issue is not just money but time. You may be working 3 jobs or caring for children or an older adult in your life and find all of this laughable. For individuals who are disempowered or spread too thin, self-care is not always a feasible option. (How can you meditate your way back to better health when you can't even pee alone?! Or when you are hustling to make ends meet?) How can you shift from survival mode to thriving given the circumstances you are facing?

I wish I had the answer to this. What I do know is that the more we connect with each other and find community resources, the better. We must address our mental health, thought patterns, relationships, beliefs, boundaries, emotional toxins, and nervous system state along the way, yet these are the things that are often viewed as an afterthought when it comes to physical healing.

436

The customized functional medicine model—while valuable—may not be an option for every patient right away. But at least half of this book described additional do-it-yourself resources available to you, and I hope that these ideas will help guide you to a foundation for further growth, regardless of the budget or time limitations you may be facing. Personalized medicine is helpful (and ideal in a best-case scenario), but I also believe that the future of fostering change (so that integrative medicine is available for all) lies in a community care model. I look forward to offering novel group-based approaches for our trifecta patient community in the coming months as part of the Origin Wellness vision, and I hope that these types of services become more commonplace and empower individuals of all socioeconomic backgrounds to find healing from chronic conditions.

Conclusions

A mentor once told me that people are going to digest information about non-mainstream treatment approaches when they are ready to, and not everyone will find themselves open-minded to some of these strategies or ready to consider them. In addition, this information can be overwhelming to the point of feeling paralyzed in terms of which direction to pursue next. It's certainly not helpful to try everything at once, but it can still be difficult to know how to prioritize the next steps in the healing journey. Hopefully the design of the Trifecta Passport and the sections that give you a template to outline things to investigate/look into in the future will be helpful in putting together a customized long-term plan.

You are on your own journey right now, and it will look very different from that of your neighbor, but I hope that you were able to extract useful and novel information from this short guide. I hope that you will stay open-minded to all sorts of possibilities, and not just the ones that you are inherently comfortable with. And I hope that you will realize how complex the human body is. Be mindful of the truth about all three conditions that make up the trifecta: there is no silver bullet treatment and no "perfect" approach. But there is so much inherent value in addressing all the angles.

I used to think that if I just focused on health stressors, nutrition, exercise and detoxification, I would find healing. These factors got me partway there, but it was not until I addressed emotional healing, hidden structural/musculoskeletal factors (that I had previously been ignoring, the classical hypocritical physical therapist!) and retraining the nervous system that I saw greater changes in my own health—and the health of my patients too. There are a variety of opinions out there on which "pillars" are essential to health and well-being, and most of them include some combination of nutrition, water (hydration), physical activity, sleep, the breath, emotional health, and connecting with others and/or with a higher being. Perhaps some folks can skate by with only addressing a few of these, but for patients with chronic illness, it is essential that these areas are addressed together simultaneously.

Never forget that you are the expert of living in your own body. Honor your intuition, prioritize self-care, filter the energy that you are exposed to (physically and emotionally) and stay open-minded to a combined Western and Eastern medicine approach. Set realistic expectations about the desired time frame for healing. Physical/mental/emotional/spiritual healing is a lifelong journey, so don't expect it to be easy, and don't expect it to be a sprint event. Practice self-compassion and give yourself grace for the bumps in the road.

Life with any of the three conditions is supremely challenging, but I encourage you to reframe these diagnoses as labels that describe dysfunctional physiological processes, as opposed to conditions that you are stuck with. While they have not identified genetic causes for hEDS yet, there's a good chance there's an inherent genetic factor. And the same could be true for MCAS and POTS (or perhaps they share a combined genetic factor, as previously theorized). Our health reality is a mixing pot of factors, and genetics is just one of the many parts of the puzzle. If genetics was the biggest factor, wouldn't we see severe disease issues immediately in infancy and youth? The truth is, most patients had issues in youth that have increased in frequency and severity over time.

Never forget that reversal of symptoms is possible. Open yourself to the possibilities that are out there. Begin with a vision. Know who you are and what your dreams are. Build an identity outside of illness. Be intentional; write out your goals, ideas and the members of your ideal multidisciplinary care team in the pages of your Trifecta Passport. Fill up your immigration/visa stamp pages with strategies to investigate and address internal/external health stressors, nervous system retraining, nutritional approaches, structural and musculoskeletal factors, meaningful movement, and physical and mental detoxification.

Remember that any information you get about a particular approach or treatment is helpful in terms of insight and knowledge, even if the outcome does not always equate to an improvement in symptoms. The process entails endurance and patience as you *gather information* to figure out which customized approach is best for your body. Ruling things out (in terms of diagnoses as well as therapeutic approaches) is extremely valuable. Keep putting one foot in front of the other with hope.

When patients get better with these types of approaches, they often remove themselves from social media support groups and go on living their lives with greater well-being. Patients who are still struggling do not always get to see this perspective from their peers, but it's one to be aware of. It's also useful to periodically remind yourself of the silver linings of chronic illness. For me, this journey has led me to new relationships with an incredible bunch of patients and colleagues, and it's enabled me to feel passionate about my career again. Despite the hardships endured in order to get here, for this I will be eternally grateful.

Holistic healing brings mind, body, emotional and spiritual factors together in the quest for optimal wellness. E pluribus unum means "out of many, one." There are many approaches out there, but make sure that you aim to cover the key bases described in this book. I wish you nothing but the best on this journey. If you've found the Trifecta Passport approach to chronic illness helpful in your own experience or if you've uncovered additional tools not discussed in this book, please reach out—I would love to hear your story!

Acknowledgments

I have so much to be thankful for and I want to start with my wonderful editor, Jennifer Leopoldt Roop. Thank you for your perspective, professionalism and patience with my ridiculous amount of over punctuation and hyphenation. I continue to learn so much from you!

Thank you to Ryan Biore, who designed the cover art, and Don Matthew, who illustrated the Trifecta Passport Workbook.

Thank you to my team of fantastic individuals who were willing to read the book in advance and provide feedback on it.

Thank you to my wonderfully supportive family and friends for continuing to believe in me, and to my partner Graham, who continues to be my positive rock and biggest cheerleader.

Thank you to my many functional and natural medicine teachers, mentors and colleagues who remind me to think outside of the box. Thank you to my fellow zebras (and healing providers) Mairead and Patty, who gave me original feedback on the passport idea. One of these days, that patient retreat will happen!

Lastly, to my patients (past and current), thank you for entrusting me with your stories. You truly teach me and inspire me every day, and my life is greatly enriched because of it.

Though my personal patient experience has been difficult, I am very grateful to God for the path that has led me to where I am today and this opportunity to share resources with others.

And to those who are still reading, this book is certainly not perfect, but I hope that these resources will empower you in some way on your own healing journey.

With deep gratitude,

Amber Walker

About the Author

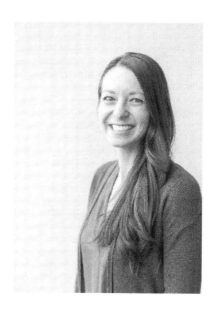

Amber Walker, PT, DPT, CFMP, CNPT, is a Doctor of Physical Therapy with advanced training in functional medicine, nutrition, and natural healing. She specializes in working with patients who suffer from mast cell activation issues, mold illness, dysautonomia/POTS, hypermobility spectrum disorders, hereditary angioedema, and other chronic conditions.

Amber utilizes the Safe & Sound Protocol with patients who have sensory processing disorders and/or a history of trauma to help restore proper autonomic nervous system regulation. She also is trained in CranioBiotic Technique, a natural method of addressing health stressors and improving immune function. She is the author of "Mast Cells United, A Holistic Approach to Mast Cell Activation Syndrome," published in 2019.

A previous Division 1 swimmer, Amber specializes in working with triathletes and has a background in coaching youth and adult swimmers. She enjoys combining functional movement analysis with hands-on manual therapy, dry needling, customized exercises and pool video analysis for the prevention and treatment of injuries.

Amber began her career as a public health volunteer in Peru and continues to be passionate about community health solutions and exploring new cultures through international travel. Originally from Alaska, she thrives on being outdoors and is particularly drawn to mountain running, hiking, camping, and exploring new hot springs. Cooking and photography are other big passions, and in summer months she teaches paddle boarding lessons.

Amber currently resides in Denver, Colorado, where, as the owner of Origin Wellness, she encourages a "root issue" approach to patient care. Amber continues to advocate for the chronic illness population with speaking engagements and special projects via the MCAS resource website www.mastcellsunited.com. Learn more about her practice, which offers telehealth and in-person services, at www.originwellnesscolorado.com.

Bibliography

PREFACE

1. Bland J. Defining function in the functional medicine model. *Integr Med.* 2017;16(1):22-25.

CHAPTER 1: MCAS

1. Haenisch B, Nöthen MM, Molderings, Gerhard J. Systemic mast cell activation disease: The role of molecular genetic alterations in pathogenesis, heritability and diagnostics. *Immunology.* 2012;137:197–205. doi:10.1111/j.1365-2567.2012.03627.x
2. Molderings GJ, Haenisch B, Bogdanow M, Fimmers R, Nöthen MM. Familial Occurrence of Systemic Mast Cell Activation Disease. *PLoS One.* 2013;8(9):e76241. doi:10.1371/journal.pone.0076241
3. Molderings GJ. The genetic basis of mast cell activation disease - looking through a glass darkly. *Crit Rev Oncol Hematol.* 2015;93(2):75-89. doi:10.1016/j.critrevonc.2014.09.001
4. Afrin L, Molderings GJ. A concise, practical guide to diagnostic assessment for mast cell activation disease. *World J Hematol.* 2014;3(1):1-7. doi:10.5315
5. Afrin L, Self S, Menk J, Lazarchick J. Characterization of mast cell activation syndrome. *Am J Med Sci.* 2017;353(3):207-215.
6. Hamilton MJ, Hornick JL, Akin C, Castells MC, Greenberger NJ. Mast cell activation syndrome: A newly recognized disorder with systemic clinical manifestations. *J Allergy Clin Immunol.* 2011;128(1)(1):147-152. doi:10.1016/j.jaci.2011.04.037
7. Arndt KK, Viswanathan RK, Mathur SK. Clinical Characteristics of Patients in Allergy Clinic with Presumed Diagnosis of Mast Cell

Activation Syndrome (MCAS). *J Allergy Clin Immunol.* 2018;141(2):AB50. doi:10.1016/J.JACI.2017.12.162

8. Mackey E, Ayyadurai S, Pohl CS, D'Costa S, Li Y, Moeser AJ. Sexual dimorphism in the mast cell transcriptome and the pathophysiological responses to immunological and psychological stress. *Biol Sex Differ.* 2016;7(1):60. doi:10.1186/s13293-016-0113-7

9. Molderings GJ, Brettner S, Homann J, Afrin LB. Mast cell activation disease: A concise practical guide for diagnostic workup and therapeutic options. J Hematol Oncol. 2011;4:10. doi:10.1186/1756-8722-4-10

10. Walker ME, Hatfield JK, Brown MA. New insights into the role of mast cells in autoimmunity: Evidence for a common mechanism of action? *Biochim Biophys Acta - Mol Basis Dis.* 2012;1822(1):57-65. doi:10.1016/j.bbadis.2011.02.009

11. St. John AL, Abraham SN. Innate Immunity and Its Regulation by Mast Cells. *J Immunol.* 2013;190:4458–4463. doi:10.4049/jimmunol.1203420

12. Soderberg M. The Mast Cell Activation Syndrome: A Mini Review. *MOJ Immunol.* 2015;2(1). doi:10.15406/moji.2015.02.00032

13. Theoharides TC, Valent P, Akin C. Mast Cells, Mastocytosis, and Related Disorders. Ingelfinger JR, ed. *N Engl J Med.* 2015;373(2):163-172. doi:10.1056/NEJMra1409760

14. Maitland A. Mast Cell Activation Syndrome. In: Jovin D, ed. Disjointed: Navigating the Diagnosis and Management of Hypermobile Ehlers-Danlos Syndrome and Hypermobility Spectrum Disorders. Hidden Stripes Publications; 2020.

15. Ratner V. Mast cell activation syndrome. *Transl Androl Urol.* 2015;4(5):587-588. doi:10.3978/j.issn.2223-4683.2015.09.03

16. Theoharides TC, Kalogeromitros D. The critical role of mast cells in allergy and inflammation. *Ann N Y Acad Sci.* 2006;1088(1):78-99. doi:10.1196/annals.1366.025

17. da Silva EZM, Jamur MC, Oliver C. Mast Cell Function: A New Vision of an Old Cell. *J Histochem Cytochem.* 2014;62(10):698–738. doi:10.1369/0022155414545334

18. González-de-Olano D, Domínguez-Ortega J, Sánchez-García S. Mast Cell Activation Syndromes and Environmental Exposures. *Curr Treat Options Allergy.* 2018;5(1):41-51. doi:10.1007/s40521-018-0151-y

19. Tsai YT, Zhou J, Weng H, Tang EN, Baker DW, Tang L. Optical imaging of fibrin deposition to elucidate participation of mast cells in foreign body responses. *Biomaterials.* 2014;35(7):2089-2096. doi:10.1016/j.biomaterials.2013.11.040

446

20. Jennings S, Russell N, Jennings B, et al. The Mastocytosis Society Survey on Mast Cell Disorders: Patient Experiences and Perceptions. *J Allergy Clin Immunol Pract.* 2014;2(1):70-76. doi:10.1016/j.jaip.2013.09.004
21. Soderberg M. The Mast Cell Activation Syndrome: A Mini Review. *MOJ Immunol.* 2015;2(1). doi:10.15406/moji.2015.02.00032
22. Coop CA, Schapira RS, Freeman TM. Are ACE Inhibitors and Beta-blockers Dangerous in Patients at Risk for Anaphylaxis? *J Allergy Clin Immunol Pract.* 2017;5(5):1207-1211. doi:10.1016/j.jaip.2017.04.033
23. Theoharides TC, Tsilioni I, Ren H. Recent advances in our understanding of mast cell activation – or should it be mast cell mediator disorders? *Expert Rev Clin Immunol.* 2019;15(6):639-656. doi:10.1080/1744666X.2019.1596800
24. Álvarez-Twose I, González de Olano D, Sánchez-Muñoz L, et al. Clinical, biological, and molecular characteristics of clonal mast cell disorders presenting with systemic mast cell activation symptoms. *J Allergy Clin Immunol.* 2010;125:1269-1278. doi:10.1016/j.jaci.2010.02.019
25. Shaker MS, Wallace DV, Golden DB, et al. Anaphylaxis – a 2020 Practice Parameter Update, Systematic Review and GRADE Analysis, *Journal of Allergy and Clinical Immunology* (2020), doi: https://doi.org/10.1016/j.jaci.2020.01.017.
26. Campbell RL, Li JTC, Nicklas RA, Sadosty AT, Members of the Joint Task Force, Practice Parameter Workgroup. Emergency department diagnosis and treatment of anaphylaxis: a practice parameter. *Ann Allergy, Asthma Immunol.* 2014;113(6):599-608. doi:10.1016/j.anai.2014.10.007
27. American College of Asthma A and I. Experts agree: Even if severe allergic reaction is in doubt, epinephrine should be used | Experts agree it's best to use epinephrine in all emergency situations. | ACAAI Public Website. https://acaai.org/news/experts-agree-even-if-severe-allergic-reaction-doubt-epinephrine-should-be-used. Published 2015. Accessed August 10, 2018.
28. Roberts LJ, Oates JA. Biochemical Diagnosis of Systemic Mast Cell Disorders. *J Invest Dermatol.* 1991;96(3):S19-S25. doi:10.1111/1523-1747.ep12468945
29. Weinstock LB, Pace LA, Rezaie A, Afrin LB, Molderings GJ. Mast Cell Activation Syndrome: A Primer for the Gastroenterologist. *Dig Dis Sci.* April 2020:1-18. doi:10.1007/s10620-020-06264-9
30. Valent P, Akin C, Arock M, et al. Definitions, criteria and global classification of mast cell disorders with special reference to mast

cell activation syndromes: A consensus proposal. *Int Arch Allergy Immunol.* 2012;157(3):215-225. doi:10.1159/000328760

31. Weiler CR, Austen KF, Akin C, et al. AAAAI Mast Cell Disorders Committee Work Group Report: Mast cell activation syndrome (MCAS) diagnosis and management. *J Allergy Clin Immunol.* 2019;144(4):883-896. doi:10.1016/j.jaci.2019.08.023

32. Tryptase - Gene By Gene. https://genebygene.com/tryptase/. Accessed May 26, 2020.

33. Vysniauskaite M, Hertfelder HJ, Oldenburg J, et al. Determination of plasma heparin level improves identification of systemic mast cell activation disease. *PLoS One.* 2015;10(4):e0124912. doi:10.1371/journal.pone.0124912

34. Zblewski D, Abdelrahman RA, Chen D, Butterfield JH, Tefferi A, Pardanani A. Patient Reported Symptoms and Tryptase Levels in WHO-Defined Systemic Mastocytosis (SM) Versus Mast Cell Activation Syndrome (MCAS) Versus Neither. *Blood.* 2014;124(21).

35. Gonzalez-Quintela A, Vizcaino L, Gude F, et al. Factors influencing serum total tryptase concentrations in a general adult population. *Clin Chem Lab Med.* 2010;48:701-706. doi:10.1515/CCLM.2010.124

36. Fellinger C, Hemmer W, Wohrl S, Sesztak-Greinecker G, Jarisch R, Wantke F. Clinical characteristics and risk profile of patients with elevated baseline serum tryptase. *Allergol Immunopathol (Madr).* 2014;42:544–552. doi:10.1016/j.aller.2014.05.002

37. Weiler CR, Alhurani RE, Butterfield JH, Divekar R. Systemic Mastocytosis (SM) and Mast Cell Activation Syndrome (MCAS); How Do They Differ? *J Allergy Clin Immunol.* 2018;141(2):AB275. doi:10.1016/j.jaci.2017.12.875

38. Van Anrooij B, Van Der Veer E, De Monchy JGR, et al. Higher mast cell load decreases the risk of Hymenoptera venom-induced anaphylaxis in patients with mastocytosis. *J Allergy Clin Immunol.* 2013;132(1):125-130. doi:10.1016/j.jaci.2012.12.1578

39. Akin C, Scott LM, Kocabas CN, et al. Demonstration of an aberrant mast-cell population with clonal markers in a subset of patients with "idiopathic" anaphylaxis. *Blood.* 2007;110:2331-2333. doi:10.1182/blood-2006-06-028100

40. Bonadonna P, Perbellini O, Passalacqua G, et al. Clonal mast cell disorders in patients with systemic reactions to Hymenoptera stings and increased serum tryptase levels. *J Allergy Clin Immunol.* 2009;123(3):680-686. doi:10.1016/J.JACI.2008.11.018

41. Lynch B. Histamine Intolerance, MTHFR and Methylation. MTHFR.net. http://mthfr.net/histamine-intolerance-mthfr-and-methylation/2015/06/11/. Published 2015. Accessed July 20, 2018.

448

42. Pinzer TC, Tietz E, Waldmann E, Schink M, Neurath MF, Zopf Y. Circadian profiling reveals higher histamine plasma levels and lower diamine oxidase serum activities in 24% of patients with suspected histamine intolerance compared to food allergy and controls. *Allergy*. 2018;73(4):949-957. doi:10.1111/all.13361

43. Bahri R, Custovic A, Korosec P, et al. Mast cell activation test in the diagnosis of allergic disease and anaphylaxis. *J Allergy Clin Immunol*. 2018;142(2):485-496.e16. doi:10.1016/J.JACI.2018.01.043

44. Molderings GJ, Haenisch B, Brettner S, et al. Pharmacological treatment options for mast cell activation disease. *Naunyn Schmiedebergs Arch Pharmacol*. 2016;389(7):671-694. doi:10.1007/s00210-016-1247-1

45. Afrin L. Ask The NY MCAS Expert: Mast Cell Activation Syndrome Questions Answered. Posted on October 16, 2017. https://www.drtaniadempsey.com/single-post/Ask-The-NY-MCAS-Expert-Mast-Cell-Activation-Syndrome-Questions-Answered. Accessed May 27, 2020.

46. Seneviratne SL, Maitland A, Afrin L. Mast cell disorders in Ehlers–Danlos syndrome. *Am J Med Genet Part C Semin Med Genet*. 2017;175(1):226-236. doi:10.1002/ajmg.c.31555

47. Theoharides T. Better Health Guy Blogcast with Scott Forsgren. Interview for episode 58: Mast Cell Master with Dr. T.C. Theoharides, PhD, MD. Aired on 1-30-18. http://www.betterhealthguy.com/episode58.

48. Nakatani K, Atsumi M, Arakawa T, et al. Inhibitions of histamine release and prostaglandin E2 synthesis by mangosteen, a Thai medicinal plant. *Biol Pharm Bull*. 2002;25(9):1137-1141. http://www.ncbi.nlm.nih.gov/pubmed/12230104. Accessed September 12, 2018.

49. Chae H-S, Oh S-R, Lee H-K, Joo SH, Chin Y-W. Mangosteen xanthones, α-and γ-mangostins, inhibit allergic mediators in bone marrow-derived mast cell. *Food Chem*. 2012;134(1):397-400. doi:10.1016/J.FOODCHEM.2012.02.075

50. Singh S, Taneja M, Majumdar DK. Biological activities of Ocimum sanctum L. fixed oil--an overview. *Indian J Exp Biol*. 2007;45(5):403-412. http://www.ncbi.nlm.nih.gov/pubmed/17569280. Accessed September 17, 2018.

51. Choudhary GP. Mast cell stabilizing activity of Ocimum sanctum leaves. *Int J Pharma Bio Sci*. 2010;1(2). https://www.cabdirect.org/cabdirect/abstract/20113372323.

52. Rahman S, Islam R, Kamruzzaman M, Alum K, Mastofa Jamal AH. Ocimum sanctum L.: A Review of Phytochemical and

Pharmacological Profile. *Am J Drug Discov Dev*. 2011:1-15. doi:10.3923/ajdd.2011

53. Sharma SC, Sharma S, Gulati OP. Pycnogenol® inhibits the release of histamine from mast cells. *Phyther Res*. 2003;17(1):66-69. doi:10.1002/ptr.1240

54. Aggarwal B, Yost D. Healing Spices: How to Use 50 Everyday and Exotic Spices to Boost Health and Beat Disease. Sterling Publishing; 2011.

55. Shealy N. Illustrated Encyclopedia of Healing Rememedies. Harper Collins; 2018.

56. Hussein A, Lobna M, Mohammed A, Mohamed G. Biochemical Effects of Chamomile Oil on Inflammatory Biomarkers in Gastroenteritis. *Int J Drug Dev Res*. 2009;9(2). http://www.ijddr.in/drug-development/biochemical-effects-of-chamomile-oil-on-inflammatory-biomarkers-ingastroenteritis.php?aid=19225. Accessed September 17, 2018.

57. Chevallier A. Encyclopedia of Herbal Medicine: 500 Herbs and Remedies for Common Ailments. 3rd Edition. Dorling Kindersley Publishing; 2016.

58. Low Dog T, Johnson R, Foster S, Kiefer D, Weil A. National Geographic Guide to Medicinal Herbs: The World's Most Effective Healing Plants. National Geographic; 2012.

59. Pursell J. The Herbal Apothecary: 100 Medicinal Herbs and How to Use Them. Timber Press; 2015.

60. Gholamnezhad Z, Keyhanmanesh R, Boskabady MH. Anti-inflammatory, antioxidant, and immunomodulatory aspects of Nigella sativa for its preventive and bronchodilatory effects on obstructive respiratory diseases: A review of basic and clinical evidence. *J Funct Foods*. 2015;17:910-927. doi:10.1016/J.JFF.2015.06.032

61. Tembhurne S, Feroz S, More B, Sakarkar D. A review on therapeutic potential of Nigella sativa (kalonji) seeds. *J Med Plants Res*. 2014;8(3):167-177. doi:10.5897/JMPR10.737

62. Shin Y-W, Bae E-A, Lee B, et al. In Vitro and In Vivo Antiallergic Effects of Glycyrrhiza glabra and Its Components. *Planta Med*. 2007;73(3):257-261. doi:10.1055/s-2007-967126

63. Thakur S, Verma A. Antihistaminic Effect of Moringa Oleifera Seed Extract. *Int J Pharm Res Allied Sci*. 2013;2(1):56-59.

64. Liu Z-Q, Li X-X, Qiu S-Q, et al. Vitamin D contributes to mast cell stabilization. *Allergy*. 2017;72(8):1184-1192. doi:10.1111/all.13110

65. Weng Z, Zhang B, Asadi S, et al. Quercetin is more effective than cromolyn in blocking human mast cell cytokine release and inhibits

contact dermatitis and photosensitivity in humans. *PLoS One.* 2012;7(3):e33805. doi:10.1371/journal.pone.0033805

66. Shaik Y, Caraffa A, Ronconi G, Lessiani G, Conti P. Impact of polyphenols on mast cells with special emphasis on the effect of quercetin and luteolin. *Cent Eur J Immunol.* 2018;43(4):476-481. doi:10.5114/ceji.2018.81347

67. Upaganlawar A, Ghule B. Pharmacological Activities of Boswellia serrata Roxb. - Mini Review. *Ethnobot Leafl.* 2009;2009(6). https://opensiuc.lib.siu.edu/ebl/vol2009/iss6/10. Accessed May 21, 2020.

68. Sharma A, Gajbhiye V, Kharya MD. *PHCOG REV.: Plant Review Phytochemical Profile of Boswellia Serrata: An Overview.* Vol 1. http://www.phcogrev.com. Accessed May 21, 2020.

69. Li GZ, Chai OH, Song CH. Inhibitory effects of epigallocatechin gallate on compound 48/80-induced mast cell activation and passive cutaneous anaphylaxis. *Exp Mol Med.* 2005;37(4):290-296. doi:10.1038/emm.2005.39

70. Maldonado MD, Garcia-Moreno H, Calvo JR. Melatonin protects mast cells against cytotoxicity mediated by chemical stimuli PMACI: Possible clinical use. *J Neuroimmunol.* 2013;262(1-2):62-65. doi:10.1016/j.jneuroim.2013.06.013

71. Carr A, Maggini S. Vitamin C and Immune Function. *Nutrients.* 2017;9(11):1211. doi:10.3390/nu9111211

72. Pareek A, Suthar M, Rathore GS, Bansal V. Feverfew (Tanacetum parthenium L.): A systematic review. *Pharmacogn Rev.* 2011;5(9):103-110. doi:10.4103/0973-7847.79105

73. Xu Y, Liu Q, Guo X, Xiang L, Zhao G. Resveratrol attenuates IL–33– induced mast cell inflammation associated with inhibition of NF–κB activation and the P38 signaling pathway. *Mol Med Rep.* 2020;21(3):1658-1666. doi:10.3892/mmr.2020.10952

74. Nakajima S, Ishimaru K, Kobayashi A, et al. Resveratrol inhibits IL-33–mediated mast cell activation by targeting the MK2/3–PI3K/Akt axis. *Sci Rep.* 2019;9(1):1-11. doi:10.1038/s41598-019-54878-5

75. Turner H. Phone interview on July 13, 2018.

76. Carnahan J. Mold is a Major Trigger of Mast Activation Cell Syndrome - Jill Carnahan, MD. https://www.jillcarnahan.com/2018/03/12/mold-is-a-major-trigger-of-mast-activation-cell-syndrome/. Accessed February 19, 2018.

77. O'Hara B. Top Tips on Environmental Mold for those with Mast Cell Activation Syndrome and Histamine Intolerance. https://mastcell360.com/top-tips-on-environmental-mold-for-

those-with-mast-cell-activation-syndrome-and-histamine-intolerance/. Accessed October 15, 2020.

78. Snow R. "Mast Cell Activation Syndrome: ID, Explanation and Treatment" presented at the 27th Annual American Herbalists Guild Symposium, September 29 – October 2, 2016, Seven Springs, PA. Accessed February 19, 2018.

79. Holt-Lunstad J, Smith TB, Layton JB. Social Relationships and Mortality Risk: A Meta-analytic Review. *PLoS Med.* 2010;7(7):e1000316. doi:10.1371/journal.pmed.1000316

CHAPTER 2: POTS

1. Mathias CJ, Low DA, Iodice V, Owens AP, Kirbis M, Grahame R. Postural tachycardia syndrome—current experience and concepts. *Nat Rev Neurol.* 2012;8(1):22-34. doi:10.1038/nrneurol.2011.187

2. Maxwell A. Dysautonomia. In: Jovin D, ed. Disjointed: Navigating the Diagnosis and Management of Hypermobile Ehlers-Danlos Syndrome and Hypermobility Spectrum Disorders. Hidden Stripes Publications; 2020.

3. Raj SR. The Postural Tachycardia Syndrome (POTS): pathophysiology, diagnosis & management. *Indian Pacing Electrophysiol J.* 2006;6(2):84-99. http://www.ncbi.nlm.nih.gov/pubmed/16943900. Accessed July 20, 2018.

4. Conner R, Sheikh M, Grubb B. Postural Orthostatic Tachycardia Syndrome (POTS): evaluation and management. *Br J Med Pract.* 2012;5(4):12-18.

5. Raj V, Haman KL, Raj SR, et al. Psychiatric profile and attention deficits in postural tachycardia syndrome. *J Neurol Neurosurg Psychiatry.* 2009;80(3):339-344. doi:10.1136/jnnp.2008.144360

6. Raj SR, Garland EM, Biaggioni I, Black BK, Robertson D. Morning heart rate surge in postural tachycardia syndrome. *Circulation.* 2005;112:U810.

7. Grubb BP. Postural Tachycardia Syndrome. *Circulation.* 2008;117(21):2814-2817. doi:10.1161/CIRCULATIONAHA.107.761643

8. Bagai K, Wakwe CI, Malow B, et al. Estimation of sleep disturbances using wrist actigraphy in patients with postural tachycardia syndrome. *Auton Neurosci Basic Clin.* 2013;177(2):260-265. doi:10.1016/j.autneu.2013.02.021

9. POTS - A World Tour, presented by Dr. Satish R. Raj on Vimeo. https://vimeo.com/72346576. Accessed May 8, 2020.
10. Schondorf R, Low PA. Idiopathic postural orthostatic tachycardia syndrome: An attenuated form of acute pandysautonomia? *Neurology.* 1993;43(1):132-137. doi:10.1212/wnl.43.1_part_1.132
11. Novak V, Novak P, Opfer-Gehrking TL, Low PA. Postural tachycardia syndrome: Time frequency mapping. *J Auton Nerv Syst.* 1996;61(3):313-320. doi:10.1016/S0165-1838(96)00101-4
12. Low PA, Sandroni P, Joyner M, Shen W-K. Postural Tachycardia Syndrome (POTS). *J Cardiovasc Electrophysiol.* 2009;20(3):352-358. doi:10.1111/j.1540-8167.2008.01407.x
13. Boris JR. Postural orthostatic tachycardia syndrome in children and adolescents. *Auton Neurosci Basic Clin.* 2018;215:97-101. doi:10.1016/j.autneu.2018.05.004
14. Boris JR, Huang J, Bernadzikowski T. Orthostatic heart rate does not predict symptomatic burden in pediatric patients with chronic orthostatic intolerance. *Clin Auton Res.* 2020;30(1):19-28. doi:10.1007/s10286-019-00622-y
15. Chelimsky G, Chelimsky T. The gastrointestinal symptoms present in patients with postural tachycardia syndrome: A review of the literature and overview of treatment. *Auton Neurosci Basic Clin.* 2018;215:70-77. doi:10.1016/j.autneu.2018.09.003
16. Olshansky B, Cannom D, Fedorowski A, et al. Postural Orthostatic Tachycardia Syndrome (POTS): A critical assessment. *Prog Cardiovasc Dis.* March 2020. doi:10.1016/j.pcad.2020.03.010
17. Postural Orthostatic Tachycardia Syndrome (POTS) - Cedars-Sinai. https://www.cedars-sinai.edu/Patients/Health-Conditions/Postural-Orthostatic-Tachycardia-Syndrome-POTS.aspx. Accessed May 6, 2020.
18. Bryarly M, Phillips LT, Fu Q, Vernino S, Levine BD. Postural Orthostatic Tachycardia Syndrome: JACC Focus Seminar. *J Am Coll Cardiol.* 2019;73(10):1207-1228. doi:10.1016/j.jacc.2018.11.059
19. Wikipedia. Median Arcuate Ligament Syndrome. https://en.wikipedia.org/wiki/Median_arcuate_ligament_syndrome. Accessed September 22, 2018.
20. Brinth LS, Pors K, Theibel AC, Mehlsen J. Orthostatic intolerance and postural tachycardia syndrome as suspected adverse effects of vaccination against human papilloma virus. *Vaccine.* 2015;33(22):2602-2605. doi:10.1016/j.vaccine.2015.03.098
21. Hineno A, Schu-ichi I, Scheinbenbogen C, Heidecke H, Schulze-Forster K, Junker. Autoantibodies against Autonomic Nerve Receptors in Adolescent Japanese Girls after Immunization with Human

Papillomavirus Vaccine OPEN ACCESS. *Ann Arthritis Clin Rheumatol.* 2019;9(2):1014.

22. Blitshteyn S, Brinth L, Hendrickson JE, Martinez-Lavin M. Autonomic dysfunction and HPV immunization: an overview. *Immunol Res.* 2018;66(6):744-754. doi:10.1007/s12026-018-9036-1

23. Jefferson T, Jorgensen L. Human papillomavirus vaccines, complex regional pain syndrome, postural orthostatic tachycardia syndrome, and autonomic dysfunction – a review of the regulatory evidence from the European Medicines Agency. *Indian J Med Ethics Online First.* 2017;2(1):30-37. http://ijme.in/pdf/a-signal-. Accessed October 15, 2020.

24. Schofield JR, Hendrickson JE. Autoimmunity, Autonomic Neuropathy, and the HPV Vaccination: A Vulnerable Subpopulation. *Clin Pediatr (Phila).* 2018;57(5):603-606. doi:10.1177/0009922817728701

25. Barboi A, Gibbons CH, Axelrod F, et al. Human papillomavirus (HPV) vaccine and autonomic disorders: a position statement from the American Autonomic Society. *Clin Auton Res.* 2020;30(1):13-18. doi:10.1007/s10286-019-00608-w

26. Tripathi R, Bernitsas E. From Postural Orthostatic Tachycardia Syndrome to Radiologically Isolated Syndrome. *Case Rep Neurol Med.* 2018;2018. doi:10.1155/2018/2956387

27. Miranda NA, Boris JR, Kouvel KM, Stiles L. Activity and exercise intolerance after concussion: Identification and management of postural orthostatic tachycardia syndrome. *J Neurol Phys Ther.* 2018;42(3):163-171. doi:10.1097/NPT.0000000000000231

28. Thomsen R, Ozturk B, Pedersen L, et al. Hospital Records of Pain, Fatigue, or Circulatory Symptoms in Girls Exposed to Human Papillomavirus Vaccination: Cohort, Self-controlled Case Serie... - PubMed - NCBI. *Am J Epidem.* 2020;3. https://www.ncbi.nlm.nih.gov/pubmed/31899791. Accessed May 8, 2020.

29. Kanjwal K, Karabin B, Kanjwal Y, Grubb BP. Autonomic dysfunction presenting as postural tachycardia syndrome following traumatic brain injury. *Cardiol J.* 2010;17(5):482-487.

30. Ponnusamy V, Owens AP, Purkayastha S, Iodice V, Mathias CJ. Orthostatic intolerance and autonomic dysfunction following bariatric surgery: A retrospective study and review of the literature. *Auton Neurosci Basic Clin.* 2016;198:1-7. doi:10.1016/j.autneu.2016.05.003

31. Nogués M, Delorme R, Saadia D, Heidel K, Benarroch E. Postural tachycardia syndrome in syringomyelia: Response to fludrocortisone and β-blockers. *Clin Auton Res.* 2001;11(4):265-267. doi:10.1007/BF02298959

32. Habek M, Krbot Skorić M, Crnošija L, Gabelić T, Barun B, Adamec I. Postural orthostatic tachycardia predicts early conversion to multiple sclerosis after clinically isolated syndrome. *Eur Neurol.* 2017;77(5-6):253-257. doi:10.1159/000469707

33. Fedorowski A. Postural orthostatic tachycardia syndrome: clinical presentation, aetiology and management. *J Intern Med.* 2019;285(4):352-366. doi:10.1111/joim.12852

34. Jacob G, Costa F, Shannon JR, et al. The Neuropathic Postural Tachycardia Syndrome. *N Engl J Med.* 2000;343(14):1008-1014. doi:10.1056/NEJM200010053431404

35. Shibao C, Arzubiaga C, Roberts ILJ, et al. Hyperadrenergic postural tachycardia syndrome in mast cell activation disorders. *Hypertension.* 2005;45(3):385-390. doi:http://dx.doi.org/10.1161/01.HYP.0000158259.68614.40

36. Strasheim C. Chapter One: Wayne Anderson, ND. In: New Paradigms in Lyme Disease Treatment: 10 Top Doctors Reveal Healing Strategies That Work. BioMed Publishing Group; 2016:40.

37. El-Sayed H, Hainsworth R. Salt supplement increases plasma volume and orthostatic tolerance in patients with unexplained syncope. *Heart.* 1996;75(2):134-140. doi:10.1136/hrt.75.2.134

38. Frey MAB, Lathers C, Davis J, Fortney S, Charles JB. Cardiovascular Responses to Standing: Effect of Hydration. *J Clin Pharmacol.* 1994;34(5):387-393. doi:10.1002/j.1552-4604.1994.tb04978.x

39. Bungo MW, Charles JB, Johnson PC. Cardiovascular deconditioning during space flight and the use of saline as a countermeasure to orthostatic intolerance. *Aviat Sp Environ Med.* 1985;56(10):985-990.

40. Sheldon RS, Grubb BP, Olshansky B, et al. 2015 heart rhythm society expert consensus statement on the diagnosis and treatment of postural tachycardia syndrome, inappropriate sinus tachycardia, and vasovagal syncope. *Hear Rhythm.* 2015;12(6):e41-e63. doi:10.1016/j.hrthm.2015.03.029

41. Thieben MJ, Sandroni P, Sletten DM, et al. Postural orthostatic tachycardia syndrome: The Mayo Clinic experience. *Mayo Clin Proc.* 2007;82(3):308-313. doi:10.4065/82.3.308

42. Plash WB, Diedrich A, Biaggioni I, et al. Diagnosing postural tachycardia syndrome: Comparison of tilt testing compared with standing haemodynamics. *Clin Sci.* 2013;124(2):109-114. doi:10.1042/CS20120276

43. Ykelenstam Y. Dr. Diana Driscoll interview: vagus nerve and POTS/mast cell activation. Healing Histamine. https://healinghistamine.com/dr-diana-driscoll-interview-vagus-nerve-and-potsmast-cell-activation/. Accessed September 22, 2018.

44. Russek LN, Stott P, Simmonds J. Recognizing and Effectively Managing Hypermobility-Related Conditions. *Phys Ther.* 2019;99(9):1189-1200. doi:10.1093/ptj/pzz078

45. George SA, Bivens TB, Howden EJ, et al. The international POTS registry: Evaluating the efficacy of an exercise training intervention in a community setting. *Hear Rhythm.* 2016;13(4):943-950. doi:10.1016/j.hrthm.2015.12.012

46. Fu Q, Vangundy TB, Shibata S, Auchus RJ, Williams GH, Levine BD. Exercise training versus propranolol in the treatment of the postural orthostatic tachycardia syndrome. *Hypertension.* 2011;58(2):167-175. doi:10.1161/HYPERTENSIONAHA.111.172262

47. Mtinangi BL, Hainsworth R. Early effects of oral salt on plasma volume, orthostatic tolerance, and baroreceptor sensitivity in patients with syncope. *Clin Auton Res.* 1998;8(4):231-235. doi:10.1007/BF02267786

48. Kerstens MN, Kobold ACM, Volmer M, Koerts J, Sluiter WJ, Dullaart RP. Reference Values for Aldosterone–Renin Ratios in Normotensive Individuals and Effect of Changes in Dietary Sodium Consumption. *Clin Chem.* 2011;57(11):1607-1611. doi:10.1373/clinchem.2011.165662

49. Claydon VE, Schroeder C, Norcliffe LJ, Jordan J, Hainsworth R. Water drinking improves orthostatic tolerance in patients with posturally related syncope. *Clin Sci.* 2006;110(3):343-352. doi:10.1042/CS20050279

50. Mathias CJ, Young TM. Water drinking in the management of orthostatic intolerance due to orthostatic hypotension, vasovagal syncope and the postural tachycardia syndrome. *Eur J Neurol.* 2004;11(9):613-619. doi:10.1111/j.1468-1331.2004.00840.x

51. Shannon JR, Diedrich A, Biaggioni I, et al. Water drinking as a treatment for orthostatic syndromes. *Am J Med.* 2002;112(5):355-360. doi:10.1016/S0002-9343(02)01025-2

52. Weinstock LB, Brook JB, Myers TL, Goodman B. Successful treatment of postural orthostatic tachycardia and mast cell activation syndromes using naltrexone, immunoglobulin and antibiotic treatment. *BMJ Case Rep.* January 2018. doi:10.1136/bcr-2017-221405

53. Wells R, Hissaria P, Elliott AD, et al. Plasma Exchange Therapy in Postural Tachycardia Syndrome: A Novel Long-Term Approach? *Am J Med.* 2020;133(4):e157-e159. doi:10.1016/j.amjmed.2019.10.016

54. Driscoll D, De A, Doherty C, Ferreira JP, Meglathery S, Pazun J. The Driscoll Theory Newly Revised: The Cause of POTS in Ehlers-Danlos Syndrome and How to Reverse the Process. Warnick Publishing; 2015.

55. Pederson CL, Brook JB. Health-related quality of life and suicide risk in postural tachycardia syndrome. *Clin Auton Res.* 2017;27(2):75-81. doi:10.1007/s10286-017-0399-5

CHAPTER 3: EDS

1. Castori M, Hakim A. Contemporary approach to joint hypermobility and related disorders. *Curr Opin Pediatr.* 2017;29(6):640-649. doi:10.1097/MOP.0000000000000541
2. Castori M, Tinkle B, Levy H, Grahame R, Malfait F, Hakim A. A framework for the classification of joint hypermobility and related conditions. *Am J Med Genet Part C Semin Med Genet.* 2017;175(1):148-157. doi:10.1002/ajmg.c.31539
3. Beighton P, De Paepe A, Steinmann B, Tsipouras P, Wenstrup RJ. Ehlers-Danlos syndromes: revised nosology, Villefranche, 1997. Ehlers-Danlos National Foundation (USA) and Ehlers-Danlos Support Group (UK). *Am J Med Genet.* 1998;77(1):31-37. http://www.ncbi.nlm.nih.gov/pubmed/9557891.
4. Laferrier J, Muldowney K, Muldowney K. A Novel Exercise Protocol for Individuals with Ehlers Danlos Syndrome: A Case Report. 2018. doi:10.4172/2165-7025.1000382
5. Miller E, Grosel JM. A review of Ehlers-Danlos syndrome. *J Am Acad Physician Assist.* 2020;33(4):23-28. doi:10.1097/01.JAA.0000657160.48246.91
6. Shirley ED, DeMaio M, Bodurtha J. Ehlers-Danlos Syndrome in Orthopaedics: Etiology, Diagnosis, and Treatment Implications. *Sports Health.* 2012;4(5):394-403. doi:10.1177/1941738112452385
7. Lee D, Mueller E. Mast Cell Activation Features in Ehlers-Danlos/Joint Hypermobility Patients: A Retrospective Analysis in Light of an Emerging Disease Cluster [abstract]. *Arthritis Rheumatol.* 2017;69(suppl 10). https://acrabstracts.org/abstract/mast-cell-activation-features-in-ehlers-danlosjoint-hypermobility-patients-a-retrospective-analysis-in-light-of-an-emerging-disease-cluster/.
8. Driscoll D, De A, Doherty C, Ferreira JP, Meglathery S, Pazun J. The Driscoll Theory Newly Revised: The Cause of POTS in Ehlers-Danlos Syndrome and How to Reverse the Process. Warnick Publishing; 2015.
9. Hamonet C, Schatz P-M, Bezire P, Ducret L, Brissot R. Cognitive and Psychopathological Aspects of Ehlers-Danlos Syndrome-Experience in a Specialized Medical Consultation. 2018. doi:10.29011/RABDT-104

10. Bennett SE, Walsh N, Moss T, Palmer S. The lived experience of Joint Hypermobility and Ehlers-Danlos Syndromes: a systematic review and thematic synthesis. *Phys Ther Rev.* 2019;24(1-2):12-28. doi:10.1080/10833196.2019.1590674

11. Block N. Physical Therapy. In: Jovin D, ed. Disjointed: Navigating the Diagnosis and Management of Hypermobile Ehlers-Danlos Syndrome and Hypermobility Spectrum Disorders. Hidden Stripes Publications; 2020.

12. Russek L, Simmonds J. The Evidence-Based Rationale for Physical Therapy Treatment of Children, Adolescents, and Adults Diagnosed With Joint Hypermobility Syndrome/Hypermobile Ehlers-Danlos Syndrome (for Non-experts) | The Ehlers Danlos Society : The Ehlers Danlos Society. https://www.ehlers-danlos.com/2017-eds-classification-non-experts/evidence-based-rationale-physical-therapy-treatment/. Accessed April 17, 2020.

13. Smith TO, Jerman E, Easton V, et al. Do people with benign joint hypermobility syndrome (BJHS) have reduced joint proprioception? A systematic review and meta-analysis. *Rheumatol Int.* 2013;33(11):2709-2716. doi:10.1007/s00296-013-2790-4

14. Scheper M, Rombaut L, de Vries J, et al. The association between muscle strength and activity limitations in patients with the hypermobility type of Ehlers–Danlos syndrome: the impact of proprioception. *Disabil Rehabil.* 2017;39(14):1391-1397. doi:10.1080/09638288.2016.1196396

15. Ericson WB, Wolman R. Orthopaedic management of the Ehlers-Danlos syndromes. *Am J Med Genet Part C Semin Med Genet.* 2017;175(1):188-194. doi:10.1002/ajmg.c.31551

16. Mitakides J. Temporomandibular Joint Dysfunction and Hypermobility Disorders. In: Jovin D, ed. Disjointed: Navigating the Diagnosis and Management of Hypermobile Ehlers-Danlos Syndrome and Hypermobility Spectrum Disorders. Hidden Stripes Publications; 2020.

17. Muldowney K. The Muldowney Protocol Part 1. Nashville; 2019. https://www.ehlers-danlos.com/pdf/2019-Nashville/Muldowney-The-Muldowney-Protocol-20.

18. Larson CM, Stone RM, Grossi EF, Giveans MR, Cornelsen GD. Ehlers-Danlos syndrome: Arthroscopic management for extreme soft-tissue hip instability. *Arthrosc - J Arthrosc Relat Surg.* 2015;31(12):2287-2294. doi:10.1016/j.arthro.2015.06.005

19. Malfait F, Francomano C, Byers P, et al. The 2017 international classification of the Ehlers-Danlos syndromes. *Am J Med Genet C Semin Med Genet.* 2017;175(1):8-26. doi:10.1002/ajmg.c.31552

20. Herman K. Genetics. In: Jovin D, ed. Disjointed: Navigating the Diagnosis and Management of Hypermobile Ehlers-Danlos Syndrome and Hypermobility Spectrum Disorders. Hidden Stripes Publications; 2020.
21. Saperstein D. Neurological Considerations in Hypermobility Disorders. In: Jovin D, ed. Disjointed: Navigating the Diagnosis and Management of Hypermobile Ehlers-Danlos Syndrome and Hypermobility Spectrum Disorders. Hidden Stripes Publications; 2020.
22. Fikree A, Chelimsky G, Collins H, Kovacic K, Aziz Q. Gastrointestinal involvement in the Ehlers-Danlos syndromes. *Am J Med Genet Part C Semin Med Genet.* 2017;175(1):181-187. doi:10.1002/ajmg.c.31546
23. Maxwell A. Dysautonomia. In: Jovin D, ed. Disjointed: Navigating the Diagnosis and Management of Hypermobile Ehlers-Danlos Syndrome and Hypermobility Spectrum Disorders. Hidden Stripes Publications; 2020.
24. Russek LN, Stott P, Simmonds J. Recognizing and Effectively Managing Hypermobility-Related Conditions. *Phys Ther.* 2019;99(9):1189-1200. doi:10.1093/ptj/pzz078
25. Chopra P. Complex Regional Pain Syndrome (CRPS) Diagnosis and Management. PowerPoint Presentation in "Often Seen, Rarely Recognized" Conference on 9-16-17 in St. Cloud, Minnesota.
26. Milhorat TH, Bolognese PA, Nishikawa M, McDonnell NB, Francomano CA. Syndrome of occipitoatlantoaxial hypermobility, cranial settling, and Chiari malformation Type I in patients with hereditary disorders of connective tissue. *J Neurosurg Spine.* 2007;7(6):601-609. doi:10.3171/SPI-07/12/601
27. Henderson FC, Austin C, Benzel E, et al. Neurological and spinal manifestations of the Ehlers-Danlos syndromes. *Am J Med Genet Part C Semin Med Genet.* 2017;175(1):195-211. doi:10.1002/ajmg.c.31549
28. Rombaut L, Malfait F, De Wandele I, et al. Medication, surgery, and physiotherapy among patients with the hypermobility type of ehlers-danlos syndrome. *Arch Phys Med Rehabil.* 2011;92(7):1106-1112. doi:10.1016/j.apmr.2011.01.016
29. Burcharth J, Rosenberg J. Gastrointestinal surgery and related complications in patients with Ehlers-Danlos syndrome: A systematic review. *Dig Surg.* 2012;29(4):349-357. doi:10.1159/000343738
30. Jesudas R, Chaudhury A, Laukaitis CM. An update on the new classification of Ehlers-Danlos syndrome and review of the causes of bleeding in this population. *Haemophilia.* 2019;25(4):hae.13800. doi:10.1111/hae.13800
31. Schubart JR, Schilling A, Schaefer E, Bascom R, Francomano C. Use of prescription opioid and other drugs among a cohort of persons with

Ehlers-Danlos syndrome: A retrospective study. *Am J Med Genet Part A.* 2019;179(3):397-403. doi:10.1002/ajmg.a.61031

32. Raj SR. The Postural Tachycardia Syndrome (POTS): pathophysiology, diagnosis & management. *Indian Pacing Electrophysiol J.* 2006;6(2):84-99. http://www.ncbi.nlm.nih.gov/pubmed/16943900.

33. Weiler CR, Austen KF, Akin C, et al. AAAAI Mast Cell Disorders Committee Work Group Report: Mast cell activation syndrome (MCAS) diagnosis and management. *J Allergy Clin Immunol.* 2019;144(4):883-896. doi:10.1016/j.jaci.2019.08.023

34. Cheung I, Vadas P. A New Disease Cluster: Mast Cell Activation Syndrome, Postural Orthostatic Tachycardia Syndrome, and Ehlers-Danlos Syndrome. *J Allergy Clin Immunol.* 2015;135(2):AB65. doi:10.1016/j.jaci.2014.12.1146

35. Goodman B, Hoffman-Snyder C, Dhawan P. Joint Hypermobility Syndrome in a Postural Orthostatic Tachycardia Syndrome (POTS) Cohort. *Neurology.* 2016;86(16 Supplement):P5.116. http://n.neurology.org/content/86/16_Supplement/P5.116.short. Accessed August 31, 2018.

36. Shibao C, Arzubiaga C, Roberts ILJ, et al. Hyperadrenergic postural tachycardia syndrome in mast cell activation disorders. *Hypertension.* 2005;45(3):385-390. doi:http://dx.doi.org/10.1161/01.HYP.0000158259.68614.40

37. Zadourian A, Doherty TA, Swiatkiewicz I, Taub PR. Postural Orthostatic Tachycardia Syndrome: Prevalence, Pathophysiology, and Management. *Drugs.* 2018;78(10):983-994. doi:10.1007/s40265-018-0931-5

38. Doherty TA, White AA. Postural orthostatic tachycardia syndrome and the potential role of mast cell activation. *Auton Neurosci Basic Clin.* 2018;215:83-88. doi:10.1016/j.autneu.2018.05.001

39. Hoffman-Snyder C, Lewis J, Harris L, Dhawan P GB. Evidence of Mast Cell Activation Disorder in Postural Tachycardia Syndrome. *Neurology.* 2015;84(14 Supplement):P1.277. http://n.neurology.org/content/84/14_Supplement/P1.277.short.

40. Kohn A, Chang C. The Relationship Between Hypermobile Ehlers-Danlos Syndrome (hEDS), Postural Orthostatic Tachycardia Syndrome (POTS), and Mast Cell Activation Syndrome (MCAS). *Clin Rev Allergy Immunol.* July 2019. doi:10.1007/s12016-019-08755-8

41. Jackson T, Rosenfeld W, Ferguson L, Maitland A, Bolognese P. Chiari malformation (CM) and/or tethered cord, idiopathic mast cell activation syndrome (MCAS), Ehlers-Danlos Syndrome (EDS), and Postural Orthostatic Tachycardia syndrome (POTS): a new pediatric

disease cluster. *Pediatrics.* 2019;144(2 MeetingAbstract):467-467. doi:10.1542/PEDS.144.2_MEETINGABSTRACT.467

42. Tinkle B, Castori M, Berglund B, et al. Hypermobile Ehlers–Danlos syndrome (a.k.a. Ehlers–Danlos syndrome Type III and Ehlers–Danlos syndrome hypermobility type): Clinical description and natural history. *Am J Med Genet Part C Semin Med Genet.* 2017;175(1):48-69. doi:10.1002/ajmg.c.31538

43. Castori M. Ehlers-Danlos Syndrome, Hypermobility Type: An Underdiagnosed Hereditary Connective Tissue Disorder with Mucocutaneous, Articular, and Systemic Manifestations. *ISRN Dermatol.* 2012;2012. doi:10.5402/2012/751768

44. Corrado B, Ciardi G. Hypermobile Ehlers-Danlos syndrome and rehabilitation: taking stock of evidence based medicine: a systematic review of the literature. *J Phys Ther Sci.* 2018;30(6):843-847. doi:10.1589/jpts.30.847

45. Bathen T, Hångmann AB, Hoff M, Andersen LØ, Rand-Hendriksen S. Multidisciplinary treatment of disability in ehlers-danlos syndrome hypermobility type/hypermobility syndrome: A pilot study using a combination of physical and cognitive-behavioral therapy on 12 women. *Am J Med Genet Part A.* 2013;161(12):3005-3011. doi:10.1002/ajmg.a.36060

46. Pennetti A. A multimodal physical therapy approach utilizing the Maitland concept in the management of a patient with cervical and lumbar radiculitis and Ehlers–Danlos syndrome-hypermobility type: A case report. *Physiother Theory Pract.* 2018;34(7):559-568. doi:10.1080/09593985.2017.1422207

47. Pacey V, Adams RD, Tofts L, Munns CF, Nicholson LL. Proprioceptive acuity into knee hypermobile range in children with Joint Hypermobility Syndrome. *Pediatr Rheumatol.* 2014;12(1):1-7. doi:10.1186/1546-0096-12-40

48. Peterson B, Coda A, Pacey V, Hawke F. Physical and mechanical therapies for lower limb symptoms in children with Hypermobility Spectrum Disorder and Hypermobile Ehlers-Danlos Syndrome: A systematic review. *J Foot Ankle Res.* 2018;11(1):1-11. doi:10.1186/s13047-018-0302-1

49. Arthur K, Caldwell K, Forehand S, Davis K. Pain control methods in use and perceived effectiveness by patients with Ehlers-Danlos syndrome: A descriptive study. *Disabil Rehabil.* 2016;38(11):1063-1074. doi:10.3109/09638288.2015.1092175

50. Brewster S. Service Dogs. In: Jovin D, ed. Disjointed: Navigating the Diagnosis and Management of Hypermobile Ehlers-Danlos Syndrome

461

and Hypermobility Spectrum Disorders. Hidden Stripes Publications; 2020.

51. Hamonet C, Brock I, Hamonet-Dewez M, Brissot R. Local Multiple Injections of Lidocaine as a Very Efficient Treatment of Intractable Pains in Ehlers-Danlos Disease. The Dysproprioception Hypothesis. *EC Anaethesia.* 2019;5(9):290-296.

52. Ehab S. Prolotherapy with 12.5% dextrose to treat temporomandibular joint dysfunction (TMD). *Int J Oral Craniofacial Sci.* April 2019:015-019. doi:10.17352/2455-4634.000039

53. Majumdar SK, Krishna S, Chatterjee A, Chakraborty R, Ansari N. Single Injection Technique Prolotherapy for Hypermobility Disorders of TMJ Using 25 % Dextrose: A Clinical Study. *J Maxillofac Oral Surg.* 2017;16(2):226-230. doi:10.1007/s12663-016-0944-0

54. Refai H. Long-term therapeutic effects of dextrose prolotherapy in patients with hypermobility of the temporomandibular joint: a single-arm study with 1-4 years' follow up. *Br J Oral Maxillofac Surg.* 2017;55(5):465-470. doi:10.1016/j.bjoms.2016.12.002

55. Mustafa R, Güngörmüş M, Mollaoğlu N. Evaluation of the Efficacy of Different Concentrations of Dextrose Prolotherapy in Temporomandibular Joint Hypermobility Treatment. *J Craniofac Surg.* 2018;29(5):e461-e465. doi:10.1097/SCS.0000000000004480

56. Cömert Kiliç S, Güngörmüş M. Is dextrose prolotherapy superior to placebo for the treatment of temporomandibular joint hypermobility? A randomized clinical trial. *Int J Oral Maxillofac Surg.* 2016;45(7):813-819. doi:10.1016/j.ijom.2016.01.006

57. Nagori SA, Jose A, Gopalakrishnan V, Roy ID, Chattopadhyay PK, Roychoudhury A. The efficacy of dextrose prolotherapy over placebo for temporomandibular joint hypermobility: A systematic review and meta-analysis. *J Oral Rehabil.* 2018;45(12):998-1006. doi:10.1111/joor.12698

58. Hauser RA, Lackner JB, Steilen-Matias D, Harris DK. A Systematic Review of Dextrose Prolotherapy for Chronic Musculoskeletal Pain. *Clin Med Insights Arthritis Musculoskelet Disord.* 2016;9:CMAMD.S39160. doi:10.4137/CMAMD.S39160

CHAPTER 5: INTERNAL HEALTH STRESSORS

1. What are microbes? - Informedhealth.org - NCBI Bookshelf. https://www.ncbi.nlm.nih.gov/books/NBK279387/. Accessed April 15, 2020.
2. O'Leary JG, Reddy KR, Wong F, et al. Long-term Use of Antibiotics and Proton Pump Inhibitors Predict Development of Infections in Patients With Cirrhosis. *Clin Gastroenterol Hepatol.* 2015;13(4):753-759.e2. doi:10.1016/j.cgh.2014.07.060
3. Biswal S. Proton Pump Inhibitors and Risk for Clostridium difficile Associated Diarrhea. doi:10.4103/2319-4170.128002
4. Lazaro-Pacheco IB, Servin-Caamano AI, Perez-Hernandez JL, Rojas-Loreiro G, Servin-Abad L, Higuera-De La Tijera F. Proton pump inhibitors increase the overall risk of developing bacterial infections in patients with cirrhosis. *Arq Gastroenterol.* 2018;55(1):28-32. doi:10.1590/S0004-2803.201800000-09
5. Khosravi A, Yáñez A, Price JG, et al. Gut microbiota promote hematopoiesis to control bacterial infection. *Cell Host Microbe.* 2014;15(3):374-381. doi:10.1016/j.chom.2014.02.006
6. Aljarallah KM. Conventional and alternative treatment approaches for Clostridium difficile infection. *Int J Health Sci (Qassim).* 2017;11(1):1.
7. Bajantri B, Venkatram S, Diaz-Fuentes G. Mycoplasma pneumoniae : A Potentially Severe Infection . *J Clin Med Res.* 2018;10(7):535-544. doi:10.14740/jocmr3421w
8. Liu Q, Meng X, Li Y, Zhao CN, Tang GY, Li H Bin. Antibacterial and antifungal activities of spices. *Int J Mol Sci.* 2017;18(6). doi:10.3390/ijms18061283
9. Bayan L, Koulivand PH, Gorji A. Garlic: a review of potential therapeutic effects. *Avicenna J phytomedicine.* 2014;4(1):1-14. doi:10.22038/ajp.2014.1741
10. Hudson J. Applications of the phytomedicine Echinacea purpurea (Purple Coneflower) in infectious diseases. *J Biomed Biotechnol.* 2012:769-896. doi:10.1155/2012/769896
11. Cech N, Junio H, Ackermann L, Kavanaugh J, Horswill A. Quorum quenching and antimicrobial activity of goldenseal (hydrastis canadensis) against methicillin-resistant staphylococcus aureus (MRSA). *Planta Med.* 2012;78(14):1556-1561. doi:10.1055/s-0032-1315042

12. Gupta S, Bhat G. Antibacterial Effect of Neem Oil on Methicillin Resistant Staphylococcus Aureus. *Journ Med Plant Studies.* 2016;4(1):1-3.
13. Mahady GB, Huang Y, Doyle BJ, Locklear T. Natural products as antibacterial agents. In: *Studies in Natural Products Chemistry.* Vol 35. Elsevier; 2008:423-444. doi:10.1016/S1572-5995(08)80011-7
14. Sienkiewicz M, Wasiela M, Głowacka A. [The antibacterial activity of oregano essential oil (Origanum heracleoticum L.) against clinical strains of Escherichia coli and Pseudomonas aeruginosa]. *Med Dosw Mikrobiol.* 2012;64(4):297-307.
15. Boskovic M, Zdravkovic N, Ivanovic J, et al. Antimicrobial Activity of Thyme (Tymus vulgaris) and Oregano (Origanum vulgare) Essential Oils against Some Food-borne Microorganisms. *Procedia Food Sci.* 2015;5:18-21. doi:10.1016/j.profoo.2015.09.005
16. Sakkas H, Papadopoulou C. Antimicrobial Activity of Basil, Oregano, and Thyme Essential Oils. *J Microbiol Biotechnol.* 2016;26(0):429-438. doi:10.4014/jmb.1608.08024
17. Dolara P, Corte B, Ghelardini C, et al. Local Anaesthetic, Antibacterial and Antifungal Properties of Sesquiterpenes from Myrrh. *Planta Med.* 2000;66(04):356-358. doi:10.1055/s-2000-8532
18. Mandal MD, Mandal S. Honey: Its medicinal property and antibacterial activity. *Asian Pac J Trop Biomed.* 2011;1(2):154-160. doi:10.1016/S2221-1691(11)60016-6
19. Carter DA, Blair SE, Cokcetin NN, et al. Therapeutic manuka honey: No longer so alternative. *Front Microbiol.* 2016;7(APR). doi:10.3389/fmicb.2016.00569
20. Rodgers BM, Kirley KM, Mounsey AM. Prescribing an Antibiotic? Pair it with probiotics. *J Fam Pract.* 2013;62(3):148-150.
21. Marshall J, King C, McCurdy J. Mast Cell Cytokine and Chemokine Responses to Bacterial and Viral Infection. *Curr Pharm Des.* 2005;9(1):11-24. doi:10.2174/1381612033392413
22. Talkington J, Nickell SP. Borrelia burgdorferi spirochetes induce mast cell activation and cytokine release. *Infect Immun.* 1999;67(3):1107-1115. http://www.ncbi.nlm.nih.gov/pubmed/10024550. Accessed September 3, 2018.
23. Carod-Artal FJ. Infectious diseases causing autonomic dysfunction. *Clin Auton Res.* 2018;28(1):67-81. doi:10.1007/s10286-017-0452-4
24. Sarwari NM, Khoury JD, Hernandez CMR. Chronic Epstein Barr virus infection leading to classical Hodgkin lymphoma. *BMC Hematol 2016 161.* 2016;16(1):19. doi:10.1186/s12878-016-0059-3

25. Cohen JI. Optimal treatment for chronic active Epstein-Barr virus disease. *Pediatr Transplant.* 2009;13(4):393-396. doi:10.1111/j.1399-3046.2008.01095.x

26. Cohen JI. Optimal treatment for chronic active Epstein-Barr virus disease. *Pediatr Transplant.* 2009;13(4):393-396. doi:10.1111/j.1399-3046.2008.01095.x

27. Chhabra A, Alyazidi R, Human A. A great masquerader: Chronic active Epstein-Barr virus for the rheumatologist. *J Rheumatol.* 2019;46(8):960-961. doi:10.3899/jrheum.180618

28. Epstein-barr | Mononucleosis | Laboratory Testing | Mono | CDC. https://www.cdc.gov/epstein-barr/laboratory-testing.html. Accessed April 15, 2020.

29. Pagano JS, Whitehurst CB, Andrei G. Antiviral drugs for EBV. *Cancers (Basel).* 2018;10(6). doi:10.3390/cancers10060197

30. Andrei G, Trompet E, Snoeck R. Novel therapeutics for Epstein–Barr virus. *Molecules.* 2019;24(5). doi:10.3390/molecules24050997

31. Lin TP, Chen SY, Duh P Der, Chang LK, Liu YN. Inhibition of the Epstein-Barr virus lytic cycle by andrographolide. *Biol Pharm Bull.* 2008;31(11):2018-2023. doi:10.1248/bpb.31.2018

32. Yiu CY, Chen SY, Yang TH, et al. Inhibition of epstein-barr virus lytic cycle by an ethyl acetate subfraction separated from polygonum cuspidatum root and its major component, emodin. *Molecules.* 2014;19(1):1258-1272. doi:10.3390/molecules19011258

33. Chang LK, Wei TT, Chiu YF, et al. Inhibition of Epstein-Barr virus lytic cycle by (-)-epigallocatechin gallate. *Biochem Biophys Res Commun.* 2003;301(4):1062-1068. doi:10.1016/S0006-291X(03)00067-6

34. Cui H, Xu B, Wu T, Xu J, Yuan Y, Gu Q. Potential antiviral lignans from the roots of saururus chinensis with activity against epstein-barr virus lytic replication. *J Nat Prod.* 2014;77(1):100-110. doi:10.1021/np400757k

35. Cho HJ, Jeong SG, Park JE, et al. Antiviral activity of angelicin against gammaherpesviruses. *Antiviral Res.* 2013;100(1):75-83. doi:10.1016/j.antiviral.2013.07.009

36. Zakaryan H, Arabyan E, Oo A, Zandi K. Flavonoids: promising natural compounds against viral infections. *Arch Virol.* 2017;162(9):2539-2551. doi:10.1007/s00705-017-3417-y

37. Hawkins J, Baker C, Cherry L, Dunne E. Black elderberry (Sambucus nigra) supplementation effectively treats upper respiratory symptoms: A meta-analysis of randomized, controlled clinical trials. *Complement Ther Med.* 2019;42:361-365. doi:10.1016/j.ctim.2018.12.004

38. Torabian G, Valtchev P, Adil Q, Dehghani F. Anti-influenza activity of elderberry (Sambucus nigra). *J Funct Foods*. 2019;54:353-360. doi:10.1016/j.jff.2019.01.031

39. Aguilar-Jimenez W, Zapata W, Rugeles MT. Antiviral molecules correlate with vitamin D pathway genes and are associated with natural resistance to HIV-1 infection. *Microbes Infect*. 2016;18(7-8):510-516. doi:10.1016/j.micinf.2016.03.015

40. Pourghanbari G, Nili H, Moattari A, Mohammadi A, Iraji A. Antiviral activity of the oseltamivir and Melissa officinalis L. essential oil against avian influenza A virus (H9N2). *VirusDisease*. 2016;27(2):170-178. doi:10.1007/s13337-016-0321-0

41. Hudson JB. The phytomedicine Echinacea Purpurea contains light dependent and light independent antiviral activities. *J Innov Pharm Biol Sci*. 2017;4(3):109-113. www.jipbs.com. Accessed April 15, 2020.

42. Ganjuri M, Darakhshan S, Taghizad F. A Review on Pharmacological and Therapeutic Properties of Echinacea. *Int Journ Pharmaco*. 2016;7(4):838-42.

43. Mardia Mohamad Nasir MMN, Abllah Z, Azura Jalaludin A, Azura Shahdan I, Hayati Wan Abd Manan WN. Virgin Coconut Oil and Its Antimicrobial Properties against Pathogenic Microorganisms: A Review. In: Atlantis Press; 2018. doi:10.2991/idcsu-17.2018.51

44. Biancatelli MRLC, Colunga Biancatelli L, Berrill M, Marik PE. The antiviral properties of vitamin C. 2019. doi:10.1080/14787210.2020.1706483

45. Srinivasan K. Ginger rhizomes (Zingiber officinale): A spice with multiple health beneficial potentials. *PharmaNutrition*. 2017;5(1):18-28. doi:10.1016/j.phanu.2017.01.001

46. Mathew D, Hsu WL. Antiviral potential of curcumin. *J Funct Foods*. 2018;40:692-699. doi:10.1016/j.jff.2017.12.017

47. Jan KN, zarafshan K, Singh S. Stinging nettle (Urtica dioica L.): a reservoir of nutrition and bioactive components with great functional potential. *J Food Meas Charact*. 2017;11(2):423-433. doi:10.1007/s11694-016-9410-4

48. Elvis AM, Ekta JS. Ozone therapy: A clinical review. *J Nat Sci Biol Med*. 2011;2(1):66-70. doi:10.4103/0976-9668.82319

49. Marshall JS, King CA, McCurdy JD. Mast cell cytokine and chemokine responses to bacterial and viral infection. *Curr Pharm Des*. 2003;9(1):11-24. doi:10.2174/1381612033392413

50. Hawman DW, Stoermer KA, Montgomery SA, et al. Chronic Joint Disease Caused by Persistent Chikungunya Virus Infection Is Controlled by the Adaptive Immune Response. *J Virol*. 2013;87(24):13878-13888. doi:10.1128/jvi.02666-13

466

51. Masuko-Hongo K, Kato T, Nishioka K. Virus-associated arthritis. *Best Pract Res Clin Rheumatol.* 2003;17(2):309-318. doi:10.1016/S1521-6942(03)00004-4

52. Bennet SMP, Ohman L, Simren M. Gut microbiota as potential orchestrators of irritable bowel syndrome. *Gut Liver.* 2015;9(3):318-331. doi:10.5009/gnl14344

53. Aminzadeh A, Sabeti Sanat A, Nik Akhtar S. Frequency of candidiasis and colonization of Candida albicans in relation to oral contraceptive pills. *Iran Red Crescent Med J.* 2016;18(10). doi:10.5812/ircmj.38909

54. Gunsalus KTW, Tornberg-Belanger SN, Matthan NR, Lichtenstein AH, Kumamoto CA. Manipulation of Host Diet To Reduce Gastrointestinal Colonization by the Opportunistic Pathogen Candida albicans. *mSphere.* 2016;1(1). doi:10.1128/mSphere.00020-15

55. Nosál R. Histamine release from isolated rat mast cells due to glycoprotein from Candida albicans in vitro. *J Hyg Epidemiol Microbiol Immunol.* 1974;18(3):377-378. http://www.ncbi.nlm.nih.gov/pubmed/4138120.

56. Yamaguchi N, Sugita R, Miki A, et al. Gastrointestinal Candida colonisation promotes sensitisation against food antigens by affecting the mucosal barrier in mice. *Gut.* 2006;55(7):954-960. doi:10.1136/gut.2005.084954

57. Omura Y, O'young B, Jones M, Pallos A, Duvvi H, Shimotsuura Y. Caprylic acid in the effective treatment of intractable medical problems of frequent urination, incontinence, chronic upper respiratory infection, root canalled tooth infection, ALS, etc., caused by Asbestos & mixed infections of Candida albicans, Helicobacter pylori & Cytomegalovirus with or without other microorganisms & mercury. *Acupunct Electro-Therapeutics Res.* 2011;36(1-2):19-64. doi:10.3727/036012911803860886

58. Khodavandi A, Alizadeh F, Harmal NS, et al. Comparison between efficacy of allicin and fluconazole against Candida albicans in vitro and in a systemic candidiasis mouse model. *FEMS Microbiol Lett.* 2011;315(2):87-93. doi:10.1111/j.1574-6968.2010.02170.x

59. Ghannoum MA. Inhibition of Candida adhesion to buccal epithelial cells by an aqueous extract of Allium sativum (garlic). *J Appl Bacteriol.* 1990;68(2):163-169. doi:10.1111/j.1365-2672.1990.tb02562.x

60. Kumar A, Dhamgaye S, Maurya IK, Singh A, Sharma M, Prasad R. Curcumin targets cell wall integrity via calcineurin-mediated signaling in candida albicans. *Antimicrob Agents Chemother.* 2014;58(1):167-175. doi:10.1128/AAC.01385-13

61. Khan N, Shreaz S, Bhatia R, et al. Anticandidal activity of curcumin and methyl cinnamaldehyde. *Fitoterapia*. 2012;83(3):434-440. doi:10.1016/j.fitote.2011.12.003

62. Sharma M, Manoharlal R, Puri N, Prasad R. Antifungal curcumin induces reactive oxygen species and triggers an early apoptosis but prevents hyphae development by targeting the global repressor TUP1 in Candida albicans. *Biosci Rep*. 2010;30(6):391-404. doi:10.1042/BSR20090151

63. Pizzo G, Giuliana G, Milici ME, Giangreco R. Effect of dietary carbohydrates on the in vitro epithelial adhesion of Candida albicans, Candida tropicalis, and Candida krusei. *New Microbiol*. 2000;23(1):63-71. http://www.ncbi.nlm.nih.gov/pubmed/10946407. Accessed April 22, 2020.

64. Sujatha G, Kumar GS, Muruganandan J, Prasad TS. Aloe Vera in Dentistry. *J Clin Diagnostic Res*. 2014;8(10):ZI01.

65. Pai MBH, Prashant GM, Murlikrishna KS, Shivakumar KM, Chandu GN. Antifungal efficacy of Punica granatum, Acacia nilotica, Cuminum cyminum and Foeniculum vulgare on Candida albicans: An in vitro study. *Indian J Dent Res*. 2010;21(3):334-336. doi:10.4103/0970-9290.70792

66. Battikh H, Chaieb K, Bakhrouf A, Ammar E. Antibacterial and Antifungal Activities of Black and Green Kombucha Teas. *J Food Biochem*. 2013;37(2):231-236. doi:10.1111/j.1745-4514.2011.00629.x

67. Futuro DO, Ferreira PG, Nicoletti CD, et al. The antifungal activity of naphthoquinones: An integrative review. *An Acad Bras Cienc*. 2018;90(1):1187-1214. doi:10.1590/0001-3765201820170815

68. Siqueira LB de O de, Matos AP dos S, Cardoso V da S, et al. Clove oil nanoemulsion showed potent inhibitory effect against Candida spp. *Nanotechnology*. 2019;30(42):425101. doi:10.1088/1361-6528/AB30C1

69. Zorić N, Kosalec I, Tomić S, et al. Membrane of Candida albicans as a target of berberine. *BMC Complement Altern Med*. 2017;17(1):268. doi:10.1186/s12906-017-1773-5

70. Dolara P, Corte B, Ghelardini C, et al. Local Anaesthetic, Antibacterial and Antifungal Properties of Sesquiterpenes from Myrrh. *Planta Med*. 2000;66(04):356-358. doi:10.1055/s-2000-8532

71. Anyanwu GO. A comparative study of the in vitro activities of *Lactobacillus Acidophilus* and two antifungal agents on *Candida Albicans*. Federal University of Technology, Owerri; 2016.

72. Mailänder-Sánchez D, Wagener J, Schaller M. Potential role of probiotic bacteria in the treatment and prevention of localised

candidosis. *Mycoses.* 2012;55(1):17-26. doi:10.1111/j.1439-0507.2010.01967.x

73. Shi D, Zhao Y, Yan H, et al. Antifungal effects of undecylenic acid on the biofilm formation of Candida albicans. *Int J Clin Pharmacol Ther.* 2016;54(5):343-353. doi:10.5414/CP202460

74. Mionić Ebersold M, Petrović M, Fong W-K, Bonvin D, Hofmann H, Milošević I. Hexosomes with Undecylenic Acid Efficient against Candida albicans. *Nanomaterials.* 2018;8(2):91. doi:10.3390/nano8020091

75. Rao A, Zhang Y, Muend S, Rao R. Mechanism of antifungal activity of terpenoid phenols resembles calcium stress and inhibition of the TOR pathway. *Antimicrob Agents Chemother.* 2010;54(12):5062-5069. doi:10.1128/AAC.01050-10

76. Tsutsumi-Arai C, Takakusaki K, Arai Y, et al. Grapefruit seed extract effectively inhibits the Candida albicans biofilms development on polymethyl methacrylate denture-base resin. *PLoS One.* 2019;14(5). doi:10.1371/journal.pone.0217496

77. Nazzaro F, Fratianni F, Coppola R, Feo V De. Essential Oils and Antifungal Activity. *Pharmaceuticals.* 2017;10(4):86. doi:10.3390/ph10040086

78. Tagoe DNA, Nyarko HD, Akpaka R. A comparison of the antifungal properties of onion (Allium cepa), ginger (Zingiber officinale) and garlic (Allium sativum) against Aspergillus flavus, Aspergillus niger and Cladosporium herbarum. *Res J Med Plant.* 2011;5(3):281-287. doi:10.3923/rjmp.2011.281.287

79. Yaya EE. Phytoalexins and other antifungal metabolites from crucifers: isolation, synthesis and biosynthesis. Dissertation: Department of Chemistry, University of Saskatchewan Saskatoon. 2013.

80. Goel N, Rohilla H, Singh G, Punia P. Antifungal Activity of Cinnamon Oil and Olive Oil against Candida Spp. Isolated from Blood Stream Infections. *J Clin DIAGNOSTIC Res.* 2016;10(8):DC09.

81. Nieto-Patlán A, Campillo-Navarro M, Rodríguez-Cortés O, et al. Recognition of Candida albicans by Dectin-1 induces mast cell activation. *Immunobiology.* 2015;220(9):1093-1100. doi:10.1016/j.imbio.2015.05.005

82. Khalique Z, Hatipoğlu S, Rosendahl U, Mohiaddin R. Unusual Complicated Fungal Endocarditis in a Patient With Vascular Ehlers-Danlos Syndrome. *Ann Thorac Surg.* 2019;107(4):e269-e271. doi:10.1016/j.athoracsur.2018.08.074

83. Zhan X, Stamova B, Sharp FR. Lipopolysaccharide associates with amyloid plaques, neurons and oligodendrocytes in Alzheimer's disease

brain: A review. *Front Aging Neurosci.* 2018;10(FEB):42. doi:10.3389/fnagi.2018.00042

84. Bach E, Møller AB, Jørgensen JOL, et al. Stress hormone release is a key component of the metabolic response to lipopolysaccharide: studies in hypopituitary and healthy subjects. *Eur J Endocrinol.* 2016;175(5):455-465. doi:10.1530/EJE-16-0444

85. Hritcu L, Gorgan LD. Intranigral lipopolysaccharide induced anxiety and depression by altered BDNF mRNA expression in rat hippocampus. *Prog Neuro-Psychopharmacology Biol Psychiatry.* 2014;51:126-132. doi:10.1016/j.pnpbp.2014.01.016

86. Maldonado RF, A-Correia IS, Valvano MA, Whitfield CE. Lipopolysaccharide modification in Gram-negative bacteria during chronic infection One sentence summary: The authors review modifications of lipopolysaccharide structure and biosynthetic pathways that occur upon bacterial adaptation to chronic respiratory and gastrointestinal infections. *FEMS Microbiol Rev.* 2016;007:480-493. doi:10.1093/femsre/fuw007

87. Nehra AK, Alexander JA, Loftus CG, Nehra V. Proton Pump Inhibitors: Review of Emerging Concerns. *Mayo Clin Proc.* 2018;93(2):240-246. doi:10.1016/j.mayocp.2017.10.022

88. Yu LY, Sun LN, Zhang XH, et al. A Review of the Novel Application and Potential Adverse Effects of Proton Pump Inhibitors. *Adv Ther.* 2017;34(5):1070-1086. doi:10.1007/s12325-017-0532-9

89. Leaky Gut: Is There a Test for That? – Naturopathic Doctor News and Review. https://ndnr.com/gastrointestinal/leaky-gut-is-there-a-test-for-that/. Accessed May 7, 2020.

90. Kucik CJ, Martin GL, Sortor B V. Common intestinal parasites. *Am Fam Physician.* 2004;69(5):1161-1168. http://www.ncbi.nlm.nih.gov/pubmed/15023017. Accessed May 7, 2020.

91. Chedid V, Dhalla S, Clarke J, et al. Herbal Therapy is Effective for Rifaximin Non-Responders with Small Intestinal Bacterial Overgrowth (SIBO) and the Irritable Bowel Syndrome (IBS). *Am J Gastroenterol.* 2012;107:s714.

92. Chedid V, Dhalla S, Clarke J, Dunbar K, Koh J, Justino E. Herbal Therapy vs. Rifaximin for Treatment of Small Intestinal Bacterial Overgrowth (SIBO). *Am J Gastroenterol.* 2012;107:s132-s133.

93. Hamilton MJ, Hornick JL, Akin C, Castells MC, Greenberger NJ. Mast cell activation syndrome: A newly recognized disorder with systemic clinical manifestations. *J Allergy Clin Immunol.* 2011;128(1)(1):147-152. doi:10.1016/j.jaci.2011.04.037

470

94. Russell N, Jennings S, Jennings B, et al. The Mastocytosis Society Survey on Mast Cell Disorders: Part 2—Patient Clinical Experiences and Beyond. *J Allergy Clin Immunol Pract.* 2019;7(4):1157-1165.e6. doi:10.1016/j.jaip.2018.07.032

95. Jennings S, Russell N, Jennings B, et al. The Mastocytosis Society Survey on Mast Cell Disorders: Patient Experiences and Perceptions. *J Allergy Clin Immunol Pract.* 2014;2(1):70-76. doi:10.1016/j.jaip.2013.09.004

96. Bischoff SC. Mast cells in gastrointestinal disorders. *Eur J Pharmacol.* 2016;778:139-145. doi:10.1016/j.ejphar.2016.02.018

97. Weinstock LB, Brook J, Kaleem Z, Afrin L, Molderings G. Small Intestinal Bacterial Overgrowth Is Common in Mast Cell Activation Syndrome. *Am J Gastroenterol.* 2019;114:S670. doi:10.14309/01.ajg.0000594304.61014.c5

98. Nelson AD, Mouchli MA, Valentin N, et al. Ehlers Danlos syndrome and gastrointestinal manifestations: a 20-year experience at Mayo Clinic. *Neurogastroenterol Motil.* 2015;27(11):1657-1666. doi:10.1111/nmo.12665

99. Beckers AB, Keszthelyi D, Fikree A, et al. Gastrointestinal disorders in joint hypermobility syndrome/Ehlers-Danlos syndrome hypermobility type: A review for the gastroenterologist. *Neurogastroenterol Motil.* 2017;29(8):e13013. doi:10.1111/nmo.13013

100. Castori M, Camerota F, Celletti C, et al. Natural history and manifestations of the hypermobility type Ehlers-Danlos syndrome: A pilot study on 21 patients. *Am J Med Genet Part A.* 2010;152A(3):556-564. doi:10.1002/ajmg.a.33231

101. Danese C, Castori M, Celletti C, et al. Screening for celiac disease in the joint hypermobility syndrome/Ehlers-Danlos syndrome hypermobility type. *Am J Med Genet Part A.* 2011;155(9):2314-2316. doi:10.1002/ajmg.a.34134

102. Fikree A, Aktar R, Grahame R, et al. Functional gastrointestinal disorders are associated with the joint hypermobility syndrome in secondary care: A case-control study. *Neurogastroenterol Motil.* 2015;27(4):569-579. doi:10.1111/nmo.12535

103. Fikree A, Aziz Q, Jafari J, Grahame R, Sifrim D. Dysphagia in patients with the joint hypermobility syndrome. *Gut.* 2011;60(Suppl 1):A181-A181. doi:10.1136/gut.2011.239301.385

104. Loavenbruck A, Iturrino J, Singer W, et al. Disturbances of Gastrointestinal transit and autonomic functions in postural orthostatic tachycardia syndrome. *Neurogastroenterol Motil.* 2015;27(1):92-98. doi:10.1111/nmo.12480

105. Sullivan SD, Hanauer J, Rowe PC, Barron DF, Darbari A, Oliva-Hemker M. Gastrointestinal Symptoms Associated with Orthostatic Intolerance. *J Pediatr Gastroenterol Nutr*. 2005;40(4):425-428. doi:10.1097/01.MPG.0000157914.40088.31

106. Siddiki H, Horsley-Silva J, Goodman B, Foxx-Orenstein A. Gastrointestinal (GI) Disease Burden in Patients with Postural Orthostatic Tachycardia : American Journal of Gastroenterology. *Am J Gastroenterol*. 2016;111:s259. https://journals.lww.com/ajg/Fulltext/2016/10001/Gastrointestinal__GI_Disease_Burden_in_Patients.566.aspx. Accessed May 7, 2020.

107. Huang KZ, Dellon ES. Increased prevalence of autonomic dysfunction due to postural orthostatic tachycardia syndrome in patients with eosinophilic gastrointestinal disorders. *J Gastrointest Liver Dis*. 2019;28(1):47-51. doi:10.15403/jgld.2014.1121.281.syd

108. Kariatsumari B. Understanding Adrenal Fatigue: Nutritional and lifestyle strategies to effectively restore proper adrenal function. *Nutr Perspect J Counc Nutr*. 2019;42(1):29-40.

109. Pirola I, Rotondi M, Cristiano A, et al. Selenium supplementation in patients with subclinical hypothyroidism affected by autoimmune thyroiditis: Results of the SETI study. *Endocrinol Diabetes y Nutr*. 2020;67(1):28-35. doi:10.1016/j.endinu.2019.03.018

110. Enríquez J, Velázquez-Cruz R, Parra-Torres A, Gutiérrez-Sagal R, Larrea F. The anti-estrogenic activity of indole-3-carbinol in neonatal rat osteoblasts is associated with the estrogen receptor antagonist 2-hydroxyestradiol. *J Endocrinol Invest*. 2016;39(10):1149-1158. doi:10.1007/s40618-016-0494-9

111. Hall DC. Nutritional Influences on Estrogen Metabolism. *Appl Nutr Sci Reports*. 2001;1.

112. Cerqueira RO, Frey BN, Leclerc E, Brietzke E. Vitex agnus castus for premenstrual syndrome and premenstrual dysphoric disorder: a systematic review. *Arch Womens Ment Health*. 2017;20(6):713-719. doi:10.1007/s00737-017-0791-0

113. Song Y, Wang H, Huang H, Zhu Z. Comparison of the efficacy between NAC and metformin in treating PCOS patients: a meta-analysis. *Gynecol Endocrinol*. 2020;36(3):204-210. doi:10.1080/09513590.2019.1689553

114. Wojciechowska A, Osowski A, Jóźwik M, Górecki R, Rynkiewicz A, Wojtkiewicz J. Inositols' Importance in the Improvement of the Endocrine–Metabolic Profile in PCOS. *Int J Mol Sci*. 2019;20(22):5787. doi:10.3390/ijms20225787

115. Li MF, Zhou XM, Li XL. The Effect of Berberine on Polycystic Ovary Syndrome Patients with Insulin Resistance (PCOS-IR): A Meta-Analysis

and Systematic Review. *Evidence-based Complement Altern Med.* 2018;2018. doi:10.1155/2018/2532935

116. Walter J, Klein C, Wehrend A. Distribution of Mast Cells in Vaginal, Cervical and Uterine Tissue of Non-pregnant Mares: Investigations on Correlations with Ovarian Steroids. *Reprod Domest Anim.* 2012;47(2). doi:10.1111/j.1439-0531.2011.01897.x

117. Haq MRU, Kapila R, Sharma R, Saliganti V, Kapila S. Comparative evaluation of cow β-casein variants (A1/A2) consumption on Th2-mediated inflammatory response in mouse gut. *Eur J Nutr.* 2014;53(4):1039-1049. doi:10.1007/s00394-013-0606-7

118. Hugon-Rodin J, Lebègue G, Becourt S, Hamonet C, Gompel A. Gynecologic symptoms and the influence on reproductive life in 386 women with hypermobility type ehlers-danlos syndrome: A cohort study. *Orphanet J Rare Dis.* 2016;11(1):124. doi:10.1186/s13023-016-0511-2

119. Maayan C, Sela O, Axelrod F, Kidron D, Hochner-Celnikier D. Gynecological aspects of female familial dysautonomia. *Isr Med Assoc J.* 2000;2(9):679-683.

120. Fu Q, VanGundy TB, Shibata S, Auchus RJ, Williams GH, Levine BD. Menstrual Cycle Affects Renal-Adrenal and Hemodynamic Responses During Prolonged Standing in the Postural Orthostatic Tachycardia Syndrome. *Hypertension.* 2010;56(1):82-90. doi:10.1161/HYPERTENSIONAHA.110.151787

121. NMT Seminars. Introduction to Neuromodulation Technique. https://www.nmt.md/p/introduction-to-nmt. Accessed October 6, 2018.

CHAPTER 6: EXTERNAL HEALTH STRESSORS

1. Nathan Neil. TOXIC: Heal your body from mold toxicity, Lyme disease, multiple chemical sensitivities, and chronic environmental illness. Victory Belt Publishing Inc. 2018.

2. Mendell MJ, Cozen M: Building-related symptoms among U.S. office workers and risk factors for moisture and contamination: Preliminary analyses of U.S. EPA BASE data. LBNL-51567, Berkeley, CA Lawrence Berkeley National Laboratory (2002).

3. Spengler J, Neas L, Nakai S, et al. Respiratory Symptoms and Housing Characteristics. *Indoor Air.* 1994;4(2):72-82. doi:10.1111/j.1600-0668.1994.t01-2-00002.x

4. Maier WC, Arrighi HM, Morray B, Liewellyn C, Redding GJ. Indoor Risk Factors for Asthma and Wheezing Among Seattle School Children. *Environ Health Perspect.* 1997;105(2):208-214.

5. Shoemaker R. Mold Illness & the Surviving Mold Official Book | Dr. Ritchie Shoemaker. https://www.survivingmold.com/. Accessed May 9, 2020.

6. Shoemaker R. VCS (Visual Contrast Senstivity) Test Q & A | Surviving Mold. https://www.survivingmold.com/physicians/dashboard/faq/vcs. Accessed May 9, 2020.

7. O'Hara B. Top Tips on Environmental Mold for those with Mast Cell Activation Syndrome and Histamine Intolerance. https://mastcell360.com/top-tips-on-environmental-mold-for-those-with-mast-cell-activation-syndrome-and-histamine-intolerance/. Accessed October 15, 2020.

8. Billings LA, Ray D. Health Hazards of Mold: Warning signs structural mold has come to visit. *Altern Med.* 2013;11:40-42.

9. Brewer J, Thrasher J, Straus D, Madison R, Hooper D. Detection of Mycotoxins in Patients with Chronic Fatigue Syndrome. *Toxins (Basel).* 2013;5(4):605-617. doi:10.3390/toxins5040605

10. Tuuminen T, Vaali K, Valtonen V. Dampness and Mold Hypersensitivity Syndrome as an Umbrella for Many Chronic Diseases: The Clinician's Point of View. *Encycl Environ Heal.* 2019;2:1-9. doi:10.1016/B978-0-12-409548-9.11454-X

11. Kritas SK, Gallenga CE, D'Ovidio C, et al. Impact of mold on mast cell-cytokine immune response. *J Biol Regul Homeost Agents.* 2018;32(4):763-768.

12. Ratnaseelan AM, Tsilioni I, Theoharides TC. Effects of Mycotoxins on Neuropsychiatric Symptoms and Immune Processes. *Clin Ther.* 2018;40(6):903-917. doi:10.1016/j.clinthera.2018.05.004

13. Bennett AT, Collins KA. An unusual case of anaphylaxis: Mold in pancake mix. *Am J Forensic Med Pathol.* 2001;22(3):292-295. doi:10.1097/00000433-200109000-00019

14. Hoffman TILT Program. What is TILT? https://tiltresearch.org/about-tilt/. Accessed September 3, 2018.

15. Pizzorno J. The Toxin Solution: How Hidden Poisons in the Air, Water, Food and Products We Use Are Destroying Our Health. Harper Collins; 2017.

16. Environmental Working Group. A Benchmark Investigation of Industrial Chemicals, Pollutants and Pesticides in Umbilical Cord Blood. Body Burden: The Pollution in Newborns.; 2005. http://www.ewg.org/research/body-burden-pollution-newborns.

17. Lang CJ. The use of neuroimaging techniques for clinical detection of neurotoxicity: a review. *Neurotoxicology.* 2000;21(5):847-855. http://www.ncbi.nlm.nih.gov/pubmed/11130290. Accessed September 3, 2018.

18. Swedenborg E, Rüegg J, Mäkelä S, Pongratz I. Endocrine disruptive chemicals: mechanisms of action and involvement in metabolic disorders. *J Mol Endocrinol.* 2009;43(1):1-10. doi:10.1677/JME-08-0132

19. Corsini E, Sokooti M, Galli CL, Moretto A, Colosio C. Pesticide induced immunotoxicity in humans: A comprehensive review of the existing evidence. *Toxicology.* 2013;307:123-135. doi:10.1016/j.tox.2012.10.009

20. Natural Resources Defense Council. NRDC Web Page. https://www.nrdc.org/. Accessed September 3, 2018.

21. Centers for Disease Control. Agency for Toxic Substances and Disease Registry. https://www.atsdr.cdc.gov/. Accessed October 1, 2018.

22. Agency for Toxic Substances and Disease Registry. Set It Up Safe: A Planning Tool | Safe Places for Child Care | ATSDR. https://www.atsdr.cdc.gov/safeplacesforECE/set_it_up_safe.html. Accessed October 1, 2018.

23. Chan K. Some aspects of toxic contaminants in herbal medicines. *Chemosphere.* 2003;52(9):1361-1371. doi:10.1016/S0045-6535(03)00471-5

24. Agency for Toxic Substances and Disease Registry. Per- and Polyfluoroalkyl Substances (PFAS) and Your Health. https://www.atsdr.cdc.gov/pfas/index.html. Accessed October 1, 2018.

25. Kempuraj D, Asadi S, Zhang B, et al. Mercury induces inflammatory mediator release from human mast cells. *J Neuroinflammation.* 2010;7:20. doi:10.1186/1742-2094-7-20

26. Agency for Toxic Substances and Disease Registry. Substance Priority List | ATSDR. https://www.atsdr.cdc.gov/spl/. Accessed September 30, 2018.

27. Ly T, Lee S. If you think you can safely ink, beware of the masking effects of tattoos. *Hong Kong J Dermatol Venereol.* 2012;20:106-110. http://medcomhk.com/hkdvb/pdf/2012v20n106-110.pdf. Accessed September 3, 2018.

28. Sweeney SM. Tattoos: a review of tattoo practices and potential treatment options for removal. *Curr Opin Pediatr.* 2006;18(4):391-395. doi:10.1097/01.mop.0000236388.64333.cd

29. Watson R. Tattooists use pigments designed as car paint. *BMJ.* 2003;327(7408):182. doi:10.1136/bmj.327.7408.182-b

30. Juhas E, English JC. Tattoo-Associated Complications. *J Pediatr Adolesc Gynecol*. 2013;26(2):125-129. doi:10.1016/J.JPAG.2012.08.005

31. Goldenberg A, Jacob SE. Paraphenylenediamine in black henna temporary tattoos: 12-year Food and Drug Administration data on incidence, symptoms, and outcomes. *J Am Acad Dermatol*. 2015;72(4):724-726. doi:10.1016/j.jaad.2014.11.031

32. Li Z, Zhang H, Li S-H, Byard RW. Fatal Phenol Toxicity Following Attempted Tattoo Removal. *J Forensic Sci*. 2016;61(4):1143-1145. doi:10.1111/1556-4029.13106

33. Sterritt RM, Lester JN. Interactions of heavy metals with bacteria. *Sci Total Environ*. 1980;14(1):5-17. http://www.ncbi.nlm.nih.gov/pubmed/6988964. Accessed September 3, 2018.

34. Bhat S, Hassan T, Majid S. Heavy metal toxicity and their harmful effects on living organisms - a review. *Int J Med Sci Diagnosis Res*. 2019;3(1):106-122. doi:10.32553/JMSDR

35. Arruti A, Fernández-Olmo I, Irabien Á. Evaluation of the contribution of local sources to trace metals levels in urban PM2.5 and PM10 in the Cantabria region (Northern Spain). *J Environ Monit*. 2010;12(7):1451-1458. doi:10.1039/b926740a

36. Beyersmann D, Hartwig A. Carcinogenic metal compounds: Recent insight into molecular and cellular mechanisms. *Arch Toxicol*. 2008;82(8):493-512. doi:10.1007/s00204-008-0313-y

37. Tomljenovic L, Shaw CA. Aluminum vaccine adjuvants: are they safe? *Curr Med Chem*. 2011;18(17):2630-2637. http://www.ncbi.nlm.nih.gov/pubmed/21568886. Accessed September 13, 2018.

38. ATSDR - Public Health Statement: Aluminum. https://www.atsdr.cdc.gov/phs/phs.asp?id=1076&tid=34. Accessed April 23, 2020.

39. Chung JY, Yu S Do, Hong YS. Environmental source of arsenic exposure. *J Prev Med Public Heal*. 2014;47(5):253-257. doi:10.3961/jpmph.14.036

40. Sakurai T, Kojima C, Ochiai M, Ohta T, Fujiwara K. Evaluation of in vivo acute immunotoxicity of a major organic arsenic compound arsenobetaine in seafood. *Int Immunopharmacol*. 2004;4(2):179-184. doi:10.1016/j.intimp.2003.11.004

41. Hong YS, Song KH, Chung JY. Health effects of chronic arsenic exposure. *J Prev Med Public Heal*. 2014;47(5):245-252. doi:10.3961/jpmph.14.035

42. Chromium (Cr) Toxicity: Where Is Chromium Found? | ATSDR - Environmental Medicine & Environmental Health Education - CSEM.

https://www.atsdr.cdc.gov/csem/csem.asp?csem=10&po=5. Accessed April 23, 2020.

43. Jacobs DE, Clickner RP, Zhou JY, et al. The prevalence of lead-based paint hazards in U.S. housing. *Environ Health Perspect.* 2002;110(10). doi:10.1289/ehp.021100599

44. Brochin R, Leone S, Phillips D, Shepard N, Zisa D, Angerio A. *The Cellular Effect of Lead Poisoning and Its Clinical Picture.* Vol 5.; 2008.

45. Trasande L, Landrigan PJ, Schechter C. Public health and economic consequences of methyl mercury toxicity to the developing brain. *Environ Health Perspect.* 2005;113(5):590-596. doi:10.1289/ehp.7743

46. Haley BE. Mercury toxicity: Genetic susceptibility and synergistic effects. *Medical Veritas Journ Med Truth.* 2005;2:535-542. doi:10.1588/medver.2005.02.00067

47. Mahboob A, Farhat SM, Iqbal G, et al. Alpha-lipoic acid-mediated activation of muscarinic receptors improves hippocampus- and amygdala-dependent memory. *Brain Res Bull.* 2016;122:19-28. doi:10.1016/j.brainresbull.2016.02.014

48. Mehrandish R, Rahimian A, Shahriary A. Heavy metals detoxification: A review of herbal compounds for chelation therapy in heavy metals toxicity. *J Herbmed Pharmacol J Herbmed Pharmacol.* 2019;8(2):69-77. doi:10.15171/jhp.2019.12

49. Qayoom A, Arif Kazmi S, Nadir Ali S. Turmeric Powder as a Natural Heavy Metal Chelating Agent: Surface Characterisation. *J Sci Ind Res Ser A Phys Sci.* 2017;60(1):1-8. https://www.researchgate.net/publication/314675376. Accessed April 23, 2020.

50. Negi R, Satpathy G, Tyagi YK, Gupta RK. Biosorption of heavy metals by utilising onion and garlic wastes. *Int J Environ Pollut.* 2012;49(3-4):179-196. doi:10.1504/IJEP.2012.050898

51. Ralston NVC, Raymond LJ. Dietary selenium's protective effects against methylmercury toxicity. *Toxicology.* 2010;278(1):112-123. doi:10.1016/j.tox.2010.06.004

52. Zhai Q, Narbad A, Chen W. Dietary strategies for the treatment of cadmium and lead toxicity. *Nutrients.* 2015;7(1):552-571. doi:10.3390/nu7010552

53. Schon EA, DiMauro S, Hirano M. Human mitochondrial DNA: roles of inherited and somatic mutations. *Nat Rev Genet.* 2012;13(12):878-890. doi:10.1038/nrg3275

54. Diaz-Sanchez D, Penichet-Garcia M, Saxon A. Diesel exhaust particles directly induce activated mast cells to degranulate and increase histamine levels and symptom severity. *J Allergy Clin Immunol.* 2000;106(6):1140-1146. doi:10.1067/mai.2000.111144

55. Bischoff SC, Barbara G, Buurman W, et al. Intestinal permeability - a new target for disease prevention and therapy. *BMC Gastroenterol.* 2014;14(1):1-25. doi:10.1186/s12876-014-0189-7

56. Potulska-Chromik A, Zakrzewska-Pniewska B, Szmidt-Sałkowska E, et al. Long lasting dysautonomia due to botulinum toxin B poisoning: Clinical- laboratory follow up and difficulties in initial diagnosis. *BMC Res Notes.* 2013;6(1):1-3. doi:10.1186/1756-0500-6-438

57. Sarasamma S, Audira G, Juniardi S, et al. Zinc Chloride Exposure Inhibits Brain Acetylcholine Levels, Produces Neurotoxic Signatures, and Diminishes Memory and Motor Activities in Adult Zebrafish. *Int J Mol Sci.* 2018;19(10):3195. doi:10.3390/ijms19103195

58. Mehpara Farhat S, Mahboob A, Ahmed T. Oral exposure to aluminum leads to reduced nicotinic acetylcholine receptor gene expression, severe neurodegeneration and impaired hippocampus dependent learning in mice. *Drug Chem Toxicol.* 2019. doi:10.1080/01480545.2019.1587452

59. Natural Resources Defense Council. Electromagnetic Fields Fact Sheet. https://www.cancer.gov/about-cancer/causes-prevention/risk/radiation/electromagnetic-fields-fact-sheet. Accessed September 3, 2018.

60. Lindén V, Rolfsen S. Video computer terminals and occupational dermatitis. *Scand J Work Environ Health.* 1981;7(1):62-64. http://www.ncbi.nlm.nih.gov/pubmed/6458886. Accessed September 3, 2018.

61. Nilsen A. Facial rash in visual display unit operators. *Contact Dermatitis.* 1982;8(1):25-28. http://www.ncbi.nlm.nih.gov/pubmed/6461488. Accessed September 3, 2018.

62. Cox R. Electromagnetic hypersensitivity – human studies in the UK. Proceedings from the International Workshop in EMF Hypersensitivity in Prague on October 24-25, 2004. Published in 2006 by the World Health Organization. http://www.who.int/peh-emf/publications/reports/EHS_Proceedings_June2006.pdf.

63. Mueller C, Schierz C. Project NEMESIS: Double Blind Study on Effects of 50 Hz EMF on Sleep Quality, Physiological Parameters and Field Perception in People Suffering from Electrical Hypersensitivity. Proceedings of International Workshop on EMF Hypersensitivity in Prague on October 24-25, 2004. http://www.who.int/peh-emf/publications/reports/EHS_Proceedings_June2006.pdf#page=121. Accessed September 3, 2018.

64. Vecchio F, Babiloni C, Ferreri F, et al. Mobile phone emission modulates interhemispheric functional coupling of EEG alpha rhythms.

Eur J Neurosci. 2007;25(6):1908-1913. doi:10.1111/j.1460-9568.2007.05405.x

65. Belyaev IY, Markovà E, Hillert L, Malmgren LOG, Persson BRR. Microwaves from UMTS/GSM mobile phones induce long-lasting inhibition of 53BP1/γ-H2AX DNA repair foci in human lymphocytes. *Bioelectromagnetics.* 2009;30(2):129-141. doi:10.1002/bem.20445

66. Khurana VG, Teo C, Kundi M, Hardell L, Carlberg M. Cell phones and brain tumors: a review including the long-term epidemiologic data. *Surg Neurol.* 2009;72(3):205-214. doi:10.1016/j.surneu.2009.01.019

67. Kesari KK, Siddiqui MH, Meena R, Verma HN, Kumar S. Cell phone radiation exposure on brain and associated biological systems. *Indian J Exp Biol.* 2013;51(3):187-200. http://www.ncbi.nlm.nih.gov/pubmed/23678539. Accessed September 3, 2018.

68. Lamech F. Self-reporting of symptom development from exposure to radiofrequency fields of wireless smart meters in Victoria, Australia: a case series. *Altern Ther Health Med.* 20(6):28-39. http://www.ncbi.nlm.nih.gov/pubmed/25478801. Accessed September 3, 2018.

69. Carpenter DO. Excessive exposure to radiofrequency electromagnetic fields may cause the development of electrohypersensitivity. *Altern Ther Health Med.* 20(6):40-42. http://www.ncbi.nlm.nih.gov/pubmed/25478802. Accessed September 3, 2018.

70. Carpenter DO. Human disease resulting from exposure to electromagnetic fields1). *Rev Environ Health.* 2013;28(4):159-172. doi:10.1515/reveh-2013-0016

71. Milham S, Morgan LL. A new electromagnetic exposure metric: High frequency voltage transients associated with increased cancer incidence in teachers in a california school. *Am J Ind Med.* 2008;51(8):579-586. doi:10.1002/ajim.20598

72. Johansson O. Disturbance of the immune system by electromagnetic fields—A potentially underlying cause for cellular damage and tissue repair reduction which could lead to disease and impairment. *Pathophysiology.* 2009;16(2-3):157-177. doi:10.1016/j.pathophys.2009.03.004

73. Sohinki D. Examining the effect of an externally-applied low-level electromagnetic field on the inductibility of atrial fibrillation. The University of Oklahoma Health Sciences Center. 2019. https://search.proquest.com/openview/60be7ab479b057b32568c72 84ba6ead2/ 1?pq-origsite=gscholar&cbl=18750&diss=y. Accessed April 23, 2020.

479

74. Laden F, Neas LM, Tolbert PE, et al. Electric blanket use and breast cancer in the Nurses' Health Study. *Am J Epidemiol.* 2000;152(1):41-49. doi:10.1093/aje/152.1.41

CHAPTER 7: NERVOUS SYSTEM RE-TRAINING

1. O'Hara B. Nervous System Balance is Essential in Mast Cell Activation Syndrome and Histamine Intolerance. https://mastcell360.com/nervous-system-balance-is-essential-in-mast-cell-activation-syndrome-and-histamine-intolerance/. Accessed May 12, 2020.
2. Maxwell A. Dysautonomia. In: Jovin D, ed. Disjointed: Navigating the Diagnosis and Management of Hypermobile Ehlers-Danlos Syndrome and Hypermobility Spectrum Disorders. Hidden Stripes Publications; 2020.
3. Bonaz B, Bazin T, Pellissier S. The vagus nerve at the interface of the microbiota-gut-brain axis. *Front Neurosci.* 2018;12(FEB):49. doi:10.3389/fnins.2018.00049
4. Rosenberg S. *Accessing the Healing Power of the Vagus Nerve.* Berkeley, California: North Atlantic Books; 2017.
5. Porges SW. Safe & Sound Protocol Training Certification. Integrative Listening. 2020. www.integratedlistening.com.
6. Lonsdale D. Is Eosinophilic Esophagitis a Sugar Sensitive Disease? *J Gastric Disord Ther (ISSN 2381-8689).* 2016;2(1). doi:10.16966/2381-8689.114
7. Schneider S, Wright CM, Heuckeroth RO. Unexpected Roles for the Second Brain: Enteric Nervous System as Master Regulator of Bowel Function. *Annu Rev Physiol.* 2019;81(1):235-259. doi:10.1146/annurev-physiol-021317-121515
8. Zhou H, Liang H, Li ZF, Xiang H, Liu W, Li JG. Vagus nerve stimulation attenuates intestinal epithelial tight junctions disruption in endotoxemic mice through α7 nicotinic acetylcholine receptors. *Shock.* 2013;40(2):144-151. doi:10.1097/SHK.0b013e318299e9c0
9. Neren D, Johnson MD, Legon W, Bachour SP, Ling G, Divani AA. Vagus Nerve Stimulation and Other Neuromodulation Methods for Treatment of Traumatic Brain Injury. *Neurocrit Care.* 2016;24(2):308-319. doi:10.1007/s12028-015-0203-0

10. Borovikova L V., Ivanova S, Zhang M, et al. Vagus nerve stimulation attenuates the systemic inflammatory response to endotoxin. *Nature*. 2000;405(6785):458-462. doi:10.1038/35013070

11. Zhu S zhi, Huang W ping, Huang L qiang, et al. Huperzine A protects sepsis associated encephalopathy by promoting the deficient cholinergic nervous function. *Neurosci Lett*. 2016;631:70-78. doi:10.1016/j.neulet.2016.07.009

12. Guideri F, Acampa M, Hayek Y, Zappella M. Effects of acetyl-L-carnitine on cardiac dysautonomia in Rett syndrome: prevention of sudden death? *Pediatr Cardiol*. 2005;26(5):574-577. doi:10.1007/s00246-005-0784-z

13. Wong A, Chernykh O, Figueroa A. Chronic L-citrulline supplementation improves cardiac sympathovagal balance in obese postmenopausal women: A preliminary report. *Auton Neurosci Basic Clin*. 2016;198:50-53. doi:10.1016/j.autneu.2016.06.005

14. Ohinata K, Takemoto M, Kawanago M, et al. Orally Administered Zinc Increases Food Intake via Vagal Stimulation in Rats. *J Nutr*. 2009;139(3):611-616. doi:10.3945/jn.108.096370

15. Goswami C, Iwasaki Y, Yada T. Short-chain fatty acids suppress food intake by activating vagal afferent neurons. *J Nutr Biochem*. 2018;57:130-135. doi:10.1016/j.jnutbio.2018.03.009

16. Speer KE, Semple S, Naumovski N, McKune AJ. Heart rate variability for determining autonomic nervous system effects of lifestyle behaviors in early life: A systematic review. *Physiol Behav*. 2020;217:112806. doi:10.1016/j.physbeh.2020.112806

17. Bravo JA, Forsythe P, Chew M V., et al. Ingestion of Lactobacillus strain regulates emotional behavior and central GABA receptor expression in a mouse via the vagus nerve. *Proc Natl Acad Sci U S A*. 2011;108(38):16050-16055. doi:10.1073/pnas.1102999108

18. Jin Z, Lee G, Kim S, Park CS, Park YS, Jin YH. Ginger and its pungent constituents non-competitively inhibit serotonin currents on visceral afferent neurons. *Korean J Physiol Pharmacol*. 2014;18(2):149-153. doi:10.4196/kjpp.2014.18.2.149

19. Mager DE, Wan R, Brown M, et al. Caloric restriction and intermittent fasting alter spectral measures of heart rate and blood pressure variability in rats. *FASEB J*. 2006;20(6):631-637. doi:10.1096/fj.05-5263com

20. Ben-Menachem E, Mañon-Espaillat R, Ristanovic R, et al. Vagus nerve stimulation for treatment of partial seizures: 1. A controlled study of effect on seizures. First International Vagus Nerve Stimulation Study Group. *Epilepsia*. 35(3):616-626. http://www.ncbi.nlm.nih.gov/pubmed/8026408.

481

21. George R, Sonnen A, Upton A, et al. A randomized controlled trial of chronic vagus nerve stimulation for treatment of medically intractable seizures. The Vagus Nerve Stimulation Study Group. *Neurology.* 1995;45(2):224-230. http://www.ncbi.nlm.nih.gov/pubmed/7854516.

22. DeGiorgio CM, Schachter SC, Handforth A, et al. Prospective long-term study of vagus nerve stimulation for the treatment of refractory seizures. *Epilepsia.* 2000;41(9):1195-1200. http://www.ncbi.nlm.nih.gov/pubmed/10999559.

23. Yuan PQ, Taché Y, Miampamba M, Yang H. Acute cold exposure induces vagally mediated Fos expression in gastric myenteric neurons in conscious rats. *Am J Physiol - Gastrointest Liver Physiol.* 2001;281(2 44-2). doi:10.1152/ajpgi.2001.281.2.g560

24. Mäkinen TM, Mäntysaari M, Pääkkönen T, et al. Autonomic nervous function during whole-body cold exposure before and after cold acclimation. *Aviat Sp Environ Med.* 2008;79(9):875-882. doi:10.3357/ASEM.2235.2008

25. Kok BE, Coffey KA, Cohn MA, et al. How Positive Emotions Build Physical Health: Perceived Positive Social Connections Account for the Upward Spiral Between Positive Emotions and Vagal Tone. *Psychol Sci.* 2013;24(7):1123-1132. doi:10.1177/0956797612470827

26. Da Silva MAH, Dorsher PT. Neuroanatomic and clinical correspondences: Acupuncture and vagus nerve stimulation. *J Altern Complement Med.* 2014;20(4):233-240. doi:10.1089/acm.2012.1022

27. He W, Wang X, Shi H, et al. Auricular Acupuncture and Vagal Regulation. *Artic ID.* 2012;2012. doi:10.1155/2012/786839

28. Bernardi L, Sleight P, Bandinelli G, et al. Effect of rosary prayer and yoga mantras on autonomic cardiovascular rhythms: Comparative study. *Br Med J.* 2001;323(7327):1446-1449. doi:10.1136/bmj.323.7327.1446

29. Khoff BV, Malmgren H, Åström R, et al. Music structure determines heart rate variability of singers music structure determines heart rate variability of singers. *Front Psychol.* 2013;4(JUL). doi:10.3389/fpsyg.2013.00334

30. Dolgoff-Kaspar R, Baldwin A, Scott Johnson M, Edling N, Sethi GK. Effect of laughter yoga on mood and heart rate variability in patients awaiting organ transplantation: A pilot study. *Altern Ther Health Med.* 2012;18(5):61-66.

31. Gerritsen RJS, Band GPH. Breath of Life: The Respiratory Vagal Stimulation Model of Contemplative Activity. *Front Hum Neurosci.* 2018;12. doi:10.3389/fnhum.2018.00397

32. Porges SW, Macellaio M, Stanfill SD, et al. Respiratory sinus arrhythmia and auditory processing in autism: Modifiable deficits of an integrated social engagement system? *Int J Psychophysiol.* 2013;88(3):261-270. doi:10.1016/j.ijpsycho.2012.11.009

33. Van Der Kolk B. The Body Keeps The Score: Brain, Mind, and Body in the Healing of Trauma. New York: Penguin Books; 2014.

CHAPTER 8: NUTRITION

1. Yun AJ, Lee PY, Bazar KA. Clinical benefits of hydration and volume expansion in a wide range of illnesses may be attributable to reduction of sympatho-vagal ratio. *Med Hypotheses.* 2005;64(3):646-650. doi:10.1016/j.mehy.2004.07.014

2. Khan N, Westfall D, Jones A, et al. The Effect of Hydration on Cognition in Children: The WITiKids Randomized Controlled Crossover Trial (OR32-08-19). *Curr Dev Nutr.* 2019;3(Supplement_1). doi:10.1093/CDN/NZZ052.OR32-08-19

3. Bethancourt HJ, Kenney WL, Almeida DM, Rosinger AY. Cognitive performance in relation to hydration status and water intake among older adults, NHANES 2011–2014. *Eur J Nutr.* November 2019:1-16. doi:10.1007/s00394-019-02152-9

4. Bryarly M, Phillips LT, Fu Q, Vernino S, Levine BD. Postural Orthostatic Tachycardia Syndrome: JACC Focus Seminar. *J Am Coll Cardiol.* 2019;73(10):1207-1228. doi:10.1016/j.jacc.2018.11.059

5. DiBaise JK, Lunsford TN, Harris LA. The POTS (Postural Tachycardia Syndrome) Epidemic: Hydration and Nutrition Issues.; 2019.

6. Zadourian A, Doherty TA, Swiatkiewicz I, Taub PR. Postural Orthostatic Tachycardia Syndrome: Prevalence, Pathophysiology, and Management. *Drugs.* 2018;78(10):983-994. doi:10.1007/s40265-018-0931-5

7. Claydon VE, Schroeder C, Norcliffe LJ, Jordan J, Hainsworth R. Water drinking improves orthostatic tolerance in patients with posturally related syncope. *Clin Sci.* 2006;110(3):343-352. doi:10.1042/CS20050279

8. Mathias CJ, Young TM. Water drinking in the management of orthostatic intolerance due to orthostatic hypotension, vasovagal syncope and the postural tachycardia syndrome. *Eur J Neurol.* 2004;11(9):613-619. doi:10.1111/j.1468-1331.2004.00840.x

9. Shannon JR, Diedrich A, Biaggioni I, et al. Water drinking as a treatment for orthostatic syndromes. *Am J Med*. 2002;112(5):355-360. doi:10.1016/S0002-9343(02)01025-2

10. Dysautonomia International: Lifestyle Adaptations for POTS. http://www.dysautonomiainternational.org/page.php?ID=44. Accessed April 26, 2020.

11. Agarwal AK, Garg R, Ritch A, Sarkar P. Postural orthostatic tachycardia syndrome. *Postgrad Med J*. 2007;83(981):478-480. doi:10.1136/pgmj.2006.055046

12. Abed H, Ball PA, Wang LX. Diagnosis and management of postural orthostatic tachycardia syndrome: A brief review. *J Geriatr Cardiol*. 2012;9(1):61-67.

13. Werpachowska E, Quasim S. Antenatal hydration in POTS – could technology help? *Int J Obstet Anesth*. 2019;37:136-137. doi:10.1016/j.ijoa.2018.10.001

14. Maintz L, Novak N. Histamine and histamine intolerance. *Am J Clin Nutr*. 2007;85(5):1185-1196. doi:10.1093/ajcn/85.5.1185

15. Komericki P, Klein G, Reider N, et al. Histamine intolerance: lack of reproducibility of single symptoms by oral provocation with histamine: A randomised, double-blind, placebo-controlled cross-over study. *Wien Klin Wochenschr*. 2011;123(1-2):15-20. doi:10.1007/s00508-010-1506-y

16. San Mauro Martin I, Brachero S, Garicano Vilar E. Histamine intolerance and dietary management: A complete review. *Allergol Immunopathol (Madr)*. 2016;44(5):475-483. doi:10.1016/j.aller.2016.04.015

17. Reese I, Ballmer-Weber B, Beyer K, et al. German guideline for the management of adverse reactions to ingested histamine. *Allergo J Int*. 2017;26(2):72-79. doi:10.1007/s40629-017-0011-5

18. Ede G. Histamine Intolerance: Why Freshness Matters. *J Evol Heal*. 2016;2(1):11. doi:10.15310/2334-3591.1054

19. Duelo A. Dietistas nutricionistas especialistas en Déficit DAO - AD Dietistas. http://www.adrianaduelo.com/. Accessed September 17, 2018.

20. de Wild-Scholten M. Understanding Histamine Intolerance & Mast Cell Activation: 3rd Edition. Create Space; 2015.

21. Ykelenstam Y. Histamine in Foods (list) | Healing Histamine. https://healinghistamine.com/histamine-in-foods-list/. Accessed September 17, 2018.

22. Paramasivam, Sadayan, Balachandar, Balakrishnan Arulkumar A. Change in Histamine Levels and Microbial Load in the Eviscerated and Uneviscerated Indian Mackerel Fish (Rastrelliger kanagurta) at

Different Storage Temperatures. *Am J Adv Food Sci Technol.* 2015;3(2):94-106.

23. Auerswald L, Morren C, Lopata AL. Histamine levels in seventeen species of fresh and processed South African seafood. *Food Chem.* 2006;98(2):231-239. doi:10.1016/J.FOODCHEM.2005.05.071

24. Cilliers JD, Van Wyk CJ. Histamine and Tyramine Content of South African Wine. *South African J Enol Vitic.* 2017;6(2):35-40. doi:10.21548/6-2-2349

25. Swiss Interest Group Histamine Intolerance (SIGHI). HIT and Introduction. https://www.histaminintoleranz.ch/en/introduction.html. Accessed September 17, 2018.

26. Wagner N, Dirk D, Peveling-Oberhag A, et al. A Popular myth - low-histamine diet improves chronic spontaneous urticaria - fact or fiction? *J Eur Acad Dermatology Venereol.* 2017;31(4):650-655. doi:10.1111/jdv.13966

27. Wöhrl S, Hemmer W, Focke M, Rappersberger K, Jarisch R. Histamine intolerance-like symptoms in healthy volunteers after oral provocation with liquid histamine. *Allergy asthma Proc.* 25(5):305-311. http://www.ncbi.nlm.nih.gov/pubmed/15603203. Accessed September 17, 2018.

28. Schwelberger HG. Histamine intolerance: a metabolic disease? *Inflamm Res.* 2010;59(S2):219-221. doi:10.1007/s00011-009-0134-3

29. Ykelenstam Y. Healing Histamine | Histamine Intolerance Research and Recipes. https://healinghistamine.com/. Accessed September 17, 2018.

30. Ykelenstam Y. *The Anti-Cookbook, 4th Edition.* LHC Productions; 2013.

31. Melgarejo E, Medina MÁ, Sánchez-Jiménez F, Urdiales JL. Targeting of histamine producing cells by EGCG: A green dart against inflammation? *J Physiol Biochem.* 2010;66(3):265-270. doi:10.1007/s13105-010-0033-7

32. Afrin L. In-person interview conducted in St. Cloud, Minnesota on 9-16-17.

33. Castells MC. Phone interview conducted on 7-20-18.

34. Paterson, J.R. & Lawrence, J.R. (2001): Salicylic acid: a link between aspirin, diet and the prevention of colorectal cancer. Q. J. Med., 94, 445–448.

35. Joneja, J. Salicylate Intolerance Forum. https://www.foodsmatter.com/allergy_intolerance/salicylate/articles/joneja-11-15.html. Accessed April 25, 2020.

36. Laher AE, Moolla M, McDonald M. Successful desensitisation of non-immune type symptoms secondary to salicylate

hypersensitivity/intolerance. *Curr Allergy Clin Immunol.* 2017;30(4):284-286. http://www.webmd.com/allergies/salicylate-allergy.

37. Malakar, S., & Bhattacharya, S. (2014). MINDING THE GREENS: ROLE OF DIETARY SALICYLATES IN COMMON BEHAVIOURAL HEALTH CONDITIONS. *Budapest Acta Alimentaria, 43*(2), 344–359. https://doi.org/10.1556/AAlim.2014.0017

38. Bolweg M. *The Three-Week Salicylate Exclusion Diet.* University of Otago, Dunedin, New Zealand.; 2010.

39. Marsh A, Eslick EM, Eslick GD. Does a diet low in FODMAPs reduce symptoms associated with functional gastrointestinal disorders? A comprehensive systematic review and meta-analysis. *Eur J Nutr.* 2016;55(3):897-906. doi:10.1007/s00394-015-0922-1

40. Halmos EP, Power VA, Shepherd SJ, Gibson PR, Muir JG. A Diet Low in FODMAPs Reduces Symptoms of Irritable Bowel Syndrome. *Gastroenterology.* 2014;146(1):67-75.e5. doi:10.1053/j.gastro.2013.09.046

41. McIntosh K, Reed DE, Schneider T, et al. FODMAPs alter symptoms and the metabolome of patients with IBS: a randomised controlled trial. *Gut.* 2017;66(7):1241-1251. doi:10.1136/gutjnl-2015-311339

42. Hill P, Muir JG, Gibson PR. Controversies and recent developments of the low-FODMAP diet. *Gastroenterol Hepatol.* 2017;13(1):36-45.

43. The Buzz about Nightshades. *Tufts Univ Heal Nutr Lett.* 2019;37:3. https://search.proquest.com/openview/317c584b27cc51f9442e1c21 54884faf/1?pq-origsite=gscholar&cbl=30886. Accessed April 24, 2020.

44. Your Health Education: Low Oxalate Diet (UPMC). https://www.upmc.com/-/media/upmc/patients-visitors/education/unique-pdfs/low-oxalate-diet.pdf. Accessed April 25, 2020.

45. Lieske JC, Tremaine WJ, De Simone C, et al. Diet, but not oral probiotics, effectively reduces urinary oxalate excretion and calcium oxalate supersaturation. *Kidney Int.* 2010;78(11):1178-1185. doi:10.1038/ki.2010.310

46. Attalla K, De S, Monga M. Oxalate content of food: A tangled web. *Urology.* 2014;84(3):555-560. doi:10.1016/j.urology.2014.03.053

47. Noori N, Honarkar E, Goldfarb DS, et al. Urinary lithogenic risk profile in recurrent stone formers with hyperoxaluria: A randomized controlled trial comparing DASH (dietary approaches to stop hypertension)-style and low-oxalate diets. *Am J Kidney Dis.* 2014;63(3):456-463. doi:10.1053/j.ajkd.2013.11.022

48. Frossi B, De Carli M, Calabrò A. Coeliac Disease and Mast Cells. *Int J Mol Sci*. 2019;20(14):3400. doi:10.3390/ijms20143400
49. Tuck CJ, Staudacher HM. The Keto Diet and The Gut: Cause for Concern? The Lancet. https://www.sochob.cl/web1/wp-content/uploads/2019/12/The-keto-diet-and-the-gut-cause-for-concern.pdf. Published 2019. Accessed April 25, 2020.
50. Joshi S, Ostfeld RJ, McMacken M. The Ketogenic Diet for Obesity and Diabetes - Enthusiasm Outpaces Evidence. *JAMA Intern Med*. 2019;179(9):1163-1164. doi:10.1001/jamainternmed.2019.2633
51. Sourbron J, Klinkenberg S, van Kuijk SMJ, et al. Ketogenic diet for the treatment of pediatric epilepsy: review and meta-analysis. *Child's Nerv Syst*. March 2020:1-11. doi:10.1007/s00381-020-04578-7
52. Davis JJ, Fournakis N, Ellison J. Ketogenic Diet for the Treatment and Prevention of Dementia: A Review. *J Geriatr Psychiatry Neurol*. January 2020:089198872090178. doi:10.1177/0891988720901785
53. Castellana M, Conte E, Cignarelli A, et al. Efficacy and safety of very low calorie ketogenic diet (VLCKD) in patients with overweight and obesity: A systematic review and meta-analysis. *Rev Endocr Metab Disord*. 2019;21(1):5-16. doi:10.1007/s11154-019-09514-y
54. Bueno NB, de Melo ISV, de Oliveira SL, da Rocha Ataide T. Very-low-carbohydrate ketogenic diet *v*. low-fat diet for long-term weight loss: a meta-analysis of randomised controlled trials. *Br J Nutr*. 2013;110(7):1178-1187. doi:10.1017/S0007114513000548
55. Noto H, Goto A, Tsujimoto T, Noda M. Low-Carbohydrate Diets and All-Cause Mortality: A Systematic Review and Meta-Analysis of Observational Studies. *PLoS One*. 2013;8(1). doi:10.1371/journal.pone.0055030
56. Meroni E, Ferraris C, Tagliabue A, et al. Impact of the ketogenic diet on human gut. *Nutr Metab Cardiovasc Dis*. 2019;29(8):881. doi:10.1016/j.numecd.2019.05.037
57. Hanson S, Thorpe G, Winstanley L, et al. Omega-3, omega-6 and total dietary polyunsaturated fat on cancer incidence: systematic review and meta-analysis of randomised trials. *Br J Cancer*. 2020;122(8):1260-1270. doi:10.1038/s41416-020-0761-6
58. Kh JK, Kh SK, Afshari A, Rezayi M, Ghayour-Mobarhan M. Dietary fatty acids-effects on cardiovascular disease. *Mini-Reviews Med Chem*. 2019;19. doi:10.2174/1389557519666190920103759
59. Shrestha N, Sleep SL, Cuffe JSM, et al. Role of omega-6 and omega-3 fatty acids in fetal programming. *Clin Exp Pharmacol Physiol*. 2020;47(5):907-915. doi:10.1111/1440-1681.13244

60. Jang H, Park K. Omega-3 and omega-6 polyunsaturated fatty acids and metabolic syndrome: A systematic review and meta-analysis. *Clin Nutr.* 2020;39(3):765-773. doi:10.1016/j.clnu.2019.03.032

61. Simopoulos AP. The importance of the ratio of omega-6/omega-3 essential fatty acids. *Biomed Pharmacother.* 2002;56(8):365-379. http://www.ncbi.nlm.nih.gov/pubmed/12442909.

62. Medawar, E., Huhn, S., Villringer, A., & Veronica Witte, A. The effects of plant-based diets on the body and the brain: a systematic review. *Translational Psychiatry* 2019;9(1). https://doi.org/10.1038/s41398-019-0552-0

63. Wells S. Specialized Nutrition for Physical Therapists. *Nutritional Physical Therapy Course.* 2020. https://www.nutritionalphysicaltherapy.com/.

64. Stone CA, Commins SP, Choudhary S, et al. Anaphylaxis after vaccination in a pediatric patient: further implicating alpha-gal allergy. *J Allergy Clin Immunol Pract.* 2019;7(1):322-324.e2. doi:10.1016/j.jaip.2018.06.005

65. Steinke JW, Platts-Mills TAE, Commins SP. The alpha-gal story: lessons learned from connecting the dots. *J Allergy Clin Immunol.* 2015;135(3):589-96; quiz 597. doi:10.1016/j.jaci.2014.12.1947

66. Commins SP. Invited Commentary: Alpha-Gal Allergy: Tip of the Iceberg to a Pivotal Immune Response. *Curr Allergy Asthma Rep.* 2016;16(9):1-3. doi:10.1007/s11882-016-0641-6

67. Cooksey K. Proposed Treatments and Therapies for Alpha-Gal Allergy Syndrome (AGAS). *Student Showc Res Creat Inq.* April 2020. https://digitalcommons.longwood.edu/spring_showcase/2020/biology/23. Accessed April 25, 2020.

68. Chen Q, Chen O, Martins IM, et al. Collagen peptides ameliorate intestinal epithelial barrier dysfunction in immunostimulatory Caco-2 cell monolayers via enhancing tight junctions. *Food Funct.* 2017;8(3):1144-1151. doi:10.1039/c6fo01347c

69. Kiss M, Kiss AA, Radics M, et al. Drosophila type IV collagen mutation associates with immune system activation and intestinal dysfunction. *Matrix Biol.* 2016;49:120-131. doi:10.1016/j.matbio.2015.09.002

70. Proksch E, Schunck M, Zague V, Segger D, Degwert J, Oesser S. Oral intake of specific bioactive collagen peptides reduces skin wrinkles and increases dermal matrix synthesis. *Skin Pharmacol Physiol.* 2014;27(3):113-119. doi:10.1159/000355523

71. Clark KL, Sebastianelli W, Flechsenhar KR, et al. 24-Week study on the use of collagen hydrolysate as a dietary supplement in athletes with activity-related joint pain. *Curr Med Res Opin.* 2008;24(5):1485-1496. doi:10.1185/030079908X291967

72. Kumar S, Sugihara F, Suzuki K, Inoue N, Venkateswarathirukumara S. A double-blind, placebo-controlled, randomised, clinical study on the effectiveness of collagen peptide on osteoarthritis. *J Sci Food Agric.* 2015;95(4):702-707. doi:10.1002/jsfa.6752

73. Asserin J, Lati E, Shioya T, Prawitt J. The effect of oral collagen peptide supplementation on skin moisture and the dermal collagen network: evidence from an *ex vivo* model and randomized, placebo-controlled clinical trials. *J Cosmet Dermatol.* 2015;14(4):291-301. doi:10.1111/jocd.12174

74. Collins H. Diet & Supplementation for Persons with Ehlers-Danlos Syndrome: You Are Not What You Eat. In: *EDS Global Learning Conference.*; 2017. https://ehlers-danlos.com/pdf/Collins-EDS-You-are-NOT-what-you-eat-S.pdf. Accessed April 25, 2020.

75. Vojdani A. Lectins, agglutinins, and their roles in autoimmune reactivities. *Altern Ther Health Med.* 2015;21:46-51.

76. Pramod SN, Venkatesh YP, Mahesh PA. Potato lectin activates basophils and mast cells of atopic subjects by its interaction with core chitobiose of cell-bound non-specific immunoglobulin E. *Clin Exp Immunol.* 2007;148(3):391-401. doi:10.1111/j.1365-2249.2007.03368.x

77. Wei Y, Lv J, Guo Y, et al. Soy intake and breast cancer risk: a prospective study of 300,000 Chinese women and a dose–response meta-analysis. *Eur J Epidemiol.* November 2019:1-12. doi:10.1007/s10654-019-00585-4

78. Sivoňov M, Kapln P, Tatarkov Z, et al. Androgen receptor and soy isoflavones in prostate cancer (Review). *Mol Clin Oncol.* 2018;10(2):191-204. doi:10.3892/mco.2018.1792

79. Paul P, Koh WP, Jin A, et al. Soy and tea intake on cervical cancer risk: the Singapore Chinese Health Study. *Cancer Causes Control.* 2019;30(8):847-857. doi:10.1007/s10552-019-01173-3

80. Orlich, M. J. et al. Vegetarian dietary patterns and mortality in Adventist Health Study 2. *JAMA Intern. Med.* 2013;173:1230–1238.

81. Le, L. T. Sabaté, J. Beyond meatless, the health effects of vegan diets: findings from the Adventist cohorts. *Nutrients.* 2014;6:2131-2147.

82. Kim, H, Caulfield, LE., Garcia-Larsen, V, et al. Plant-Based Diets Are Associated With a Lower Risk of Incident Cardiovascular Disease, Cardiovascular Disease Mortality, and All-Cause Mortality in a General Population of Middle-Aged Adults. *Journal of the American Heart Association.* 2019;8(16). https://doi.org/10.1161/JAHA.119.012865

83. Lara, KM, Levitan, EB, Gutierrez, OM, et al. Dietary Patterns and Incident Heart Failure in U.S. Adults Without Known Coronary

Disease. *Journal of the American College of Cardiology.* 2019;73(16): 2036.

84. Rahmani, J, Fakhri, Y, Shahsavani, A, et al. A systematic review and meta-analysis of metal concentrations in canned tuna fish in Iran and human health risk assessment. *Food and Chemical Toxicology.* 2019;118:753–765. https://doi.org/10.1016/j.fct.2018.06.023

85. Fakhri, Y, Mohseni-Bandpei, A, Oliveri Conti, G, et al. Systematic review and health risk assessment of arsenic and lead in the fished shrimps from the Persian gulf. *Food and Chemical Toxicology.* 2018;113:278–286. https://doi.org/10.1016/j.fct.2018.01.046

86. Morcillo, P, Angeles Esteban, M, Cuesta, A. Mercury and its toxic effects on fish. *AIMS Environmental Science.* 2017;4(3):386-402. https://doi.org/10.3934/environsci.2017.3.386

87. Bonito, LT, Hamdoun, A, Sandin, SA. Evaluation of the global impacts of mitigation on persistent, bioaccumulative and toxic pollutants in marine fish. *PeerJ.* 2016(1). https://doi.org/10.7717/peerj.157

88. Santana, MS, Sandrini-Neto, L, Filipak Neto, F, et al. Biomarker responses in fish exposed to polycyclic aromatic hydrocarbons (PAHs): Systematic review and meta-analysis. *Environmental Pollution.* 2018;*242*:449–461. https://doi.org/10.1016/j.envpol.2018.07.004

89. U.S. Food & Drug Administration. Food Additives and Ingredients - Overview of Food Ingredients, Additives and Colors. 2010. https://www.fda.gov/Food/IngredientsPackagingLabeling/FoodAddit ivesIngredients/ucm094211.htm. Accessed September 17, 2018.

90. Vieira T, Cunha S, Casal S. Mycotoxins in Coffee. *Coffee Heal Dis Prev.* January 2015:225-233. doi:10.1016/B978-0-12-409517-5.00025-5

91. Smith A. CranioBiotic Technique: Educational Material. In: CBT Training; 2019.

92. Kresser C. 9 Steps to Perfect Health - #1: Don't Eat Toxins. https://chriskresser.com/9-steps-to-perfect-health-1-dont-eat-toxins/. Published 2019. Accessed October 24, 2020.

93. Lomer MCE. Review article: the aetiology, diagnosis, mechanisms and clinical evidence for food intolerance. *Aliment Pharmacol Ther.* 2015;41(3):262-275. doi:10.1111/apt.13041

94. Hibi M, Hachimura S, Hashizume S, Obata T, Kaminogawa S. Amaranth Grain Inhibits Antigen-Specific IgE Production Through Augmentation of the IFN-gamma Response in vivo and in vitro. *Cytotechnology.* 2003;43(1-3):33-40. doi:10.1023/B: CYTO.0000039908.34387.d3

95. Patil SD, Patel MR, Patel SR, Surana SJ. *Amaranthus spinosus* Linn. inhibits mast cell-mediated anaphylactic reactions. *J Immunotoxicol.* 2012;9(1):77-84. doi:10.3109/1547691X.2011.631609

96. Shealy N. Illustrated Encyclopedia of Healing Rememedies. Harper Collins; 2018.

97. Tokura T, Nakano N, Ito T, et al. Inhibitory effect of polyphenol-enriched apple extracts on mast cell degranulation in vitro targeting the binding between IgE and FcepsilonRI. *Biosci Biotechnol Biochem.* 2005;69(10):1974-1977. doi:10.1271/bbb.69.1974

98. Kanda T, Akiyama H, Yanagida A, et al. Inhibitory Effects of Apple Polyphenol on Induced Histamine Release from RBL-2H3 Cells and Rat Mast Cells. *Biosci Biotechnol Biochem.* 1998;62(7):1284-1289. doi:10.1271/bbb.62.1284

99. Fratianni F, Pepe R, Nazzaro F. Polyphenol Composition, Antioxidant, Antimicrobial and Quorum Quenching Activity of the "Carciofo di Montoro" (Cynara cardunculus var. scolymus) Global Artichoke of the Campania Region, Southern Italy. *Food Nutr Sci.* 2014;5:2053-2062. doi:10.4236/fns.2014.521217

100. Jain S, Garg VK, Sharma PK. Anti-inflammatory activity of aqueous extract of Beta vulgaris L. *J basic Clin Pharm.* 2011;2(2):83-86. http://www.ncbi.nlm.nih.gov/pubmed/24826006. Accessed September 17, 2018.

101. Nagase H, Hojima Y, Moriwaki C, Moriya H. Anti-bradykinin activity found in beet (Beta vulgaris L. var rapa Dumort. f. rubra DC.). *Chem Pharm Bull (Tokyo).* 1975;23(5):971-979. doi:10.1248/CPB.23.971

102. Martinez RM, Longhi-Balbinot DT, Zarpelon AC, et al. Anti-inflammatory activity of betalain-rich dye of Beta vulgaris: effect on edema, leukocyte recruitment, superoxide anion and cytokine production. *Arch Pharm Res.* 2015;38(4):494-504. doi:10.1007/s12272-014-0473-7

103. Choi SP, Kim SP, Kang MY, Nam SH, Friedman M. Protective effects of black rice bran against chemically-induced inflammation of mouse skin. *J Agric Food Chem.* 2010;58(18):10007-10015. doi:10.1021/jf102224b

104. Kim CD, Lee W-K, No K-O, et al. Anti-allergic action of buckwheat (Fagopyrum esculentum Moench) grain extract. *Int Immunopharmacol.* 2003;3(1):129-136. http://www.ncbi.nlm.nih.gov/pubmed/12538043. Accessed September 17, 2018.

105. Imaoka K, Ushijima H, Inouye S, Takahashi T, Kojima Y. Effects of Celosia argentea and Cucurbita moschata extracts on anti-DNP IgE antibody production in mice. *Arerugi.* 1994;43(5):652-659. http://www.ncbi.nlm.nih.gov/pubmed/8031259. Accessed September 17, 2018.

491

106. Trombetta D, Occhiuto F, Perri D, et al. Antiallergic and antihistaminic effect of two extracts of Capparis spinosa L. flowering buds. *Phyther Res.* 2005;19(1):29-33. doi:10.1002/ptr.1591

107. Das S, Vasudeva N, Sharma S. Cichorium intybu: A concise report on its ethnomedicinal, botanical, and phytopharmacological aspects. *Drug Dev Ther.* 2016;7(1):1. doi:10.4103/2394-6555.180157

108. Verma C. Applications and Utilization of Coriander-A. *Int J Res Eng Appl Sci.* 2014;4(3):85-94. http://www.euroasiapub.orghttp//www.euroasiapub.org86. Accessed September 17, 2018.

109. Kumar D, Kumar S, Singh J, et al. Free Radical Scavenging and Analgesic Activities of Cucumis sativus L. Fruit Extract. *J Young Pharm.* 2010;2(4):365-368. doi:10.4103/0975-1483.71627

110. Agatemor UM-M, Okwesili FCN, Anosike CA. Anti-inflammatory Activity of Cucumis sativus L. *Br J Pharm Res.* 2015;8(2):1-8. doi:10.9734/BJPR/2015/19700

111. Kyo E, Uda N, Kasuga S, Itakura Y. Immunomodulatory Effects of Aged Garlic Extract. *J Nutr.* 2001;131(3):1075S-1079S. doi:10.1093/jn/131.3.1075S

112. Kim JH, Nam SH, Rico CW, Kang MY. A comparative study on the antioxidative and anti-allergic activities of fresh and aged black garlic extracts. *Int J Food Sci Technol.* 2012;47(6):1176-1182. doi:10.1111/j.1365-2621.2012.02957.x

113. Hwang S-L, Shih P-H, Yen G-C. Neuroprotective Effects of Citrus Flavonoids. *J Agric Food Chem.* 2012;60(4):877-885. doi:10.1021/jf204452y

114. Nakatani K, Atsumi M, Arakawa T, et al. Inhibitions of histamine release and prostaglandin E2 synthesis by mangosteen, a Thai medicinal plant. *Biol Pharm Bull.* 2002;25(9):1137-1141. http://www.ncbi.nlm.nih.gov/pubmed/12230104. Accessed September 12, 2018.

115. Chae H-S, Oh S-R, Lee H-K, Joo SH, Chin Y-W. Mangosteen xanthones, α-and γ-mangostins, inhibit allergic mediators in bone marrow-derived mast cell. *Food Chem.* 2012;134(1):397-400. doi:10.1016/J.FOODCHEM.2012.02.075

116. Chatuevedi N, Yadav S, Shukla K. *Diversified Therapeutic Potential of Avena Sativa: An Exhaustive Review.* Vol 1.; 2011. www.pelagiaresearchlibrary.com. Accessed September 17, 2018.

117. Aggarwal B, Yost D. Healing Spices: How to Use 50 Everyday and Exotic Spices to Boost Health and Beat Disease. Sterling Publishing; 2011.

118. Cardile V, Frasca G, Rizza L, Rapisarda P, Bonina F. Antiinflammatory effects of a red orange extract in human keratinocytes treated with interferon-gamma and histamine. *Phyther Res.* 2010;24(3):414-418. doi:10.1002/ptr.2973

119. Al-Khazraji SM. Studying the Analgesic, Anti-inflammatory and Antipyretic Properties of The Aqueous Extract of Petroselinum crispum in Experimental Animal Models. *IOSR Journal of Pharmacy.* 2015;5(9):17-23. www.iosrphr.org. Accessed September 17, 2018.

120. Liu H, Chen Y, Hu T, et al. The influence of light-emitting diodes on the phenolic compounds and antioxidant activities in pea sprouts. *J Funct Foods.* 2016;25:459-465. doi:10.1016/J.JFF.2016.06.028

121. Kim GJ, Choi HG, Kim JH, Kim SH, Kim JA, Lee SH. Anti-allergic inflammatory effects of cyanogenic and phenolic glycosides from the seed of Prunus persica. *Nat Prod Commun.* 2013;8(12):1739-1740. http://www.ncbi.nlm.nih.gov/pubmed/24555287. Accessed September 17, 2018.

122. Shin T-Y, Park S-B, Yoo J-S, et al. Anti-allergic inflammatory activity of the fruit of Prunus persica: Role of calcium and NF-κB. *Food Chem Toxicol.* 2010;48(10):2797-2802. doi:10.1016/j.fct.2010.07.009

123. Miguel MG, Neves MA, Antunes MD. Pomegranate (Punica granatum L.): A medicinal plant with myriad biological properties - A short review. *J Med Plants Res.* 2010;4(25):2836-2847. https://academicjournals.org/journal/JMPR/article-abstract/46EEE0023212. Accessed September 17, 2018.

124. Barwal S, Sunil A, Dhasade V, Patil M, Pal S, Subhash C. Antihistaminic effect of various extracts of Punica granatum Linn. flower buds. *J Young Pharm.* 2009;1(4):322. doi:10.4103/0975-1483.59321

125. Lee C-J, Chen L-G, Liang W-L, Wang C-C. Anti-inflammatory effects of Punica granatum Linne invitro and in vivo. *Food Chem.* 2010;118(2):315-322. doi:10.1016/J.FOODCHEM.2009.04.123

126. Meira M, Pereira Da Silva E, David JM, David JP. Review of the genus Ipomoea: traditional uses, chemistry and biological activities. *Rev Bras Farmacogn Brazilian J Pharmacogn.* 2012;22(3):682-713. doi:10.1590/S0102

127. Sadeghi H, Mostafazadeh M, Sadeghi H, et al. Anti-inflammatory properties of aerial parts of Nasturtium officinale. *Pharm Biol.* 2014;52(2):169-174. doi:10.3109/13880209.2013.821138

128. Karpagam T, Varalakshmi B, Suguna Bai J, Gomathi S. Effect of different doses of Cucurbita pepo linn extract as an anti-Inflammatory and analgesic nutraceautical agent on inflamed rats. *Int J Pharm Res Dev.* 2011;3:184-192.

https://www.researchgate.net/publication/281304533. Accessed September 17, 2018.

129. Wang R, Wu G, Du L, et al. Semi-bionic extraction of compound turmeric protects against dextran sulfate sodium-induced acute enteritis in rats. *J Ethnopharmacol.* 2016;190:288-300. doi:10.1016/j.jep.2016.05.054

130. Subramanian VS, Priya VV, Gayathri R. Antiallergic activity of alpha-lipoic acid. *Drug Interv Today.* 2019;11(6):1499-1501.

131. Upaganlawar A, Ghule B. Pharmacological Activities of Boswellia serrata Roxb. - Mini Review. *Ethnobot Leafl.* 2009;(6). https://opensiuc.lib.siu.edu/ebl/vol2009/iss6/10. Accessed May 21, 2020.

132. Sharma A, Gajbhiye V, Kharya MD. *PHCOG REV.: Plant Review Phytochemical Profile of Boswellia Serrata: An Overview.* Vol 1. http://www.phcogrev.com. Accessed May 21, 2020.

133. Carr A, Maggini S. Vitamin C and Immune Function. *Nutrients.* 2017;9(11):1211. doi:10.3390/nu9111211

134. Li GZ, Chai OH, Song CH. Inhibitory effects of epigallocatechin gallate on compound 48/80-induced mast cell activation and passive cutaneous anaphylaxis. *Exp Mol Med.* 2005;37(4):290-296. doi:10.1038/emm.2005.39

135. Pareek A, Suthar M, Rathore GS, Bansal V. Feverfew (Tanacetum parthenium L.): A systematic review. *Pharmacogn Rev.* 2011;5(9):103-110. doi:10.4103/0973-7847.79105

136. Zhang T, Finn DF, Barlow JW, Walsh JJ. Mast cell stabilisers. *Eur J Pharmacol.* 2016;778:158-168. doi:10.1016/j.ejphar.2015.05.071

137. Shaik Y, Caraffa A, Ronconi G, Lessiani G, Conti P. Impact of polyphenols on mast cells with special emphasis on the effect of quercetin and luteolin. *Cent Eur J Immunol.* 2018;43(4):476-481. doi:10.5114/ceji.2018.81347

138. Maldonado MD, Garcia-Moreno H, Calvo JR. Melatonin protects mast cells against cytotoxicity mediated by chemical stimuli PMACI: Possible clinical use. *J Neuroimmunol.* 2013;262(1-2):62-65. doi:10.1016/j.jneuroim.2013.06.013

139. Weng Z, Zhang B, Asadi S, et al. Quercetin is more effective than cromolyn in blocking human mast cell cytokine release and inhibits contact dermatitis and photosensitivity in humans. *PLoS One.* 2012;7(3):e33805. doi:10.1371/journal.pone.0033805

140. Xu Y, Liu Q, Guo X, Xiang L, Zhao G. Resveratrol attenuates IL–33–induced mast cell inflammation associated with inhibition of NF–κB activation and the P38 signaling pathway. *Mol Med Rep.* 2020;21(3):1658-1666. doi:10.3892/mmr.2020.10952

494

141. Nakajima S, Ishimaru K, Kobayashi A, et al. Resveratrol inhibits IL-33–mediated mast cell activation by targeting the MK2/3–PI3K/Akt axis. *Sci Rep.* 2019;9(1):1-11. doi:10.1038/s41598-019-54878-5

142. Tiralongo E, Wee S, Lea R. Elderberry Supplementation Reduces Cold Duration and Symptoms in Air-Travellers: A Randomized, Double-Blind Placebo-Controlled Clinical Trial. *Nutrients.* 2016;8(4):182. doi:10.3390/nu8040182

143. Hawkins J, Baker C, Cherry L, Dunne E. Black elderberry (Sambucus nigra) supplementation effectively treats upper respiratory symptoms: A meta-analysis of randomized, controlled clinical trials. *Complement Ther Med.* 2019;42:361-365. doi:10.1016/j.ctim.2018.12.004

144. Sidor A, Gramza-Michałowska A. Advanced research on the antioxidant and health benefit of elderberry (Sambucus nigra) in food - a review. *J Funct Foods.* 2015;18:941-958. doi:10.1016/j.jff.2014.07.012

145. Liu Z-Q, Li X-X, Qiu S-Q, et al. Vitamin D contributes to mast cell stabilization. *Allergy.* 2017;72(8):1184-1192. doi:10.1111/all.13110

146. Yong YK, Zakaria ZA, Kadir AA, Somchit MN, Ee Cheng Lian G, Ahmad Z. Chemical constituents and antihistamine activity of Bixa orellana leaf extract. *BMC Complement Altern Med.* 2013;13:32. doi:10.1186/1472-6882-13-32

147. Lee W, Kim TH, Ku S-K, et al. Barrier protective effects of withaferin A in HMGB1-induced inflammatory responses in both cellular and animal models. *Toxicol Appl Pharmacol.* 2012;262(1):91-98. doi:10.1016/j.taap.2012.04.025

148. Chevallier A. Encyclopedia of Herbal Medicine: 500 Herbs and Remedies for Common Ailments. 3rd Edition. Dorling Kindersley Publishing; 2016.

149. Dharmananda S. Reducing inflammation with diet and supplements: the story of eicosanoid inhibition. Institute for Traditional Medicine (Portland, Oregon). http://www.itmonline.org/arts/lox.htm. Accessed June 23, 2017.

150. Gholamnezhad Z, Keyhanmanesh R, Boskabady MH. Anti-inflammatory, antioxidant, and immunomodulatory aspects of Nigella sativa for its preventive and bronchodilatory effects on obstructive respiratory diseases: A review of basic and clinical evidence. *J Funct Foods.* 2015;17:910-927. doi:10.1016/J.JFF.2015.06.032

151. Tembhurne S, Feroz S, More B, Sakarkar D. A review on therapeutic potential of Nigella sativa (kalonji) seeds. *J Med Plants Res.* 2014;8(3):167-177. doi:10.5897/JMPR10.737

152. Low Dog T, Johnson R, Foster S, Kiefer D, Weil A. National Geographic Guide to Medicinal Herbs: The World's Most Effective Healing Plants. National Geographic; 2012.

153. Sachan AK, Das DR, Kumar M. Carum carvi-An important medicinal plant. *J Chem Pharm Res.* 2016;8(3):529-533. www.jocpr.com. Accessed September 17, 2018.

154. Hussein A, Lobna M, Mohammed A, Mohamed G. Biochemical Effects of Chamomile Oil on Inflammatory Biomarkers in Gastroenteritis. *Int J Drug Dev Res.* 2009;9(2). http://www.ijddr.in/drug-development/biochemical-effects-of-chamomile-oil-on-inflammatory-biomarkers-ingastroenteritis.php?aid=19225. Accessed September 17, 2018.

155. Bhat SP, Rizvi W, Kumar A. Coriandrum Sativum on Pain and Inflammation. *International journal of Research in Pharmacy and Chemistry.* 2014;4(4):939-945.

156. Park HJ, Park JS, Hayek MG, Reinhart GA, Chew BP. Dietary fish oil and flaxseed oil suppress inflammation and immunity in cats. *Vet Immunol Immunopathol.* 2011;141(3-4):301-306. doi:10.1016/J.VETIMM.2011.02.024

157. Zaidi SF, Kim J-H, Tomoe Y, Usmanghani K, Kadowaki M. Effect of Pakistani medicinal plants on IgE/antigen- and ionophore-induced mucosal mast cells degranulation. *Pak J Pharm Sci.* 2014;27(4 Suppl):1041-1048. http://www.ncbi.nlm.nih.gov/pubmed/25016264. Accessed September 17, 2018.

158. Ravindran PN, Pillai GS, Balachandran I, Divakaran M. Galangal. *Handb Herbs Spices.* January 2012:303-318. doi:10.1533/9780857095688.303

159. Kiuchi F, Iwakami S, Shibuya M, Hanaoka F, Sankawa U. Inhibition of prostaglandin and leukotriene biosynthesis by gingerols and diarylheptanoids. *Chem Pharm Bull (Tokyo).* 1992;40(2):387-391. http://www.ncbi.nlm.nih.gov/pubmed/1606634. Accessed September 17, 2018.

160. Pursell J. The Herbal Apothecary: 100 Medicinal Herbs and How to Use Them. Timber Press; 2015.

161. Singh S, Taneja M, Majumdar DK. Biological activities of Ocimum sanctum L. fixed oil--an overview. *Indian J Exp Biol.* 2007;45(5):403-412. http://www.ncbi.nlm.nih.gov/pubmed/17569280. Accessed September 17, 2018.

162. Choudhary GP. Mast cell stabilizing activity of Ocimum sanctum leaves. *Int J Pharma Bio Sci.* 2010;1(2). https://www.cabdirect.org/cabdirect/abstract/20113372323. Accessed September 17, 2018.

163. Rahman S, Islam R, Kamruzzaman M, Alum K, Mastofa Jamal AH. Ocimum sanctum L.: A Review of Phytochemical and Pharmacological Profile. *Am J Drug Discov Dev.* 2011:1-15. doi:10.3923/ajdd.2011

164. Asha'ari ZA, Ahmad MZ, Wan Din WSJ, Che Hussin CM, Leman I. Ingestion of honey improves the symptoms of allergic rhinitis: evidence from a randomized placebo-controlled trial in the East Coast of Peninsular Malaysia. *Ann Saudi Med.* 2013;33(5):469-475. doi:10.5144/0256-4947.2013.469

165. Birdane YO, Büyükokurog -lu ME, Birdane FM, Cemek M, Yavuz H, Emin Büyükokurog -lu M. *Anti-Inflammatory and Antinociceptive Effects of Melissa Officinalis L. in Rodents.* Vol 158.; 2007. https://pdfs.semanticscholar.org/5878/238e3799fa869d5fa8add813 b46e3da796ca.pdf. Accessed September 17, 2018.

166. Cheel J, Theoduloz C, Rodríguez J, Schmeda-Hirschmann G. Free Radical Scavengers and Antioxidants from Lemongrass (Cymbopogon citratus (DC.) Stapf.). *J Agric Food Chem.* 2005;53(7):2511-2517. doi:10.1021/jf0479766

167. Shin Y-W, Bae E-A, Lee B, et al. In Vitro and In Vivo Antiallergic Effects of Glycyrrhiza glabra and Its Components. *Planta Med.* 2007;73(3):257-261. doi:10.1055/s-2007-967126

168. Mukherjee D, Biswas A, Bhadra S, et al. Exploring the potential of Nelumbo nucifera rhizome on membrane stabilization, mast cell protection, nitric oxide synthesis, and expression of costimulatory molecules. *Immunopharmacol Immunotoxicol.* 2010;32(3):466-472. doi:10.3109/08923970903514830

169. Sharma BR, Gautam LNS, Adhikari D, Karki R. A Comprehensive Review on Chemical Profiling of Nelumbo Nucifera : Potential for Drug Development. *Phyther Res.* 2017;31(1):3-26. doi:10.1002/ptr.5732

170. Lecomte J. General pharmacologic properties of silybine and silymarine in the rat. *Arch Int Pharmacodyn Ther.* 1975;214(1):165-176. http://www.ncbi.nlm.nih.gov/pubmed/50765. Accessed September 17, 2018.

171. Thakur S, Verma A. Antihistaminic Effect of Moringa Oleifera Seed Extract. *Int J Pharm Res Allied Sci.* 2013;2(1):56-59. www.ijpras.com. Accessed September 17, 2018.

172. Atawodi SE, Atawodi JC. Azadirachta indica (neem): a plant of multiple biological and pharmacological activities. *Phytochem Rev.* 2009;8(3):601-620. doi:10.1007/s11101-009-9144-6

173. Sonika G, Manubala R, Deepak J. Comparative Studies on Anti-Inflammatory Activity of Coriandrum Sativum, Datura Stramonium and Azadirachta Indica. *Asian J Exp Biol Sci.* 2010;1(1):151-154.

174. Chandak R, Devdhe S, Changediya V. Evaluation of anti-histaminic activity of aqueous extract of ripe olives of olea-europea. *J Pharm Res.* 2009;2. http://jprsolutions.info/files/final-file-5691ddee522e91.46302541.pdf. Accessed September 17, 2018.

175. Persia FA, Mariani ML, Fogal TH, Penissi AB. Hydroxytyrosol and oleuropein of olive oil inhibit mast cell degranulation induced by immune and non-immune pathways. *Phytomedicine.* 2014;21(11):1400-1405. doi:10.1016/j.phymed.2014.05.010

176. Silva F V., Guimarães AG, Silva ERS, et al. Anti-Inflammatory and Anti-Ulcer Activities of Carvacrol, a Monoterpene Present in the Essential Oil of Oregano. *J Med Food.* 2012;15(11):984-991. doi:10.1089/jmf.2012.0102

177. Baser KHC. Chapter Four: The Turkish Origanum species. In: Kintzios SE, ed. *Oregano: The Genera Origanum and Lippia.* CRC Press; 2003:123-140. doi:10.1201/B12591-11

178. Grigoleit H-G, Grigoleit P. Pharmacology and preclinical pharmacokinetics of peppermint oil. *Phytomedicine.* 2005;12(8):612-616. doi:10.1016/j.phymed.2004.10.007

179. Inoue T, Sugimoto Y, Masuda H, Kamei C. Effects of peppermint (Mentha piperita L.) extracts on experimental allergic rhinitis in rats. *Biol Pharm Bull.* 2001;24(1):92-95. http://www.ncbi.nlm.nih.gov/pubmed/11201253. Accessed September 17, 2018.

180. Sharma SC, Sharma S, Gulati OP. Pycnogenol® inhibits the release of histamine from mast cells. *Phyther Res.* 2003;17(1):66-69. doi:10.1002/ptr.1240

181. Boskabady MH, Ghasemzadeh Rahbardar M, Nemati H, Esmaeilzadeh M. Inhibitory effect of Crocus sativus (saffron) on histamine (H1) receptors of guinea pig tracheal chains. *Pharmazie.* 2010;65(4):300-305. http://www.ncbi.nlm.nih.gov/pubmed/20432629. Accessed September 17, 2018.

182. Kang OH, Chae H-S, Choi J-H, et al. Effects of the Schisandra Fructus Water Extract on Cytokine Release from a Human Mast Cell Line. *J Med Food.* 2006;9(4):480-486. doi:10.1089/jmf.2006.9.480

183. Wilson L. Review of adaptogenic mechanisms: Eleuthrococcus senticosus, Panax ginseng, Rhodiola rosea, Schisandra chinensis and Withania somnifera. *Aust J Med Herbal.* 2007;19(3):126-138. https://search.informit.com.au/documentSummary;dn=406522201744304;res=IELHEA. Accessed September 16, 2018.

184. Kim HM, Lee EH, Cho HH, Moon YH. Inhibitory effect of mast cell-mediated immediate-type allergic reactions in rats by spirulina.

Biochem Pharmacol. 1998;55(7):1071-1076. http://www.ncbi.nlm.nih.gov/pubmed/9605430. Accessed September 17, 2018.

185. Yang HN, Lee EH, Kim HM. Spirulina platensis inhibits anaphylactic reaction. *Life Sci.* 1997;61(13):1237-1244. http://www.ncbi.nlm.nih.gov/pubmed/9324065. Accessed January 26, 2019.

186. Eidi A, Oryan S, Zaringhalam J, Rad M. Antinociceptive and anti-inflammatory effects of the aerial parts of *Artemisia dracunculus* in mice. *Pharm Biol.* 2016;54(3):549-554. doi:10.3109/13880209.2015.1056312

187. Maham M, Moslemzadeh H, Jalilzadeh-Amin G. Antinociceptive effect of the essential oil of tarragon (Artemisia dracunculus). *Pharm Biol.* 2014;52(2):208-212. doi:10.3109/13880209.2013.824007

188. Russell N, Jennings S, Jennings B, et al. The Mastocytosis Society Survey on Mast Cell Disorders: Part 2-Patient Clinical Experiences and Beyond. *J allergy Clin Immunol Pract.* 2018;0(0). doi:10.1016/j.jaip.2018.07.032

189. Turner H. Phone interview on July 13, 2018.

CHAPTER 9: STRUCTURAL & MUSCULOSKELETAL ISSUES

1. Henderson Sr FC, Henderson FC. Cranio-cervical Instability in Patients with Hypermobility Connective Disorders. *J Spine.* 2016;5:299. doi:10.4172/2165-7939.1000299

2. Saperstein D. Neurological Considerations in Hypermobility Disorders. In: Jovin D, ed. Disjointed: Navigating the Diagnosis and Management of Hypermobile Ehlers-Danlos Syndrome and Hypermobility Spectrum Disorders. Hidden Stripes Publications; 2020.

3. Klinge P, McElroy A. Neurosurgical Considerations. In: Jovin D, ed. Disjointed: Navigating the Diagnosis and Management of Hypermobile Ehlers-Danlos Syndrome and Hypermobility Spectrum Disorders. Hidden Stripes Publications; 2020.

4. Piccin CF, Pozzebon D, Scapini F, Corrêa ECR. Craniocervical Posture in Patients with Obstructive Sleep Apnea. *Int Arch Otorhinolaryngol.* 2016;20(3):189-195. doi:10.1055/s-0036-1584295

5. Chopra P. Fatigue and Hypermobility Disorders. In: Jovin D, ed. Disjointed: Navigating the Diagnosis and Management of Hypermobile

Ehlers-Danlos Syndrome and Hypermobility Spectrum Disorders. Hidden Stripes Publications; 2020.

6. Block N. Physical Therapy. In: Jovin D, ed. Disjointed: Navigating the Diagnosis and Management of Hypermobile Ehlers-Danlos Syndrome and Hypermobility Spectrum Disorders. Hidden Stripes Publications; 2020.

7. Mitakides J. Temporomandibular Joint Dysfunction and Hypermobility Disorders. In: Jovin D, ed. *Disjointed: Navigating the Diagnosis and Management of Hypermobile Ehlers-Danlos Syndrome and Hypermobility Spectrum Disorders.* Hidden Stripes Publications; 2020.

8. Centeno C. Craniocervical Instability Series: Understanding CCI Measurements. https://centenoschultz.com/craniocervical-instability-measurements/. Accessed May 11, 2020.

9. Klekamp J. Neurological deterioration after foramen magnum decompression for Chiari malformation Type I: Old or new pathology? Clinical article. *J Neurosurg Pediatr.* 2012;10(6):538-547. doi:10.3171/2012.9.PEDS12110

10. Centeno C. C1-C2 Fusion - Complications are Common | Centeno-Schultz Clinic. https://centenoschultz.com/c1-c2-fusion/. Accessed May 11, 2020.

11. Rectenwald RJ, DeSimone CM, Sweat RW. Vascular Ultrasound Measurements After Atlas Orthogonal Chiropractic Care in a Patient With Bow Hunter Syndrome. *J Chiropr Med.* 2018;17(4):231-236. doi:10.1016/j.jcm.2018.07.002

12. Abbaszadeh-Amirdehi M, Ansari NN, Naghdi S, Olyaei G, Nourbakhsh MR. Therapeutic effects of dry needling in patients with upper trapezius myofascial trigger points. *Acupunct Med.* 2017;35(2):85-92. doi:10.1136/acupmed-2016-011082

13. Rosenberg S. *Accessing the Healing Power of the Vagus Nerve.* Berkeley, California: North Atlantic Books; 2017.

14. Goldstein I. Pelvic Floor Muscle Dysfunction | San Diego Sexual Medicine. http://sandiegosexualmedicine.com/female-issues/pelvic-floor-muscle-dysfunction. Accessed May 14, 2020.

15. Fletcher E. Differential Diagnosis of High-Tone and Low-Tone Pelvic Floor Muscle Dysfunction. *J Wound Ostomy Cont Nurs.* 2005;32(3s):s10-s11. https://journals.lww.com/jwocnonline/fulltext/2005/05001/differen tial_diagnosis_of_high_tone_and_low_tone.3.aspx. Accessed May 23, 2020.

16. Faubion SS, Shuster LT, Bharucha AE. Recognition and management of nonrelaxing pelvic floor dysfunction. *Mayo Clin Proc.* 2012;87(2):187-193. doi:10.1016/j.mayocp.2011.09.004

17. Tufo A, Desai GJ, Joshua Cox W. Psoas syndrome: A frequently missed diagnosis. *J Am Osteopath Assoc.* 2012;112(8):522-528. doi:10.7556/jaoa.2012.112.8.522
18. Yemm T. Alternative Approach to Psoas Release in Posterior Pelvic Pain. *PM&R.* 2019;11(S1):S118-S119. doi:10.1002/pmrj.12169
19. Lima CD, Ruas C V., Behm DG, Brown LE. Acute Effects of Stretching on Flexibility and Performance: A Narrative Review. *J Sci Sport Exerc.* 2019;1(1):29-37. doi:10.1007/s42978-019-0011-x
20. Coppieters, I., Meeus, M., Kregel, J., Caeyenberghs, K., De Pauw, R., Goubert, D., & Cagnie, B. (2016). Relations Between Brain Alterations and Clinical Pain Measures in Chronic Musculoskeletal Pain: A Systematic Review. In Journal of Pain (Vol. 17, Issue 9, pp. 949–962). Churchill Livingstone Inc. https://doi.org/10.1016/j.jpain.2016.04.005
21. Tishler J. Medical Cannabis & Pain Management. In: Jovin D, ed. Disjointed: Navigating the Diagnosis and Management of Hypermobile Ehlers-Danlos Syndrome and Hypermobility Spectrum Disorders. Hidden Stripes Publications; 2020.

CHAPTER 10: MOVEMENT

1. American Heart Association. American Heart Association Recommendations for Physical Activity in Adults. https://www.heart.org/en/healthy-living/fitness/fitness-basics/aha-recs-for-physical-activity-in-adults#.WpHn8ainHIU. Accessed May 23, 2020.
2. Donaldson PR. Does generalized joint hypermobility predict joint injury in sport? A review. *Clin J Sport Med.* 2012;22(1):77-78. doi:10.1097/01.jsm.0000410964.68476.f8
3. Pacey V, Nicholson LL, Adams RD, Munn J, Munns CF. Generalized Joint Hypermobility and Risk of Lower Limb Joint Injury During Sport: A Systematic Review With Meta-Analysis. *Am J Sport Med.* 2010. doi:https://doi.org/10.1177/0363546510364838
4. Oddy C, Johnson MI, Jones G. The effect of generalised joint hypermobility on rate, risk and frequency of injury in male university-

level rugby league players: A prospective cohort study. *BMJ Open Sport Exerc Med.* 2017;2(1). doi:10.1136/bmjsem-2016-000177

5. Junge T, Larsen LR, Juul-Kristensen B, Wedderkopp N. The extent and risk of knee injuries in children aged 9-14 with Generalised Joint Hypermobility and knee joint hypermobility - The CHAMPS-study Denmark Rehabilitation, physical therapy and occupational health. *BMC Musculoskelet Disord.* 2015;16(1). doi:10.1186/s12891-015-0611-5

6. Russek L, Simmonds J. The Evidence-Based Rationale for Physical Therapy Treatment of Children, Adolescents, and Adults Diagnosed With Joint Hypermobility Syndrome/Hypermobile Ehlers-Danlos Syndrome (for Non-experts) | The Ehlers Danlos Society : The Ehlers Danlos Society. https://www.ehlers-danlos.com/2017-eds-classification-non-experts/evidence-based-rationale-physical-therapy-treatment/. Accessed April 17, 2020.

7. Hain TC, DiLiberto F. Physical therapy for POTS. http://dizziness-and-balance.com/treatment/rehab/pots training.html. Accessed May 15, 2020.

8. Dysautonomia International: Exercises for Dysautonomia Patients. http://www.dysautonomiainternational.org/page.php?ID=43. Accessed May 15, 2020.

9. Russek LN, Stott P, Simmonds J. Recognizing and Effectively Managing Hypermobility-Related Conditions. *Phys Ther.* 2019;99(9):1189-1200. doi:10.1093/ptj/pzz078

10. Engelbert RH, Juul-Kristensen B, Pacey V, et al. The evidence-based rationale for physical therapy treatment of children, adolescents and adults diagnosed with joint hypermobility syndrome/hypermobile Ehlers Danlos syndrome. *Am J Med Genet.* 2017;175:158–167.

11. Lee JH. Effects of forward head posture on static and dynamic balance control. *J Phys Ther Sci.* 2016;28(1):274-277. doi:10.1589/jpts.28.274

12. Yeom H, Lim J, Yoo SH, Lee W. A new posture-correcting system using a vector angle model for preventing forward head posture. *Biotechnol Biotechnol Equip.* 2014;28(sup1):S6-S13. doi:10.1080/13102818.2014.949040

13. Spanos A. *Physical Therapy, Exercise and Braces for People with EDS Section 1: For Patients.*; 2016. https://alanspanosmd.com/wp-content/uploads/2016/09/PT-Exercise-for-People-with-EDS.pdf. Accessed May 15, 2020.

14. Dupuy EG, Leconte P, Vlamynck E, et al. Ehlers-Danlos syndrome, hypermobility type: impact of somatosensory orthoses on postural control: a pilot study. Front Hum Neurosci. 2017;11:283.

15. Ericson WB, Wolman R. Orthopaedic management of the Ehlers-Danlos syndromes. *Am J Med Genet Part C Semin Med Genet*. 2017;175(1):188-194. doi:10.1002/ajmg.c.31551
16. Block N. Physical Therapy. In: Jovin D, ed. Disjointed: Navigating the Diagnosis and Management of Hypermobile Ehlers-Danlos Syndrome and Hypermobility Spectrum Disorders. Hidden Stripes Publications; 2020.
17. Reina-Bueno M, Vázquez-Bautista C, Palomo-Toucedo IC, Domínguez-Maldonado G, Castillo-López JM, Munuera-Martínez P V. Custom-Made Foot Orthoses Reduce Pain and Fatigue in Patients with Ehlers-Danlos Syndrome. A Pilot Study. *Int J Environ Res Public Health*. 2020;17(4):1359. doi:10.3390/ijerph17041359
18. Muldowney K. *The Muldowney Protocol Part 1*. Nashville; 2019. https://www.ehlers-danlos.com/pdf/2019-Nashville/Muldowney-The-Muldowney-Protocol-20
19. Laferrier JZ, Muldowney K, Muldowney K. A Novel Exercise Protocol for Individuals with Ehlers Danlos Syndrome: A Case Report. *J Nov Physiother*. 2018;08(02). doi:10.4172/2165-7025.1000382
20. Palmer S, Bailey S, Barker L, Barney L, Elliott A. The effectiveness of therapeutic exercise for joint hypermobility syndrome: A systematic review. *Physiother (United Kingdom)*. 2014;100(3):220-227. doi:10.1016/j.physio.2013.09.002
21. Barton LM, Bird HA: Improving pain by the stabilization of hyperlax joints, *Journal of Orthopaedic Rheumatology*. 9:46-51, 1996.
22. Ferrell WR, Tennant N, Sturrock RD, et al. Amelioration of symptoms by enhancement of proprioception in patients with joint hypermobility syndrome. *Arthritis Rheum*. 2004;50(10):3323-3328. doi:10.1002/art.20582
23. Kerr A, Macmillan CE, Uttley WS, Luqmani RA. Physiotherapy for children with hypermobility syndrome. *Physiotherapy*. 2000;86(6):313-317. doi:10.1016/S0031-9406(05)61005-X
24. What is the Alexander Technique and what are its Benefits? – The Complete Guide to the Alexander Technique. https://www.alexandertechnique.com/at. Accessed May 29, 2020.
25. Muldowney K. Living Life to the Fullest with Ehlers-Danlos Syndrome: Guide to Living a Better Quality of Life While Having EDS. Outskirts Press; 2015.
26. Arthur K, Caldwell K, Forehand S, Davis K. Pain control methods in use and perceived effectiveness by patients with Ehlers-Danlos syndrome: A descriptive study. *Disabil Rehabil*. 2016;38(11):1063-1074. doi:10.3109/09638288.2015.1092175

27. Simmonds JV, Keer RJ. Hypermobility and the hypermobility syndrome. Man Ther. 2007;12:298–309.

28. Pacey V, Adams RD, Tofts L, Munns CF, Nicholson LL. Proprioceptive acuity into knee hypermobile range in children with joint hypermobility syndrome. Pediatr Rheumatol Online J. 2014;12:40.

29. Chopra P, Tinkle B, Hamonet C, et al. Pain management in the Ehlers–Danlos syndromes. *Am J Med Genet Part C Semin Med Genet.* 2017;175(1):212-219. doi:10.1002/ajmg.c.31554

30. Keer R. Physical therapy for hypermobility – The Ehlers-Danlos Support UK. https://www.ehlers-danlos.org/information/physical-therapy-for-hypermobility/. Accessed May 15, 2020.

31. Seneviratne SL, Maitland A, Afrin L. Mast cell disorders in Ehlers–Danlos syndrome. *Am J Med Genet Part C Semin Med Genet.* 2017;175(1):226-236. doi:10.1002/ajmg.c.31555

32. Luttrell MJ, Halliwill JR. The Intriguing Role of Histamine in Exercise Responses. *Exerc Sport Sci Rev.* 2017;45(1):16-23. doi:10.1249/JES.0000000000000093

33. Schott C, Fozard J. Chapter 8: Hypotension and Shock. In: Murugan R, Darby J, eds. *Rapid Response System: A Practical Guide.* Oxford University Press; 2018:80.

34. Phungphong S, Kijtawornrat A, Wattanapermpool J, Bupha-Intr T. Regular exercise modulates cardiac mast cell activation in ovariectomized rats. *J Physiol Sci.* 2016;66(2):165-173. doi:10.1007/s12576-015-0409-0

35. Abera Tessema T. Significance of yoga in modern life. *Int J Yoga, Physiother Phys Educ.* 2017;2(5):123-125.

36. Vempati R, Bijlani RL, Deepak KK. The efficacy of a comprehensive lifestyle modification programme based on yoga in the management of bronchial asthma: a randomized controlled trial. *BMC Pulm Med.* 2009;9:37. doi:10.1186/1471-2466-9-37

37. Ifeoma OJ, Uchenna CU, Chukwuemeka EO. Effects of Yoga in Health and Aging: A Knowledge-Based Descriptive Study of Health Educators in Universities of Nigeria. *Am J Educ Res.* 2017;5(4):443-452. doi:10.12691/education-5-4-14

38. Tripathi S, Sharma P, Singh A, Sharma A. Ayurveda and Yoga Therapy for Allergy and Asthma. In: Vedanthan P, Nelson H, Agashe S, Mahesh P, eds. *Textbook of Allergy for the Clinician.* CRC Press; 2014:421.

39. Uno Y. Irritable bowel syndrome-how a low-FODMAP diet or yoga might help. *Aliment Pharmacol Ther.* 2018;47(3):444-445. doi:10.1111/apt.14433

40. Alikiani Z, Toloee ME, Jafari AK. The effects of Pilates exercise and caraway supplementation on the levels of prostaglandin E2 and

perception dysmenorrhea in adolescent girls non-athlete. *Asian Exerc Sport Sci J.* 2017;1(1):11-16.

41. Mazzarino M, Kerr D, Wajswelner H, Morris ME. Pilates Method for Women's Health: Systematic Review of Randomized Controlled Trials. *Arch Phys Med Rehabil.* 2015;96(12):2231-2242. doi:10.1016/j.apmr.2015.04.005

42. Curi VS, Vilaça J, Haas AN, Fernandes HM. Effects of 16-weeks of Pilates on health perception and sleep quality among elderly women. *Arch Gerontol Geriatr.* 2018;74:118-122. doi:10.1016/j.archger.2017.10.012

43. Lin H-C, Lin H-P, Yu H-H, et al. Tai-Chi-Chuan Exercise Improves Pulmonary Function and Decreases Exhaled Nitric Oxide Level in Both Asthmatic and Nonasthmatic Children and Improves Quality of Life in Children with Asthma. 2017. doi:10.1155/2017/6287642

44. Lashkari M, Taghian F. The Effect of 12 Weeks of Tai Chi Exercise on IL-6 and CRP of Obese and Lean Middle-Aged Women. *Sci Arena Publ Spec J Sport Sci.* 2019;4(2):7-15. www.sciarena.com. Accessed May 15, 2020.

45. Weisgerber MC, Guill M, Weisgerber JM, Butler H. Benefits of swimming in asthma: Effect of a session of swimming lessons on symptoms and PFTs with review of the literature. *J Asthma.* 2003;40(5):453-464. doi:10.1081/JAS-120018706

46. Ramos JS, Dalleck LC, Tjonna AE, Beetham KS, Coombes JS. The Impact of High-Intensity Interval Training Versus Moderate-Intensity Continuous Training on Vascular Function: a Systematic Review and Meta-Analysis. *Sport Med.* 2015;45(5):679-692. doi:10.1007/s40279-015-0321-z

47. Milanović Z, Sporiš G, Weston M. Effectiveness of High-Intensity Interval Training (HIT) and Continuous Endurance Training for VO2max Improvements: A Systematic Review and Meta-Analysis of Controlled Trials. *Sport Med.* 2015;45(10):1469-1481. doi:10.1007/s40279-015-0365-0

48. Pearson SJ, Hussain SR. A Review on the Mechanisms of Blood-Flow Restriction Resistance Training-Induced Muscle Hypertrophy. *Sport Med.* 2015;45(2):187-200. doi:10.1007/s40279-014-0264-9

CHAPTER 11: DETOXIFICATION

1. Pizzorno J. The Toxin Solution: How Hidden Poisons in the Air, Water, Food and Products We Use Are Destroying Our Health. Harper Collins. 2017.
2. Pizzorno J. Glutathione! *Integr Med.* 2014;13(1):8-12. https://www.ncbi.nlm.nih.gov/pmc/articles/PMC4684116/. Accessed May 19, 2020.
3. Paris L. Functional Medicine Explains Detox Phases 1, 2, and 3 | Paris Healing Arts. https://www.parishealingarts.com/functional-medicine-phase-detox/. Accessed May 19, 2020.
4. Bajpai VK, Kim N-H, Kim J-E, Kim K, Kang SC. Protective Effect of Heat-Treated Cucumber (Cucumis Sativus L.) Juice on Alcohol Detoxification in Experimental Rats. *Pak J Pharm Sci.* 2016;29(3):1005-1009. https://pubmed-ncbi-nlm-nih-gov.dml.regis.edu/27383492/. Accessed May 19, 2020.
5. Esfahani A, Wong JMW, Truan J, et al. Health Effects of Mixed Fruit and Vegetable Concentrates: A Systematic Review of the Clinical Interventions. *J Am Coll Nutr.* 2011;30(5):285-294. doi:10.1080/07315724.2011.10719971
6. Hussain J, Cohen M. Clinical Effects of Regular Dry Sauna Bathing: A Systematic Review. *Evid Based Complement Alternat Med.* 2018;2018. doi:10.1155/2018/1857413
7. Wass T, Gallagher K. Evaluation of heavy metals levels in levels in relation to ionic foot bath sessions with Ioncleanse®. *Center for Research Strategies.*; 2008. www.crsllc.orgwww.crsllc.org2. Accessed May 19, 2020.
8. Lee M-J. The Study of Enema Therapy as One of the Detoxification Therapy. *J Orient Neuropsychiatry.* 2004;15(2):23-36. http://www.koreascience.or.kr/article/JAKO200403039814862.page. Accessed May 19, 2020.
9. Hodges RE, Minich DM, Biesalski HK. Modulation of Metabolic Detoxification Pathways Using Foods and Food-Derived Components: A Scientific Review with Clinical Application. 2015. doi:10.1155/2015/760689
10. Metagenics. RingCentral Webinar: Detox and GI Health. May 8th, 2020.
11. List of lymph nodes of the human body - Wikipedia. https://en.wikipedia.org/wiki/List_of_lymph_nodes_of_the_human_body. Accessed June 23, 2020.
12. Jin H, Xiang Y, Feng Y, et al. Effectiveness and Safety of Acupuncture Moxibustion Therapy Used in Breast Cancer-Related Lymphedema: A

Systematic Review and Meta-Analysis. *Evidence-Based Complement Altern Med.* 2020:1-10. doi:https://doi.org/10.1155/2020/3237451

13. 10 Ways To Cleanse A Clogged Lymphatic System. https://synergyhealthassociates.com/blog/cleanse-clogged-lymphatic-system/. Accessed May 21, 2020.

14. Herbs that Promote Lymphatic Drainage. https://herbalismroots.com/herbs-promote-lymphatic-drainage/. Accessed May 21, 2020.

15. Six ways to love your lymph - Urban Moonshine. https://www.urbanmoonshine.com/blogs/blog/six-ways-to-love-your-lymph. Accessed May 21, 2020.

16. University of Pennsylvania School of Medicine. "One in four Americans develop insomnia each year: 75 percent of those with insomnia recover." ScienceDaily. ScienceDaily, 5 June 2018. <www.sciencedaily.com/releases/2018/06/180605154114.htm>.

17. Hashimoto S, Kohsaka M, Nakamura K, Honma H, Honma S, Honma K. Midday exposure to bright light changes the circadian organization of plasma melatonin rhythm in humans. *Neurosci Lett.* 1997;221(2-3):89-92. doi:10.1016/s0304-3940(96)13291-2

18. Brainspotting – Where you look affects how you feel. https://brainspotting.com/. Accessed June 23, 2020.

19. Billot M, Daycard M, Wood C, Tchalla A. Reiki therapy for pain, anxiety and quality of life. *BMJ Support Palliat Care.* 2019;9(4):434-438. doi:10.1136/bmjspcare-2019-001775

20. Jones J. Use of Reiki for pain control in post-surgical patients: a critical review of the literature. *Carolina Digit Repos.* 2018. https://cdr.lib.unc.edu/concern/masters_papers/nz8061379. Accessed May 20, 2020.

21. Demir Doğan M. The effect of reiki on pain: A meta-analysis. *Complement Ther Clin Pract.* 2018;31:384-387. doi:10.1016/j.ctcp.2018.02.020

22. McManus DE. Reiki Is Better Than Placebo and Has Broad Potential as a Complementary Health Therapy. *J Evid Based Complementary Altern Med.* 2017;22(4):1051-1057. doi:10.1177/2156587217728644

23. Goldsby TL, Goldsby ME, McWalters M, Mills PJ. Effects of Singing Bowl Sound Meditation on Mood, Tension, and Well-being: An Observational Study. *J Evid Based Complementary Altern Med.* 2017;22(3):401-406. doi:10.1177/2156587216668109

24. Oschman JL. Traditional Sound Healing with High-Tech Enrichments. *Int J Adv Complement Tradit Med.* 2018;4(1):83-93. doi:10.23953/cloud.ijactm.389

25. Sung H-C, Lee W-L, Li H-M, et al. Familiar Music Listening with Binaural Beats for Older People with Depressive Symptoms in Retirement Homes. *Neuropsychiatry (London)*. 2017;7(4):347-353. doi:10.4172/Neuropsychiatry.1000221

26. Colzato LS, Barone H, Sellaro R, Hommel B. More attentional focusing through binaural beats: evidence from the global-local task. *Psychol Res*. 2017;81(1):271-277. doi:10.1007/s00426-015-0727-0

27. Isik BK, Esen A, Büyükerkmen B, Kilinç A, Menziletoglu D. Effectiveness of binaural beats in reducing preoperative dental anxiety. *Br J Oral Maxillofac Surg*. 2017;55(6):571-574. doi:10.1016/j.bjoms.2017.02.014

28. Oschman JL, Chevalier G, Ober AC. Chapter 38: Biophysics of Earthing (Grounding) the Human Body. In: Rosch P, ed. *Bioelectromagnetic and Subtle Energy Medicine, 2nd Edition*. 2014:427-456.

29. Lakhan SE, Sheafer H, Tepper D. The Effectiveness of Aromatherapy in Reducing Pain: A Systematic Review and Meta-Analysis. *Pain Res Treat*. 2016;2016. doi:10.1155/2016/8158693

30. Lin PC, Lee PH, Tseng SJ, Lin YM, Chen SR, Hou WH. Effects of aromatherapy on sleep quality: A systematic review and meta-analysis. *Complement Ther Med*. 2019;45:156-166. doi:10.1016/j.ctim.2019.06.006

31. Kim ME, Jun JH, Hur MH. Effects of aromatherapy on sleep quality: A systematic review and meta-analysis. *J Korean Acad Nurs*. 2019;49(6):655-676. doi:10.4040/jkan.2019.49.6.655

32. Isabel Sánchez-Vidaña D, Pui-Ching Ngai S, He W, Ka-Wing Chow J, Wui-Man Lau B, Wing-Hong Tsang H. The Effectiveness of Aromatherapy for Depressive Symptoms: A Systematic Review. 2017. doi:10.1155/2017/5869315

33. Asay K, Olson C, Donnelly J, Perlman E. The Use of Aromatherapy in Postoperative Nausea and Vomiting: A Systematic Review. *J Perianesthesia Nurs*. 2019;34(3):502-516. doi:10.1016/j.jopan.2018.08.006

34. Song JA, Lee M kyoung, Min E, Kim ME, Fike G, Hur MH. Effects of aromatherapy on dysmenorrhea: A systematic review and meta-analysis. *Int J Nurs Stud*. 2018;84:1-11. doi:10.1016/j.ijnurstu.2018.01.016

35. O'Hara B. Must Have Essential Oils for Mast Cell Activation Syndrome and Histamine Intolerance. https://mastcell360.com/must-have-essential-oils-for-mast-cell-activation-syndrome-and-histamine-intolerance/. Accessed October 23, 2020.

36. Silva J, Abebe W, Sousa SM, Duarte VG, Machado MIL, Matos FJA. Analgesic and anti-inflammatory effects of essential oils of Eucalyptus.

J Ethnopharmacol. 2003;89(2-3):277-283. doi:10.1016/j.jep.2003.09.007

37. Frank MB, Yang Q, Osban J, et al. Frankincense oil derived from Boswellia carteri induces tumor cell specific cytotoxicity. *BMC Complement Altern Med.* 2009;9:6. doi:10.1186/1472-6882-9-6

38. Iram F, Khan SA, Husain A. Phytochemistry and potential therapeutic actions of Boswellic acids: A mini-review. *Asian Pac J Trop Biomed.* 2017;7(6):513-523. doi:10.1016/j.apjtb.2017.05.001

39. Kobayashi Y, Sato H, Yorita M, et al. Inhibitory effects of geranium essential oil and its major component, citronellol, on degranulation and cytokine production by mast cells. *Biosci Biotechnol Biochem.* 2016;80(6):1172-1178. doi:10.1080/09168451.2016.1148573

40. Dongre PR, Bhujbal SS, Kumar D. Bronchodilatory activity of Curcuma longa, Zingiber officinale and Alpinia galanga based herbal formulation (AHF). *Orient Pharm Exp Med.* 2015;15(4):341-346. doi:10.1007/s13596-015-0205-7

41. Kuttan R, Jeena K, Liju VB. Antioxidant, anti-inflammatory and antinociceptive activities of essential oil from ginger. *Indian J Physiol Pharmacol.* 2013;57(1):51-62.

42. Mao Q-Q, Xu X-Y, Cao S-Y, et al. Bioactive Compounds and Bioactivities of Ginger (Zingiber officinale Roscoe). *Foods.* 2019;8(6):185. doi:10.3390/foods8060185

43. Alam K, Hena MA, Jamal M. *Ocimum Sanctum L.: A Review of Phytochemical and Pharmacological Profile.*; 2011. https://www.researchgate.net/publication/215692097. Accessed October 8, 2020.

44. Bhasha S, Sahukari R, Korivi M, Subbaiah VG, Reddy SK. Ocimum sanctum: a review on the pharmacological properties IJBCP International Journal of Basic & Clinical Pharmacology Ocimum sanctum: a review on the pharmacological properties. *www.ijbcp.com Int J Basic Clin Pharmacol.* 2016;3. doi:10.18203/2319-2003.ijbcp20161491

45. Chu CJ, Kemper KJ, Lavender M. The Longwood Herbal Task Force (Http://Www.Mcp.Edu/Herbal/) and The Center for Holistic Pediatric Education and Research (Http://Www.Childrenshospital.Org/Holistic/) Lavender (Lavandula Spp.).; 2001. http://www.mcp.edu/herbal/. Accessed October 8, 2020.

46. Ueno-Iio T, Shibakura M, Yokota K, et al. Lavender essential oil inhalation suppresses allergic airway inflammation and mucous cell hyperplasia in a murine model of asthma. *Life Sci.* 2014;108(2):109-115. doi:10.1016/j.lfs.2014.05.018

47. Cardia GFE, Silva-Filho SE, Silva EL, et al. Effect of Lavender (Lavandula angustifolia) Essential Oil on Acute Inflammatory Response . *Evidence-Based Complement Altern Med.* 2018;2018:1-10. doi:10.1155/2018/1413940

48. Hajhashemi V, Ghannadi A, Sharif B. Anti-inflammatory and analgesic properties of the leaf extracts and essential oil of Lavandula angustifolia Mill. *J Ethnopharmacol.* 2003;89(1):67-71. doi:10.1016/S0378-8741(03)00234-4

49. Su S, Wang T, Duan JA, et al. Anti-inflammatory and analgesic activity of different extracts of Commiphora myrrha. *J Ethnopharmacol.* 2011;134(2):251-258. doi:10.1016/j.jep.2010.12.003

50. Shin J, Che D, Cho B, Kang H, Kim J, Jang S. Commiphora myrrha inhibits itch-associated histamine and IL-31 production in stimulated mast cells. *Exp Ther Med.* 2019;18(3):1914-1920. doi:10.3892/etm.2019.7721

51. Sharma S, Rasal VP, Patil PA, Joshi RK. Mentha arvensis essential oil suppressed airway changes induced by histamine and ovalbumin in experimental animals. *Nat Prod Res.* 2018;32(4):468-472. doi:10.1080/14786419.2017.1311891

52. Inoue T, Sugimoto Y, Masuda H, Kamei C. Effects of peppermint (Mentha piperita L.) extracts on experimental allergic rhinitis in rats. *Biol Pharm Bull.* 2001;24(1):92-95. http://www.ncbi.nlm.nih.gov/pubmed/11201253. Accessed September 17, 2018.

53. Işcan G, Kirimer N, Kürkcüoğlu M, Başer KHC, Demirci F. Antimicrobial screening of Mentha piperita essential oils. *J Agric Food Chem.* 2002;50(14):3943-3946. doi:10.1021/jf011476k

54. Liju VB, Jeena K, Kuttan R. An evaluation of antioxidant, anti-inflammatory, and antinociceptive activities of essential oil from Curcuma longa. L. *Indian J Pharmacol.* 2011;43(5):526-531. doi:10.4103/0253-7613.84961

55. Faurot K (Kim) R, Gaylord S, Palsson OS, Garland EL, Mann JD, Whitehead WE. 715 Mindfulness Meditation Has Long-Term Therapeutic Benefits in Women With Irritable Bowel Syndrome (IBS): Follow-Up Results From a Randomized Controlled Trial. *Gastroenterology.* 2014;146(5):S-124. doi:10.1016/S0016-5085(14)60447-9

56. Banks SJ, Eddy KT, Angstadt M, Nathan PJ, Luan Phan K. Amygdala-frontal connectivity during emotion regulation. *Soc Cogn Affect Neurosci.* 2007;2(4):303-312. doi:10.1093/scan/nsm029

57. Van Der Kolk B. The Body Keeps The Score: Brain, Mind, and Body in the Healing of Trauma. New York: Penguin Books; 2014.

58. Lin H, Li Y. Using EEG data analytics to measure meditation. In: Lecture Notes in Computer Science (Including Subseries Lecture Notes in Artificial Intelligence and Lecture Notes in Bioinformatics). Vol 10287 LNCS. Springer Verlag; 2017:270-280. doi:10.1007/978-3-319-58466-9_25

59. Gauthier T, Meyer RML, Grefe D, Gold JI. An On-the-Job Mindfulness-based Intervention For Pediatric ICU Nurses: A Pilot. *J Pediatr Nurs.* 2015;30(2):402-409. doi:10.1016/j.pedn.2014.10.005

60. Goyal M, Singh S, Sibinga EMS, et al. Meditation programs for psychological stress and well-being: a systematic review and meta-analysis. *JAMA Intern Med.* 2014;174(3):357-368. doi:10.1001/jamainternmed.2013.13018

61. Wilkins L. The Research on Prayer and Healing: Past, Present and Future Challenges. *Baylor BEARdocs.* May 2015. https://baylor-ir.tdl.org/baylor-ir/handle/2104/9453.

CHAPTER 12: SUMMARY & CASE EXAMPLES

1. Maskell J. The Community Cure: Transforming Health Outcomes Together. Austin, Texas: Lioncrest Publishing; 2020.

Index

A

acupuncture, 108, 238, 329, 345, 385, 396, 482, 506

allostatic load, 37, 38

alpha gal, 129, 133, 288, 289

alternative medicine, v

aluminum, 201, 476

anaphylaxis, 5, 8, 9, 11, 13, 14, 15, 16, 21, 26, 36, 40, 111, 192, 262, 264, 274, 278, 279, 289, 308, 310, 314, 315, 373, 401, 447, 448, 449, 451, 474, 494

angioedema, 10, 14, 25, 138, 443

anxiety, 9, 11, 14, 21, 25, 27, 35, 45, 49, 52, 70, 76, 78, 94, 96, 102, 111, 112, 123, 132, 142, 147, 160, 173, 174, 184, 223, 231, 255, 268, 276, 305, 308, 346, 351, 375, 397, 399, 401, 402, 403, 411, 412, 413, 416, 417, 426, 430, 470, 507, 508

arsenic, 199, 201

autism spectrum disorders, 131, 146, 192, 202, 203, 232, 295, 402, 403

autoimmune, 44, 46, 132, 295

autonomic nervous system, 43, 47, 55, 71, 88, 136, 140, 165, 166, 206, 212, 224, 227, 228, 234, 235, 257, 262, 265, 323, 326, 327, 348, 364, 365, 375, 402, 419, 443, 481

B

bacterial infections, vi, 6, 125, 127, 129, 130, 131, 135, 136, 139, 140, 145, 165, 167, 169, 380, 401, 463

Barre-Lieou syndrome, 86, 97

Beighton evaluation, 80, 81

binaural beats, 252, 400, 413, 422, 508

bracing, 74, 91, 92, 93, 97, 326, 363, 365, 366, 368, 370, 377

breathing exercises, 62, 245, 345, 399

C

cadmium, 202

candida, vi, 36, 37, 131, 141, 142, 143, 144, 145, 182, 185, 192, 282, 288, 387, 397, 427, 428, 431, 432, 467

cannabis, 346

cardiovascular exercise, 358

513

castor oil, 186, 385, 400

cauda equina syndrome, 87, 97

celiac disease, 24, 35, 36, 149, 156, 157, 169, 283, 471

Chiari malformation, 46, 71, 73, 77, 84, 85, 86, 89, 97, 226, 227, 234, 324, 325, 368, 459, 460, 500

chromium, 202, 476

chronic streptococcus, 132

CIRS

chronic inflammatory response syndrome, 13, 167, 172, 173, 175, 176, 177, 180, 184, 185, 188, 191, 397

clostridium difficile, 129, 131, 463

collagen, 68, 69, 70, 71, 80, 87, 89, 94, 95, 96, 97, 157, 206, 289, 290, 405, 410, 488, 489

complementary medicine, v

constipation, 10, 21, 49, 57, 78, 142, 151, 153, 154, 155, 157, 158, 161, 174, 190, 216, 283, 285, 287, 387, 426, 434

conventional medicine, iv, 132, 161, 346

CranioBiotic Technique, 165, 166, 443, 490

craniocervical instability, 71, 73, 86, 227, 321, 354, 368, 434

craniosacral therapy, 108, 190, 222

D

degranulation, 4

depression, 9, 11, 25, 35, 49, 76, 78, 114, 131, 138, 142, 147, 161, 173, 184, 211, 223, 232, 234, 251, 255, 257, 276, 277, 283, 305, 323, 346, 351, 401, 402, 403, 411, 412, 413, 414, 417, 426, 430, 431, 433, 470

detoxification, 1, 205, 248, 302, 379, 381, 383, 388, 389, 391, 393, 506

diabetes, iv, 24, 53, 64, 147, 158, 162, 201, 286, 293, 413

diamine oxidase

DAO, 267, 272, 311, 449

dislocation, 74, 91, 97, 362, 372

Dynamic Neural Retraining System, 250, 387, 429

dysautonomia, ii, 25, 38, 43, 44, 47, 60, 61, 62, 63, 64, 70, 71, 75, 76, 78, 86, 88, 89, 90, 95, 96, 128, 130, 136, 145, 165, 191, 193, 207, 212, 226, 237, 241, 242, 246, 256, 266, 324, 388, 396, 443, 473, 478, 481

E

Eagle syndrome, 86

Ehlers-Danlos syndrome

EDS, ii, 13, 67, 89, 96, 116, 191, 207, 212, 457, 458, 459, 460, 461, 471, 502, 503

elimination diet, 306, 307, 308

514

emergency plan, 40, 111, 125

EMF, 167, 208, 209, 210, 211, 212, 217, 219, 254, 478

Emotional Freedom Technique, 244, 247, 399, 416

endometriosis, 46, 159

enteric nervous system, 156, 225, 235, 236

Environmental Relative Moldiness Index, 175

eosinophilic esophagitis, 146, 148

epsom salt baths, 345, 386, 395, 422

Epstein-Barr virus, 46, 128, 137, 138, 165, 169, 397, 435, 465

essential oils, 131, 132, 133, 144, 187, 347, 398, 408, 414, 508, 510

estrogen dominance, 160

F

fasting, v, 181, 237, 284, 385, 386, 399, 411, 422, 481

fibromyalgia, 13, 46

functional medicine, i, iv, v, vi, vii, viii, 36, 37, 38, 60, 65, 95, 97, 108, 121, 122, 130, 136, 138, 142, 145, 149, 162, 163, 167, 182, 282, 316, 397, 427, 431, 433, 436, 437, 443, 445

fungal infections, 6, 140, 145

G

gastroesophageal reflux disease, 24, 146

gluten, 24, 30, 38, 61, 149, 155, 278, 283, 291, 296, 303, 304, 426, 429, 432

grounding, 255, 413, 508

Gupta Program, 251, 387, 435

H

heart rate variability, 241, 481

heavy metals, 64, 125, 127, 161, 167, 171, 189, 193, 199, 203, 204, 205, 206, 207, 214, 222, 227, 263, 283, 299, 300, 385, 476, 477, 506

heparin, 5, 23

hereditary alpha tryptasemia, 20, 21, 26, 89

histamine, 5, 22, 27, 164, 267, 268, 269, 374, 448, 451, 455, 467, 474, 480, 484, 485, 491, 504, 508

histamine intolerance, 27, 484, 485

holistic medicine, iv

hydration, 34, 41, 54, 60, 62, 65, 144, 155, 170, 184, 205, 222, 249, 264, 265, 266, 296, 301, 383, 421, 422, 428, 432, 438, 483, 484

Hymenoptera venom, 15, 26, 448

hyperbaric oxygen, 133, 190, 385

hypothalamic-pituitary-adrenal axis, 234

hypothyroidism, 161

I

ileocecal valve, 10, 148, 155, 321, 331, 333, 340, 341
integrative medicine, vi
intracranial hypertension, 85
irritable bowel syndrome, 13, 46, 78, 323, 504

K

ketogenic diet, 284, 487
Kounis syndrome, 13, 25

L

lead, 202, 477
leaky gut, 28, 36, 37, 91, 130, 141, 146, 147, 151, 152, 170, 207, 226, 227, 236, 280, 288, 289, 427
lectins, 290
leukotriene, 5, 23
limbic system, 247, 250, 416
Loeys-Dietz syndrome, 80, 83
low-FODMAP, 279
low-histamine diet, 261, 267, 271, 272, 274, 275, 485
low-oxalate diet, 281
low-salicylate diet, 275
low-toxin diet, 296, 302, 306, 319

Lyme disease, 53, 65, 129, 130, 133, 136, 166, 169, 174, 180, 227, 289, 397, 430, 473
lymphatic system, 393, 394, 507

M

Marfan syndrome, 68, 80, 83
mastocytosis, 2, 3, 4, 20, 26, 39, 448
MCAS
    mast cell activation syndrome, 1, i, ii, iii, iv, 1, 2, 3, 6, 7, 8, 9, 12, 15, 16, 17, 18, 19, 20, 22, 23, 24, 25, 26, 27, 28, 29, 32, 33, 34, 35, 36, 37, 39, 40, 41, 43, 46, 54, 61, 62, 68, 71, 78, 80, 87, 88, 89, 90, 93, 95, 128, 130, 156, 160, 163, 170, 191, 192, 193, 206, 223, 227, 228, 261, 262, 264, 266, 268, 272, 273, 274, 275, 276, 278, 279, 280, 283, 289, 290, 309, 311, 312, 316, 319, 351, 363, 372, 373, 375, 376, 377, 380, 388, 397, 401, 405, 411, 419, 425, 434, 435, 438, 444, 445, 446, 448, 449, 460
median arcuate ligament syndrome, 46
meditation, 108, 112, 190, 222, 234, 244, 248, 249, 252, 256, 259, 344, 355, 383, 410, 412, 416, 417, 418, 419, 423, 436, 511

mercury, 203, 293, 475, 477, 490

mindfulness, 248, 383, 416, 417, 510, 511

mitochondria, 386

mold, vi, 7, 34, 41, 62, 125, 127, 128, 171, 172, 173, 174, 175, 176, 177, 178, 179, 180, 181, 182, 184, 185, 186, 187, 188, 189, 190, 191, 192, 204, 205, 212, 213, 214, 216, 221, 222, 223, 263, 268, 283, 300, 319, 379, 381, 385, 391, 397, 401, 426, 427, 428, 443, 451, 473, 474

monoclonal, 3

multiple chemical sensitivity, 13, 235

myalgic encephalomyelitis/chronic fatigue syndrome, 13

mycoplasma pneumoniae, 134

N

naturopathic medicine, v

nightshades, 144, 280, 281, 290, 303

nutritionist, 316

O

ozone, v, 133, 139, 191, 222, 385

P

parasite, 147, 153, 155

passport, ii, 101, 102, 103, 104, 105, 107, 109, 113, 115, 119, 120, 124, 128, 441

pelvic floor, 70, 76, 82, 96, 233, 259, 321, 328, 329, 330, 341, 348, 434, 500

polycystic ovarian syndrome, 159, 162

Polyvagal Theory, 228, 231

post-traumatic stress disorder, 227, 402

postural training, 361

POTS

postural orthostatic tachycardia syndrome, 1, ii, iii, iv, 13, 25, 35, 38, 43, 44, 45, 47, 48, 50, 51, 52, 53, 54, 55, 57, 58, 59, 60, 61, 62, 63, 64, 65, 71, 77, 78, 80, 85, 86, 88, 89, 90, 93, 128, 129, 157, 158, 160, 165, 167, 170, 174, 191, 192, 228, 231, 234, 242, 261, 265, 266, 273, 275, 283, 290, 316, 319, 346, 351, 355, 356, 357, 358, 359, 360, 361, 362, 372, 377, 380, 388, 399, 406, 411, 419, 430, 432, 438, 443, 452, 453, 455, 456, 457, 460, 483, 484, 502

probiotics, 34, 155, 237, 435, 464, 486

prolapse, 76, 78, 82, 328

prolotherapy, 94, 95, 97, 462

proprioception, 72, 75, 92, 93, 333, 354, 366, 367, 369, 370, 371, 377, 434, 458, 503 prostaglandin, 5, 22

psoas, 331, 332, 333, 334, 335, 336, 339, 341, 348, 354

ptosis, 77

R

reiki, v, 346, 411, 507

S

Safe & Sound Protocol, 254, 255, 259, 387, 432, 443, 480

sauna, v, 182, 384, 385

serotonin, 5

Sjögren's syndrome, 45, 47, 53, 65

sleep hygiene, 344, 386, 396, 432

small intestinal bacterial overgrowth, 13, 47

sound healing, 108, 412, 423

strength training, 360

T

Tension & Trauma Releasing Exercise, 251

tethered cord syndrome, 85

The Driscoll Theory®, 61

toxicant-induced loss of tolerance, 192

toxin binders, 188, 189, 190, 192, 203, 204, 385, 400, 422

toxins, 192, 194, 196, 206, 213, 263, 380, 381, 474, 490

tryptase, 6, 39, 448

V

vagus nerve, 58, 62, 71, 86, 90, 207, 225, 226, 228, 230, 231, 232, 233, 234, 236, 237, 238, 244, 252, 253, 258, 259, 263, 326, 329, 330, 332, 365, 387, 455, 480, 481, 482

viral infections, 34, 36, 41, 54, 62, 127, 137, 139, 140, 165, 198, 319, 465

visceral manipulation, 108, 191, 222, 333, 341

W

WFPB diet

whole food plant based diet, 291, 294

Wim Hoff Method, 251

Made in the USA
Columbia, SC
05 November 2024

45682738R00293